Joe P. Morgan · Alida Wind · Autumn P. Davidson

**Hereditary Bone and
Joint Diseases in the Dog**

Osteochondroses · Hip dysplasia · Elbow dysplasia

Joe P. Morgan · Alida Wind · Autumn P. Davidson

# Hereditary Bone and Joint Diseases in the Dog

Osteochondroses · Hip dysplasia · Elbow dysplasia

Joe P. Morgan, DVM, Vet. med. dr., DACVR
Emeritus Professor, Department of Surgical and Radiological Sciences,
School of Veterinary Medicine, University of California, Davis, California

Alida Wind, DVM
Emeritus Lecturer, Department of Surgical and Radiological Sciences,
School of Veterinary Medicine, University of California, Davis, California

Autumn P. Davidson, DVM, DACVIM
Associate Clinical Professor, Veterinary Medical Teaching Hospital,
School of Veterinary Medicine, University of California, Davis, California

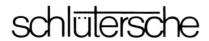

Morgan, Joe P.:
Hereditary bone and joint diseases in the dog:
osteochondroses, hip dysplasia, elbow dysplasia
Joe P. Morgan; Alida Wind; Autumn P. Davidson.
Hannover: Schlütersche, 2000
ISBN 3-87706-548-1

© 2000, Schlütersche GmbH & Co. KG, Verlag und Druckerei,
Hans-Böckler-Allee 7, 30173 Hannover, Germany

U.S.A. and Canada: PO Box 30, Williston, VT 05495-0030,
Toll free number 888-880-0328

Printed by Schlütersche GmbH & Co. KG, Verlag und Druckerei,
Hannover.

All rights reserved. The contents of this book both photographic and textual, may not be reproduced in any form by print, photoprint, phototransparency, microfiches, video disc, or any other means, nor may it be included in any computer retrieval system, without written permission from the publisher.

Any person who does any unauthorised act in relation to this publication may be liable to criminal prosecution and civil claims for damages.

# Preface

This book offers the reader, whether owner, breeder, or veterinarian, information on common skeletal lesions that affect the growing dog of many of the larger breeds. These diseases include the osteochondroses of the humeral head, distal humeral condyle, distal ulna, sacrum, distal femoral condyle, and tarsal bones. In addition, the important features of both elbow and hip dysplasia are discussed. The methods of most accurate diagnosis are clearly explained with detailed information on what to expect in gait abnormalities and what can be found on physical examination. The changes noted on radiographic examination are clearly illustrated as are the various techniques recommended for the examination procedure. The prognosis for a pet dog, athletic dog, or working dog is explained when a disease is detected. Osteoarthrosis or degenerative joint disease is explained as the consequence of the diseases regardless of anatomic location and its affect on athletic performance is described. Various treatments are offered that may control the progression of osteoarthrosis in an affected joint and include conservative measures that an owner can control that may offer a pet a relatively happy life. These treatments are compared with the use of drug therapy and surgery so that the reader has a concept of the wide range of treatment available. The relative costs of surgery are listed. The reader is acquainted with the goals of various forms of therapy and an effort is made to offer recommendations of the appropriatness of treatment for the various forms of developmental diseases.

The reader is offered information from a large study of Labrador Retrievers that indicates the frequency of the diseases as well as the possibility of disease in several anatomical sites in one dog. Because these diseases are inherited, their control is dependent on selection of sound breeding stock. The last chapter of the book is a lengthy review of the history of attempts to control some of these diseases throughout the world. These are written by experts who explain the principles of registration of both diseased and normal dogs and how this information can be utilized in disease control. The value of progeny evaluation is especially stressed.

Davis, October 1999　　　　　　　　　　　　　　　　　　　Joe P. Morgan

# Table of contents

## Chapter 1
## Introduction

Normal growth and ossification of the skeleton . . . 3
Definition of osteochondrosis (OC) and
osteochondritis dissecans (OCD) . . . . . . . . . . . . . 4
   Epiphyseal growth plate . . . . . . . . . . . . . . . . 5
   Metaphyseal growth plate . . . . . . . . . . . . . . 8
Definition of dysplasia . . . . . . . . . . . . . . . . . . . . . 9
Definition of osteoarthrosis (OA) . . . . . . . . . . . . 10
Influence of diet and growth rate . . . . . . . . . . . 12
Heritability of hip dysplasia, elbow dysplasia,
and osteochondrosis in the dog . . . . . . . . . . . . 14
Sites of disease predilection in the dog . . . . . . . 15
Diagnosis . . . . . . . . . . . . . . . . . . . . . . . . . . . . . . 16
Treatment and prognosis . . . . . . . . . . . . . . . . . . 16
Significance of osteochondrosis and dysplasia . . . . 16
Goals of the monograph . . . . . . . . . . . . . . . . . . 17
References . . . . . . . . . . . . . . . . . . . . . . . . . . . . . 18

## Chapter 2
## Osteochondrosis of the humeral head

Introduction . . . . . . . . . . . . . . . . . . . . . . . . . . . . 21
History . . . . . . . . . . . . . . . . . . . . . . . . . . . . . . . 21
Course of the disease . . . . . . . . . . . . . . . . . . . . 22
Gross lesion . . . . . . . . . . . . . . . . . . . . . . . . . . . . 23
Clinical signs . . . . . . . . . . . . . . . . . . . . . . . . . . . 24
Physical examination . . . . . . . . . . . . . . . . . . . . . 26
Anatomy and development of the shoulder joint . 27
Radiographic diagnosis . . . . . . . . . . . . . . . . . . . 27
Radiographic grading of lesions . . . . . . . . . . . . . 29
Differential radiographic diagnosis . . . . . . . . . . . 34
Treatment . . . . . . . . . . . . . . . . . . . . . . . . . . . . . 35
   Conservative treatment . . . . . . . . . . . . . . . . 35
   Surgical treatment . . . . . . . . . . . . . . . . . . . . 36
Prognosis . . . . . . . . . . . . . . . . . . . . . . . . . . . . . . 37
Heritability . . . . . . . . . . . . . . . . . . . . . . . . . . . . 37
References . . . . . . . . . . . . . . . . . . . . . . . . . . . . . 39

## Chapter 3
## Elbow dysplasia

Introduction . . . . . . . . . . . . . . . . . . . . . . . . . . . . 41
History . . . . . . . . . . . . . . . . . . . . . . . . . . . . . . . 41
   Proposed etiologies . . . . . . . . . . . . . . . . . . . 46
Clinical signs . . . . . . . . . . . . . . . . . . . . . . . . . . . 48
Physical examination . . . . . . . . . . . . . . . . . . . . . 51
Anatomy and development of the
elbow joint . . . . . . . . . . . . . . . . . . . . . . . . . . . . 51
Radiographic diagnosis . . . . . . . . . . . . . . . . . . . 54
   Radiographic views . . . . . . . . . . . . . . . . . . . 54
   Purpose of study . . . . . . . . . . . . . . . . . . . . . 56
   Techniques for evaluation . . . . . . . . . . . . . . 57
Radiographic appearance of the
normal elbow joint . . . . . . . . . . . . . . . . . . . . . . 57
Radiographic appearance of the
dysplastic elbow joint . . . . . . . . . . . . . . . . . . . . 58
Differential radiographic diagnosis . . . . . . . . . . . 61
Treatment . . . . . . . . . . . . . . . . . . . . . . . . . . . . . 63
   Conservative treatment . . . . . . . . . . . . . . . . 65
   Surgical treatment . . . . . . . . . . . . . . . . . . . . 65
Prognosis . . . . . . . . . . . . . . . . . . . . . . . . . . . . . . 67
   Non-operated dogs . . . . . . . . . . . . . . . . . . . 67
   Operated dogs . . . . . . . . . . . . . . . . . . . . . . 67
   Immature dogs . . . . . . . . . . . . . . . . . . . . . . 67
   Mature dogs . . . . . . . . . . . . . . . . . . . . . . . . 68
Heritability . . . . . . . . . . . . . . . . . . . . . . . . . . . . 68

**Ununited anconeal process (UAP)** . . . . . . . . 69
Introduction . . . . . . . . . . . . . . . . . . . . . . . . . . . . 69
History . . . . . . . . . . . . . . . . . . . . . . . . . . . . . . . 71
Clinical signs . . . . . . . . . . . . . . . . . . . . . . . . . . . 73
Physical examination . . . . . . . . . . . . . . . . . . . . . 74
Radiographic diagnosis . . . . . . . . . . . . . . . . . . . 74
Differential radiographic diagnosis . . . . . . . . . . . 76
Treatment . . . . . . . . . . . . . . . . . . . . . . . . . . . . . 76
   Conservative treatment . . . . . . . . . . . . . . . . 76
   Surgical treatment . . . . . . . . . . . . . . . . . . . . 76
Prognosis . . . . . . . . . . . . . . . . . . . . . . . . . . . . . .77
Heritability . . . . . . . . . . . . . . . . . . . . . . . . . . . . .77

**Medial coronoid process disease (MCPD)** .. 77
Introduction . . . . . . . . . . . . . . . . . . . . . . . . 77
History . . . . . . . . . . . . . . . . . . . . . . . . . . . 77
Clinical signs . . . . . . . . . . . . . . . . . . . . . . . 79
Physical examination . . . . . . . . . . . . . . . . . 80
Radiographic diagnosis . . . . . . . . . . . . . . . 80
  Diagnosis using other radiographic
  imaging techniques . . . . . . . . . . . . . . . . . 83
Differential radiographic diagnosis . . . . . . . 84
Treatment . . . . . . . . . . . . . . . . . . . . . . . . 85
  Conservative treatment . . . . . . . . . . . . . . 85
  Surgical treatment . . . . . . . . . . . . . . . . . 85
Prognosis . . . . . . . . . . . . . . . . . . . . . . . . 85
Heritability . . . . . . . . . . . . . . . . . . . . . . . 86

**Osteochondrosis of the medial aspect
of the humeral condyle** . . . . . . . . . . . . . 87
Introduction . . . . . . . . . . . . . . . . . . . . . . 87
History . . . . . . . . . . . . . . . . . . . . . . . . . 87
Clinical signs . . . . . . . . . . . . . . . . . . . . . 88
Physical examination . . . . . . . . . . . . . . . 88
Radiographic diagnosis . . . . . . . . . . . . . . 89
Differential radiographic diagnosis . . . . . . 89
Treatment . . . . . . . . . . . . . . . . . . . . . . . 90
Prognosis . . . . . . . . . . . . . . . . . . . . . . . 90
Heritability . . . . . . . . . . . . . . . . . . . . . . 90
References . . . . . . . . . . . . . . . . . . . . . . 91

# Chapter 4
# Retained cartilage core

Introduction . . . . . . . . . . . . . . . . . . . . . . 95
History . . . . . . . . . . . . . . . . . . . . . . . . . 95
Course of the disease . . . . . . . . . . . . . . . 96
Clinical signs . . . . . . . . . . . . . . . . . . . . . 97
Physical examination . . . . . . . . . . . . . . . 97
Anatomy and development of the distal ulna . . . . 97
Radiographic diagnosis . . . . . . . . . . . . . . 98
Differential radiographic diagnosis . . . . . . . 106
Treatment . . . . . . . . . . . . . . . . . . . . . . . 106
  Conservative treatment . . . . . . . . . . . . . 106
  Surgical treatment . . . . . . . . . . . . . . . . 106
Prognosis . . . . . . . . . . . . . . . . . . . . . . . 107
Heritability . . . . . . . . . . . . . . . . . . . . . . 107
References . . . . . . . . . . . . . . . . . . . . . . 107

# Chapter 5
# Hip dysplasia

Introduction . . . . . . . . . . . . . . . . . . . . . 109
History . . . . . . . . . . . . . . . . . . . . . . . . 109
Affected breeds . . . . . . . . . . . . . . . . . . . 112

Prevalence of hip dysplasia . . . . . . . . . . . . . 112
Clinical signs . . . . . . . . . . . . . . . . . . . . . . 113
  Clinical signs in the puppy . . . . . . . . . . . . 113
  Clinical signs in the preadolescent . . . . . . 115
  Clinical signs in the young dog . . . . . . . . . 116
  Clinical signs in the adult dog . . . . . . . . . 117
  Clinical signs of lumbosacral disease . . . . . . . 117
  Clinical signs of transitional
  lumbosacral vertebral segment . . . . . . . . . 118
Physical examination . . . . . . . . . . . . . . . . 118
  Joint laxity as an indicator of hip dysplasia . . . . 118
  Bardens' technique . . . . . . . . . . . . . . . . 120
  Ortolani technique . . . . . . . . . . . . . . . . 121
  Anatomy and development of the hip joint . . . 125
  Femoral head . . . . . . . . . . . . . . . . . . . 126
  Acetabulum . . . . . . . . . . . . . . . . . . . . 126
  Hip joint . . . . . . . . . . . . . . . . . . . . . . 128
  Femoral neck . . . . . . . . . . . . . . . . . . . 130
  Greater trochanter . . . . . . . . . . . . . . . . 131
Radiographic views . . . . . . . . . . . . . . . . . 131
  Ventrodorsal view . . . . . . . . . . . . . . . . . 133
  Ventrodorsal „frog leg" view . . . . . . . . . . 136
  Ventrodorsal wedge view . . . . . . . . . . . . 138
  Standing position . . . . . . . . . . . . . . . . . 139
  Badertscher view . . . . . . . . . . . . . . . . . 140
  Flückiger view . . . . . . . . . . . . . . . . . . . 140
  Compression-distraction views . . . . . . . . . 141
  Dorsal acetabular rim view . . . . . . . . . . . 143
Radiographic diagnosis . . . . . . . . . . . . . . . 143
  Patterns of radiographic change . . . . . . . . 146
    Joint laxity . . . . . . . . . . . . . . . . . . . . 147
    Secondary bony changes . . . . . . . . . . . 149
    Subchondral sclerosis . . . . . . . . . . . . . 154
    Bilabiation . . . . . . . . . . . . . . . . . . . 155
    Modeling patterns . . . . . . . . . . . . . . . 156
    Acetabular margin . . . . . . . . . . . . . . 156
    Ilial and ischial new bone . . . . . . . . . . 156
    Femoral head and neck . . . . . . . . . . . 157
    Inclination of the femoral neck . . . . . . . 158
    Anteversion/retroversion . . . . . . . . . . . 162
    Greater trochanter . . . . . . . . . . . . . . 163
    Pelvic conformation . . . . . . . . . . . . . 165
Grading radiographic changes . . . . . . . . . . 168
  Systems of grading . . . . . . . . . . . . . . . . 171
  Breed influence on radiographic changes . . . . 171
Influence of age on diagnosis . . . . . . . . . . . 171
Differential radiographic diagnosis . . . . . . . . 175
  Hip luxation . . . . . . . . . . . . . . . . . . . . 176
  Aseptic necrosis of the femoral head . . . . . 176
  Acute fracture . . . . . . . . . . . . . . . . . . . 179
  Healed fracture of the femoral head or
  acetabulum . . . . . . . . . . . . . . . . . . . . 180
  Infectious arthritis in the older dog . . . . . . . 180
  Primary arthrosis . . . . . . . . . . . . . . . . . 183

Treatment .............................. 184
  Conservative treatment in the immature dog .. 184
  Conservative treatment in the mature dog .... 184
  Medical treatment ....................... 185
  Surgical treatment ...................... 186
  Surgical treatment in the immature dog ..... 187
    Tension relief procedures ............... 188
    Triple pelvic osteotomy ................ 189
    Intertrochanteric derotational varus osteotomy 192
    Neck lengthening or intertrochanteric
    lateralization of the proximal femur ....... 193
    Greater trochanteric repositioning ........ 193
    Acetabuloplasty ...................... 193
  Surgical treatment in the mature dog ....... 194
    Femoral head and neck ostectomy ....... 194
    Total hip replacement ................. 196
Prognosis ................................ 197
Heritability .............................. 197
References ............................... 203

# Chapter 6
# Lumbosacral disease

Introduction ............................. 209
History .................................. 210
Clinical signs ............................ 212
Physical examination ..................... 214
Anatomy and development of
the lumbosacral region ................... 215
Radiographic diagnosis ................... 216
  Survey radiography .................... 216
  Stress radiography ..................... 216
  Epidurography ........................ 217
  Discography .......................... 218
  Myelography .......................... 218
Examination protocol .................... 220
Differential radiographic diagnosis ......... 220
Treatment ............................... 220
  Medical treatment ..................... 220
  Chemonucleolysis ..................... 221
  Surgical treatment ..................... 221
Prognosis ................................ 223
Transitional lumbosacral vertebrae ........ 223
Definition ............................... 223
Radiographic diagnosis ................... 223
Heritability .............................. 226
Osteochondrosis of the sacrum ........... 227
Definition ............................... 226
Radiographic diagnosis ................... 227
Heritability .............................. 227
Spinal canal stenosis .................... 227
Definition ............................... 227

Radiographic diagnosis ................... 228
Heritability .............................. 228
References ............................... 229

# Chapter 7
# Osteochondrosis of the femoral condyle

Introduction ............................. 231
Clinical signs ............................ 231
Physical examination ..................... 232
Anatomy and development of the
femoral condyles ......................... 233
Radiographic diagnosis ................... 233
Differential radiographic diagnosis ......... 236
Treatment ............................... 236
  Conservative treatment ................. 236
  Surgical treatment ..................... 237
Prognosis ................................ 237
Heritability .............................. 237
References ............................... 238

# Chapter 8
# Osteochondrosis of the talus

Introduction ............................. 239
Clinical signs ............................ 239
Physical examination ..................... 239
Anatomy and development of the talus ..... 240
Radiographic diagnosis ................... 241
Differential radiographic diagnosis ......... 243
Treatment ............................... 244
  Conservative treatment ................. 244
  Surgical treatment ..................... 244
Prognosis ................................ 244
Heritability .............................. 244
References ............................... 245

# Chapter 9
# Bone dysplasias in the Labrador Retriever: A radiographic study

Introduction ............................. 247
Materials and methods ................... 247
Radiographic studies ..................... 247
Results .................................. 248
Discussion ............................... 250
Conclusions ............................. 251
References ............................... 252

# Chapter 10
## Schemes for control of disease

Introduction to control of dysplasia
through use of registries . . . . . . . . . . . . . . . . . 253

Control of hip dysplasia in Sweden
JOE P. MORGAN and LARS AUDELL . . . . . . . . . . 255

Fédération Cynologigue Internationale (FCI)
SAKI PAATSAMA . . . . . . . . . . . . . . . . . . . . . . . 263

Hip dysplasia and its control in Great Britain
DONALD D. LAWSON . . . . . . . . . . . . . . . . . . . 267

Orthopedic Foundation for Animals, Inc.
E. A. CORLEY . . . . . . . . . . . . . . . . . . . . . . . . . 284

Control of CHD in Switzerland
MARK FLÜCKIGER . . . . . . . . . . . . . . . . . . . . . 289

The Institute for Genetic Disease Control
in Animals (GDC)
P. W. POULOS . . . . . . . . . . . . . . . . . . . . . . . . . 295

Hip dysplasia diagnosis
– the use of distraction radiography
G. K. SMITH . . . . . . . . . . . . . . . . . . . . . . . . . . 301

Control of elbow dysplasia in Sweden
LARS AUDELL . . . . . . . . . . . . . . . . . . . . . . . . 305

International Elbow Working Group (IEWG)
MARK FLÜCKIGER . . . . . . . . . . . . . . . . . . . . . 309

**Index** . . . . . . . . . . . . . . . . . . . . . . . . . 313

# Chapter 1

# Introduction

This monograph presents information concerning a clinically important group of hereditary diseases of the skeleton occurring during growth in the larger sized breeds of dog. One group of these diseases is the result of osteochondrosis (OC) and affects several parts of the skeletal system. Another group affects the elbow and hip joints. One of these, elbow dysplasia, includes specific diseases known earlier as: (1) ununited anconeal process, (2) medial coronoid disease, and (3) osteochondrosis of the medial humeral condyle. Hip dysplasia (CHD) is the other severe joint disease that results in incorrect development of the hip joint. A discussion of certain specific congenital and developmental diseases of the lumbosacral joint is included because of similar clinical signs shared with hip dysplasia, and because they also appear to be hereditary.

As we consider the problems of these skeletal diseases, it is appropriate to consider how we, as owners and breeders, have been instrumental in causing dogs to be indiscriminately inbred without regard to the presence of hereditary disease. In addition, we have also encouraged over feeding resulting in too rapid growth. The result is that man has dramatically and widely changed the inherited physical characteristics of the dog. Most of today's working dogs, including the herding and sporting breeds generally weigh more than the ancestral dog and are discussed at greatest length in this monograph.

In an effort to achieve a larger dog, we have become victims of the adage "bigger is better." Certainly, the dog has not escaped this philosophy that seems to pervade the world. Today, over-nutrition is common in the industrialized countries and young animals are fed in a manner leading to a maximum growth rate. Because rapid growth is an important economic factor in animal husbandry, there has been for many years a genetic selection for individuals that demonstrates rapid growth, particularly in pigs, turkeys, and broilers, and, to some extent, in beef cattle and horses. The economic gains have been considerable, but an increasing incidence of osteochondrosis and joint dysplasia is correlated with the rapid growth. This is especially noticeable in the pig (Reiland 1978 e). The main clinical problems resulting from this change in animal husbandry have been lameness and pain. Contrary to the long-living dog, this problem can be better tolerated in pigs because of the practice of slaughtering at such a young age (Reiland 1978 b).

The average weight of popular male German Shepherd Dogs seen in shows has increased in the last 30 years from 32 kg in the male and 30 kg in the female to a weight today of over 50 kg in the male and over 40 kg in the female. This has been accompanied by a great increase in depth of the thorax and a marked decrease in forelimb length, and has not been without cost in the form of an increase in bone and joint disease. This problem with over-nutrition and selection for rapid growth is evidenced by the general absence of orthopedic disease in wild dogs when compared with the high prevalence of orthopedic disease in modern breeds of domesticated dogs. Further, it offers evidence that bone disease in the dog at least in part reflects the high cost of its domestication (Riser 1985). Reference will be made throughout this monograph to studies that positively confirm the fact that breeding for increased size, in addition to an increased rate of early body growth and the prerequisite increased energy intake, positively influences the frequency of developmental bone and joint disease.

It is the purpose of this monograph to describe in detail the osteochondroses as they affect:

1 the caudal central aspect of the humeral head (the shoulder joint),
2 the medial aspect of the distal humeral condyle (the elbow joint),
3 both medial and lateral distal femoral condyles (the stifle joint),
4 both medial and lateral trochlear ridges of the talus (the hock joint),
5 the distal ulnar growth plate, and
6 the sacrum,
along with the resulting joint disease.

Another pattern of disease affects elbow and hip joints that are dysplastic and develop abnormally. The reader is provided information concerning the history of the lesions as described in the medical literature. The lesions are presented from the standpoint of the individual dog including: (1) clinical signs, (2) physical diagnosis, (3) radiographic diagnosis, (4) conservative treatment, (5) medical treatment, (6) surgical treatment, and (7) prognosis. Etiology, pathophysiology, histopathology, and pathogenesis of the conditions are presented in some detail when it is felt that the information can be of value to the reader. The heritability of the conditions is described when information concerning this important feature is known and it is the authors' opinion that anecdotal expirience of disease occurrence within families or breeds should not be ignored when considering heritability.

Within the first chapter is a discussion of normal growth and ossification of the skeleton, which is important to the understanding of how these hereditary diseases develop.

In an effort to learn more of the significance of these conditions within a single breed, one chapter in particular (Chapter 9) discusses the frequency of the diseases within over 1000 members of the Labrador Retriever breed. The final chapter (Chapter 10) is a most important one as it considers the consequence of these diseases worldwide and discusses the results of actions that have been taken to reduce the disease frequency. This chapter includes the history of programs, some of which resulted in reduction of the frequency of hip dysplasia, and includes early results derived from programs aimed at gaining control of elbow dysplasia.

Accurate diagnosis of bone disease has potential importance for many reasons. Pet dogs are commonly presented for evaluation of lameness. The owner has an obvious interest in discovering the cause of the lameness, the treatments that are possible, and the prognosis relative to the disease. This can be learned through observation of the dog and physical and radiographic examination. If the dog is to be a working or performance dog, determination of the cause of the lameness increases in importance and early screening is advisable before the investment of time and trainer fees. The situation is more critical if the dog is to be used in a breeding program where knowledge of both the phenotype and genotype is important. Information concerning the presence of disease in parents, littermates, and siblings in addition to knowing if the individual dog is affected, is necessary in an effort to ascertain what is the risk for transmission of a particular disease. Finding the dogs to be free of disease means that sales can be made with a higher expectation that a puppy will also be free of that disease. While freedom of these diseases influences the value of the puppies and makes them more salable, distribution of affected off-spring results in a perpetuation of the problems.

This book is directed to the individual pet owner, who discovers a pet to be affected by one of these painful, physically limiting diseases; to the performance dog owner, who has lost an investment in time and money because of limited capabilities caused by an inherited orthopedic disease; and to the dog breeder who is disappointed with the production of affected puppies.

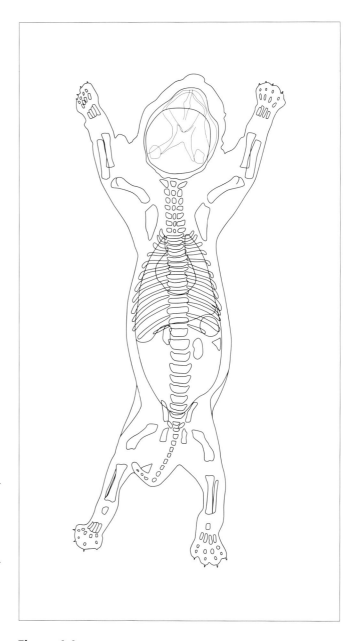

**Figure 1-1**
A drawing made from a dorsoventral whole body radiograph of a newborn puppy showing the portions of the skeleton that are ossified at birth. Ends of the long bones and many small bones are cartilaginous at this time and are not identified on the radiograph.

In particular, information is provided to all potential dog owners to make them aware that care in selection of any dog, regardless of its intended use, has a positive consequence and that careful selection can help in preventing personal grief and avoiding veterinary cost. Therefore, beginning with a healthy dog is advantageous to all. The following chapters offer help in gaining an understanding that careful selection of dogs to be used for breeding can bring a better future for all concerned.

Further it is hoped that the veterinary clinician finds the information in this monograph helpful in educating all dog owners and breeders about specific orthopedic diseases, including: (1) clinical signs, (2) different diagnostic techniques, (3) clinical significance, (4) available treatments, (5) ultimate prognosis, whether a pet or a working dog, and (6) heritability of disease.

## Normal growth and ossification of the skeleton

Developmental bone disease and secondary osteoarthrosis can be best understood if the reader has some basic knowledge of the mechanisms of skeletal development. The majority of the bones of the dog are originally formed of a cartilage model which passes through stages of ossification, that begin in utero, and continue following birth eventually leading to complete ossification. This process begins at certain sites within the bones which are referred to as primary ossification centers that are present within the midshaft, or diaphyses, of long bones. Later, the cartilaginous ends of the long bones, or epiphyses, begin to ossify. The major length of the bones results from growth within the metaphyseal growth plates located between the epiphyses and the metaphyses. Once ossification has begun, it proceeds in a specific and orderly pattern for that breed until the length of the long bones is determined, between 10 and 12 months of age in most large dogs (Figure 1-1).

During the time of skeletal growth, especially during the first six months of life, the dog is athletically active. At this time, the ends of the bones include the most important articular surfaces that remain in a cartilaginous form (Figure 1-2). This causes the joint spaces on the radiographs to appear greatly widened. The rapid increase in size and weight of the dog occurs when the ends of the bone are still cartilaginous and thus are more potentially vulnerable to injury. The presence of the cartilage model makes radiographic diagnosis of the skeleton of the immature dog difficult since the cartilage that is potentially damaged is radiolucent and cannot be identified on the radiograph. (Figure 1-3).

Between the diaphysis and the epiphysis are cartilaginous plates that are referred to as metaphyseal growth plates (Figures 1-2, 1-3). These growth areas furnish most of the length of the long bones. On the side of the growth plate nearest the epiphysis, cartilage cells multiply and grow in columns toward the diaphysis. As the cartilage cells extend into the diaphyseal side of the growth plate. They become vesiculated, die, and their intercellar matrix is calcified. At the same time, a specialized cell population (osteoclasts) that is derived from mononuclear cells within the bone marrow removes some of the calcified matrix. These cells open channels into which vessels penetrate.

A second population of bone forming cells originates from osteoprogenitor cells that lie adjacent to bone surfaces. They are capable of cell division and produce osteoblasts that synthesize bone matrix. They deposit osteoid on the walls of the channels in the cartilage, followed by deposition of mineral salts within the osteoid matrix, resulting in formation of immature bone tissue. Once

**Figure 1-2**
Radiographs of specimens of the femoral head from an immature puppy (A) and a mature dog (B). The femoral head is referred to as an epiphyseal ossification center that contains an ossified center surrounded by growth cartilage that is radiolucent (small arrows). The black line between the femoral head and the shaft of the bone represents another area of bone growth with the radiolucent cartilage (large arrow) referred to as the metaphyseal growth plate. It provides the greater part of longitudinal growth for the long bone.

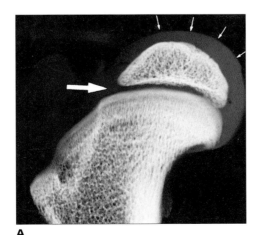
A

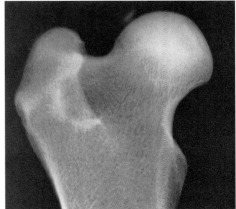
B

formed, the early bone becomes more mature in character by forming trabecular and cortical bone that supports the increasing weight of the growing dog. This mechanism of bone growth is referred to as endochondral ossification (bone formation from an earlier cartilage model). Skeletal maturity continues with an increase in the width of bones by a different process called appositional bony growth that continues during the second year of life.

During growth of the dog when it is becoming heavier and being encouraged to be athletic, the epiphyses of the long bones have an outer cartilage that serves as the articular cartilage, with an inner cartilage that serves as a growth cartilage. Thus, two functions are satisfied (Figures 1-2, 1-3). As a growth cartilage, it enables a minimal increase in the length of the bone to occur by endochondral ossification within the epiphyseal growth plate that covers the end of the bone. As an articular cartilage, it provides a smooth surface that articulates with the opposing cartilage on the other side of the joint.

## Definition of osteochondrosis (OC) and osteochondritis dissecans (OCD)

Osteochondrosis (OC) is a developmental bone disease of major clinical consequence that is seen in various anatomical locations (Olsson, 1973, 1975 a, b, 1976, 1986). The basic feature of OC is an error in the manner by which the body converts cartilage to bone during the growth process (Table 1-1). Olsson (1978) has defined the condition rather clearly as a disturbance of cell differentiation in metaphyseal growth plates and joint cartilage (epiphyseal growth cartilage). The cartilage cells divide at a normal or increased rate and rapid growth is maintained, but the cells do not mature and vesiculate, and matrix does not calcify. This leads to retention of cartilage, which may necrotize or die. In the surrounding bone, secondary changes, such as marrow fibrosis and thickening of the trabeculae, may be seen. The lesions occur in specific sites throughout the body and may be seen as unilateral or bilateral disease at one site or may be present as a more generalized disease. Not all lesions have a similar clinical importance.

While the growth zones of both the diaphysis and the epiphysis may be involved in this disease, the lesions in the epiphyses have a more direct clinical consequence because they result in alteration of the articular surfaces and, thus initiate the early development of osteoarthrosis. Metaphyseal growth zone disruption can affect the length of bones (metaphyseal chondrosis), but this is of import principally within the distal ulna.

Use of the term osteochondrosis in the description of this growth disturbance is not exactly accurate since osteochondrosis implies disease in both bone (osteo) and cartilage (chondro) while the lesions of osteochondrosis

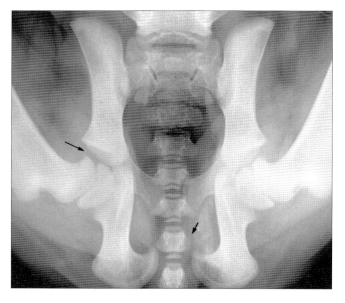

**Figure 1-3**
Radiographs of a normal pelvis of an immature dog made using two separate techniques for positioning illustrate the incomplete development of the skeletal system shortly after birth. The pelvic bones remain separated by growth cartilage (short arrows). The femoral heads are separated from the femoral necks by the metaphyseal growth plates. The joints are covered by cartilage that is radiolucent making the joint spaces appear widened (long arrows).

are primarily located in the cartilage and only secondarily affect the development of bony tissue. However, the name is widely accepted and there is little reason to consider altering it at this time. A better term is dyschondroplasia because it makes a stronger reference to a lesion within the cartilage that is the result of incorrect development. Both osteochondrosis and dyschondroplasia are used to describe pathologic conditions in man, using definitions somewhat different than the ones used in the veterinary literature. Because of this, the reader should be cautioned when examining references from the literature about human disease. A complete review of this problem in terminology is given in a monograph edited by Olsson (1978).

The lesions noted in osteochondrosis are those of a disturbance of endochondral ossification. The techniques used primarily for diagnosis of these lesions are routine diagnostic radiology, arthrography, and arthroscopy. Additional information can be obtained from tissues removed from the lesion that are examined using microradiography or microangiography, in conjunction with intravital staining of bone, as well as conventional staining of decalcified bone (Craig and Riser 1965; Paatsama, et al 1971; Carrig and Morgan 1974). An exhaustive report on diagnosis and the histopathology of canine joint disease is included in a review of osteochondrosis and osteochondritis dissecans (Pedersen and Pool 1978).

## Epiphyseal growth plate

The earliest phase of the epiphyseal disease of osteochondrosis is evident histologically with the delay in bone formation resulting only in a thickened cartilage (Figure 1-4). The cartilage is otherwise nearly normal histologically and viable chondrocytes are identified indicating a healthy cartilage. At this stage, the lesion is not recognized radiographically. At a somewhat later stage, the lesion is characterized by delay in ossification of the bone and this abnormal shape can be noted radiographically where it is characterized by a slight flattening and a slight increase in density of the surrounding subchondral bone. The thickened articular cartilage is not identified on the conventional radiograph because the cartilage is radiolucent. At this time arthroscopy allows for more detailed evaluation of the articular cartilage and demonstrates a chondromalacia and indentation that are probable precursors (van Bree and Van Ryssen 1995).

As the cartilage continues to grow without being normally converted to bone, it loses part of its nutrition because of its increased thickness. Importantly, cartilage has no blood vessels within its matrix and relies on nutrition from the surrounding synovial fluid in the joint and blood vessels from the underlying epiphysis, which normally penetrate the calcifying cartilage matrix at the cartilage-bone junction. Some studies suggest that vascular

**Table 1-1: Definition of osteochondrosis (OC) and osteochondritis dissecans (OCD)**

| Osteochondrosis (OC) - an error in ossification within a cartilaginous growth area characterized by: | Osteochondritis dissecans (OCD) - progression of an osteochondrosis characterized by: |
|---|---|
| 1. Persistence of a normal contour of the bony epiphysis with an area of<br>   a. Thickened cartilage<br>   b. Necrotic cartilage<br><br>2. Clinically<br>   a. A non-painful lesion<br>   b. Affects epiphyseal growth<br>   c. Unimpaired limb length<br><br>3. Healing or progression to an OCD | 1. Fissure formation between thickened cartilage and subchondral bone<br><br>2. Separation of cartilage fragment that<br>   a. Remains partially attached or<br>   b. Becomes a free joint body<br><br>3. A painful lesion<br>   a. An inflammatory synovitis<br><br>4. Healing<br>   a. Somewhat dependent on location of cartilage flap<br>   b. Resulting from filling of the defect by fibrous tissue<br>   c. With epiphyseal shape that<br>      1. Forms abnormally<br>      2. Forms normally<br><br>5. Osteoarthrosis<br><br>6. Unimpaired limb length |

channels (cartilage canals) of the epiphysis may permit vascularization to a part of the cartilage layer (Kincaid, et al 1985). Where the deficiency in the blood supply becomes severe enough, the cartilage becomes necrotic in its deepest portion (next to the bony epiphysis). The cancellous spicules of bone surrounding the subchondral triangular area become thickened in response to an alteration in weight-bearing that occurs as a result of the absence of functional articular cartilage (Figure 1-4).

Following cartilage necrosis, the overlying cartilage can separate from the underlying bone, possibly influenced by traumatic forces occurring as the result of a puppy's normal activities. Extension of the cleft from the depth of the lesion to the articular cartilage surface permits the entrance of synovial fluid with pain resulting from the hyperemia and from mediators released in the exposed epiphyseal spongiosa. These changes also initiate a sterile inflammatory process within the synovium. Beneath the cleft, an intense mesenchymal reaction occurs with granulation tissue, active fibrogenesis, fiberbone formation, and osteoclastic activity. Cartilage necrosis is seen at the depth of the lesion. Surrounding the lesion, the cancellous spicules of bone thicken. As the fissure increases in size, the cartilaginous fragment loosens to the degree that it may be called a "flap" (Figure 1-4). The larger subchondral lesions are more likely associated with rupture and separation of the articular cartilage causing the first clinical signs of pain and lameness to appear (van Bree 1994). The lesion is now referred to as an osteochondritis dissecans.

A similarity in the pathophysiology of the epiphyseal lesion is present despite the bone involved. Local ischemia leads to zones of epiphyseal cartilage that are particularly prone to stress-induced necrosis. Therefore, the weight of the dog, the joint in question, the congruity or incongruity of opposing articular surfaces, and the types of activities all effect the final outcome. Trauma, whether major or minor, to the overlying articular cartilage leads to separation and cleft formation, clinical signs of pain and lameness, and other chronic sequelae (Ekman and Carlson 1998).

Because a noticeable difference can exist in the size of the lesion and its clinical severity, two closely related terms have evolved and are used in descriptions of this developmental bone disease: (1) osteochondrosis (OC) and (2) osteochondritis dissecans (OCD). During its early stages of development, the lesion is referred to as an osteochondrosis. This describes the failure of ossification of the epiphysis that leaves a section of thickened cartilage that may contain necrotic cartilage and debris. If the fragment of cartilage that forms a lesion of osteochondrosis partially separates from the articular surface, material from the degenerating cartilage now can easily flow into the joint cavity. This causes a sterile inflammatory reaction within the synovium resulting in a swollen, hot, and painful joint, permitting the use of the word ending, "itis," as in osteochondritis, to indicate an inflammatory disease. The term dissecans refers to the separation of the overlying diseased cartilage from the underlying epiphysis. Regardless of the future status of the "flap" of cartilage, irritation of the synovium perpetuates the inflammatory process and the resulting clinical signs. It is possible for the "flap" to become separated completely and form a loose body within the joint capsule (Table 1-1).

In summary, OC is a non-clinical condition that may resolve or may progress to an OCD, which is the clinical form of the disease causing pain and lameness and an eventual osteoarthrosis. However, both presentations are part of an inheritable disease. The terms are used separately throughout this monograph when reference is made

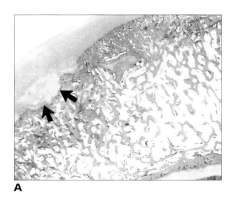
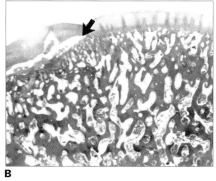
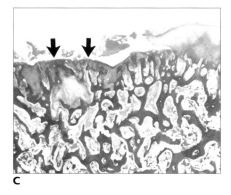

A  B  C

**Figure 1-4**
Photomicrographs of histological sections showing a progression of change as an osteochondrosis progresses to an osteochondritis dissecans within the humeral head. (A) The delay in epiphyseal bone formation results in a thickened cartilage that is otherwise nearly normal histologically. The cancellous spicules of bone thicken in the area surrounding the lesion (arrows). (B) Following cartilage necrosis, a fissure (arrow) can develop separating the overlying necrotic cartilage from the underlying bone forming a "flap." (C) With further time, the cartilaginous fragment loosens and separates leaving a necrotic cartilage bed (arrow).

to a specific form of the disease. In some instances, "osteochondrosis" within quote marks is used as a general term making reference to both stages of the disease when the exact stage cannot be determined.

An important feature of OCD is the cartilaginous "flap." It can become unattached and remain as a single loose body within the joint capsule, or upon detachment, may break into several loose bodies. These cause an acute synovitis. In addition, any of these loose bodies can migrate into a connecting tendon sheath causing tendosynovitis. The loose bodies may also attach to the synovium, gain nourishment, and increase in size often forming what are referred to as synovial osteochondromas. The cartilaginous "flap," whatever its course, strongly influences the course of the clinical signs.

Complete separation of the fragment may be beneficial since removal of the "flap" permits healing of the "bed" of the lesion, with the result that some repair of the defect within the articular cartilage can take place. This is the reason why surgical removal of the lesion is an important goal in treatment (Figure 1-5). While the "flap" remains in position, no healing of the cartilage defect by fibrogenesis can occur, and no scar tissue can fill the defect.

An early lesion of osteochondrosis can: (1) progress to a clinically important OCD, (2) remain unchanged, or (3) heal through restoration of the process of ossification. The lesion that remains unchanged or heals may develop a minimal osteoarthrosis while the lesions that progress to an OCD will develop a prominent osteoarthrosis.

The presence of the lesion of OC can be the basis for a diagnostic error. This can happen in the case of a forelimb lameness in which only the shoulder is radiographed, demonstrating this type of early osteochondrosis lesion of the humeral head. The lameness noted in such a dog may not be caused by the early humeral head osteochondrosis, but it may be caused by a co-existing elbow dysplasia not detected clinically and not radiographed. In this patient, the shoulder osteochondrosis is only an incidental finding. A thorough physical examination of the shoulder joint should have shown an absence of pain on flexion suggesting the OC lesion to be only incidental. Because these early lesions are not associated with clinical signs, it is uncertain how frequently the process of their early healing may occur. However, this dog, while not clinically lame, should still be considered genetically affected.

It is possible for the depth of the necrosis of the thickened cartilage to be so extensive that a subchondral bone cyst is formed. This occurs more commonly in OCD in the horse. Only a small defect remains within the articular surface with more healthy bone forming a partial bridge or covering over the necrotic tissue contained within the cyst. While this pattern is rarely seen in osteochondrosis in dogs, it can be found within the femoral condyle. These lesions are of less clinical importance since only a minimal portion of the articular surface may be affected and the secondary osteoarthrosis is minimal. Still, the necrotic lesion cannot provide normal support to the overlying articular cartilage. An opening into the cyst provides for the influx of synovial fluid and the possibility for synovitis and joint pain (Figure 1-6). All lesions of osteochondrosis, whether ultimately forming a "flap" or "cyst," are similar in that an accumulation of necrotic cartilage prevents the outgrowth of a healthy blood supply from deep within the epiphysis and thus the synovial fluid provides nutrition only to the surface layers of cartilage. This creates

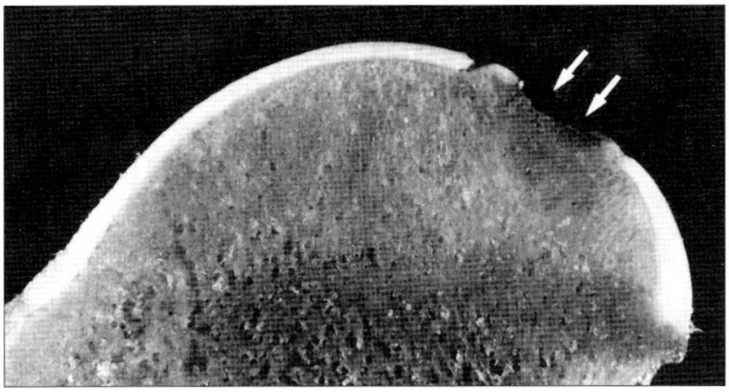

**Figure 1-5**
Photograph of a slab section of the humeral head with OCD that illustrates separation of the cartilage fragment leaving open the cavity within the epiphysis (arrows). Following separation of the cartilage "flap," healing of the lesion can progress under some circumstances.

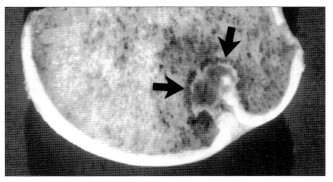

**Figure 1-6**
Photograph of a slab section of the femoral condyle from a horse that illustrates a "subchondral cyst." This form of osteochondrosis does not create a cartilage "flap" but forms a cavity of necrotic cartilage deep to the articular surface (arrows). The size of articular surface that is affected is relatively small and the lesions may not be as painful. This type of OC lesion is uncommon in the dog.

a zone of cartilage that dies, preventing the orderly conversion of the epiphysis into trabecular bone.

Smaller cysts may also be found in association with the more commonly noted "flap" formation and seem to be dependent on the manner in which the separating cleft has formed. These cysts are located deep within the epiphysis, actually beneath the primary defect and their formation probably is highly dependent on the tissue secondary reaction to invading synovial fluid.

## Metaphyseal growth plate

While the most clinically obvious lesions of OC occur either centrally or peripherally within an epiphyseal growth area, OC lesions do occur within metaphyseal growth plates and may disturb growth of a long bone to such a degree that the shape or length of the bone may be altered. This rather uncommon clinical finding may assume separate forms. A common primary form of metaphyseal OC occurs without an associated epiphyseal lesion within the distal ulna where the unique shape of the growth plate is that of an inverted cone (Figure 1-7). Because of this shape, central cartilage nutrition may be impaired resulting in a delay in skeletal maturation. Instead of normal conversion of cartilage to bone, a delay in removal of the necrotic cartilage cells leads to the persistence of large columns of cartilage cells that stream into the distal metaphysis. This error in skeletal maturation results in a delayed growth and a shortened ulna that may have a marked effect on growth of the adjacent radius and may affect the congruity of the antebrachiocarpal elbow joint (see Chapter 4).

A less commonly seen metaphyseal lesion occurs independently in the transverse growth area of the femoral neck where abnormal growth of the cartilage may cause weakness that paves the way for epiphysiolysis, or slippage of both femoral heads. This is contrary to the unilateral physeal fracture that may occur in the skeletally immature dog following trauma (Lee 1976). This is an uncommon occurrence in the dog, but is devastating clinically. Separation of the capital femoral epiphysis from the femoral neck has been reported most commonly in swine where it has been suggested to result from a defect in the growth cartilage (dyschondroplasia) (Duthie and Lancaster 1964, Grøndalen 1974). The condition in swine has been suggested to result from increased body weight causing a bending and weakening of the metaphyseal trabeculae (Yamasaki, et al 1989). The condition has been reported in humans: in adolescents as a complication of renal disease in which both rickets and secondary hyperparathyroidism produced gross and microscopic changes in the proximal femur that maximized the effect of mechanical shearing stresses on the cartilaginous growth plate (Goldman, et al 1978); and in children who received radiotherapy to the pelvis including the non-fused capital femoral epiphyseal plate (Silverman, et al 1981).

In one report of this condition in two dogs, both were of excessive weight (Dupruis, et al 1997). Both dogs had been castrated with the possibility of a resulting extended period of skeletal growth attributable to a lack of the gonadal hormones (testosterone and estradiol 17-B) that normally hasten maturation of physeal cartilage (Salmeri, et al 1991). Tissue used for histological examination is usually removed quite some time following the onset of the condition and it is difficult to know whether any abnormality that is noted represents a primary cartilaginous defect (dyschondroplasia) or a stage of repair after the separation of the epiphysis. Because of its uncommon appearance, it is difficult to characterize these lesions with accuracy, to speculate on the prognosis with or without surgical treatment, or to determine any particular feature of heritability.

A more distant effect of an epiphyseal osteochondrosis may result in premature closure of an adjacent metaphyseal growth plate. This has been noticed most often in the proximal humerus in conjunction with a humeral head OCD. It is most easily seen when comparing radiographs of both shoulders in which the OC is more prominent on one limb than the other. In this situation, the premature closure of the physis can be detected. The total effect on the limb length is clinically insignificant (see Chapter 2).

OCD has been incorrectly described to be the result of an osteochondral fracture (a fracture that extends through cartilage and bone). One reason that osteochondral fractures have been considered a cause of OCD is that bony tissue is often found as a part of the cartilage flap or within a joint body. It has been assumed that presence of the bony tissue is the result of both bone and cartilage tissue being separated from the epiphysis at the time of injury. Thus, a fracture is thought to have occurred through both bone and cartilage. Pathogenesis of this type has been considered by researchers, but support for an osteochondral fracture has not been noted in the dog (Olsson 1976), pig (Reiland 1978 c), horse (Rejnö and Strömberg 1978), or bull calves (Reiland, et al 1978 b). In all situations, early histological examination of tissue has shown that the original lesion is within the cartilage and not within bone. The more plausible explanation for the appearance of bony tissue within the free cartilaginous fragment is to consider that after separation of the cartilaginous fragment, the fragment gained an attach-

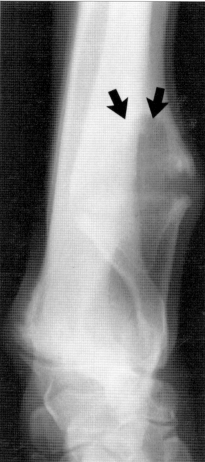 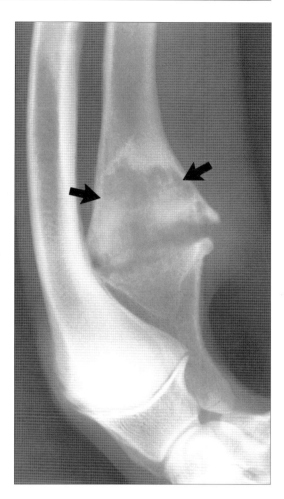

**Figure 1-7**
Radiographs of the distal antebrachium of an immature dog in which an osteochondrosis of the distal ulnar metaphysis has lead to the presence of a large metaphyseal cartilaginous mass (arrows). This interferes with normal endochondral ossification and results in shortening of the ulna and a curvature within the adjacent radius. This type of lesion, when minimal, may be clinically unimportant with recovery permitting an eventual normal bone maturation. However, in this patient, the forelimb abnormalities are characterized by the shortened ulna with curvature and the associated curvature of the radius with the probability of either elbow or antebrachiocarpal joint osteoarthrosis.

ment to the synovium and a blood supply was established. It then proceeded to undergo endochondral ossification resulting in the formation of bony tissue in what was previously a pure cartilaginous fragment. Many detached cartilage fragments reattach in this manner and increase in size and ossify.

## Definition of dysplasia

Dysplasia of the hip joint and elbow joint are additional inherited developmental diseases of bone. The term dysplasia means literally a faulty development and is formed from the Greek "dys," meaning abnormal, and "plassein," meaning to form. Dysplasia of the hip joint was the first of the developmental bone and joint diseases to be recognized and thus has been most widely studied in the dog. Dysplasia is not a congenital disease and the joints are normal at birth but uneven growth between the skeletal and muscular systems in the hip joint results in a femoral head that is forced out of the acetabular cup dorsally and laterally. Elbow dysplasia results in the development of an ulnar trochlear notch that is too small in circumference to encompass the humeral trochlea, thus creating incongruity within the joint. Depending partially on the breed of dog, the effect of this incongruity may result in different forms of dysplasia including the clinically important: (1) ununited anconeal process (UAP), (2) medial coronoid process disease (MCPD), and (3) osteochondritis dissecans (OCD) of the medial humeral condyle. If the incongruity is minor, the only result may be a minimal osteoarthrosis causing no obvious clinical signs. This abnormal development occurs at an early age when the joint components are cartilaginous and thus soft and malleable resulting in deformation of the acetabulum ("shallow" acetabulum) or deformation of the trochlear notch leading to the development of a painful osteoarthrosis. The impact of hip and elbow dysplasia on the dog world can be noticed by talking with owners who have seen the life of a promising field or show dog cut short by the disease.

The early phase of joint dysplasia is typically asymptomatic and is characterized by a mild nonsuppurative synovitis with: (1) an increased volume of synovial fluid, (2) thickening of synovium, (3) thickening of the joint

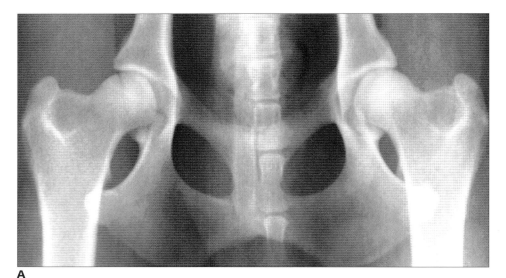
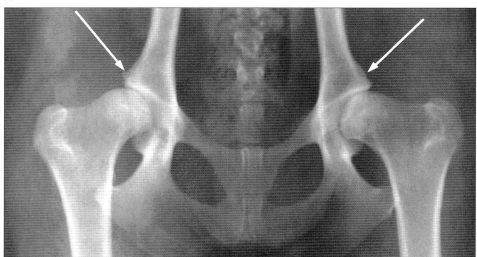

**Figure 1-8**
Radiographs of the hip joints of a 2-year-old male Australian Shepherd Dog (A) show normal hip joints characterized by smooth articular surfaces of the femoral heads that articulate with the opposing acetabula. Compare the normal hips with those of a 2-year-old female Australian Shepherd Dog (B) with hip dysplasia indicated by joint laxity and secondary osteoarthrosis that is characterized by: (1) femoral heads that have lost their round contour, (2) thickened femoral necks, (3) shallow acetabular cups, and (4) new bony spurs that have formed adjacent to the acetabular margin (arrows). These changes seen radiographically are evidence that the bones do not articulate normally and are characteristic of the early changes of osteoarthrosis, a non-inflammatory joint disease. This form of painful joint disease in the dog is often secondary to inherited developmental disease, such as osteochondrosis and elbow or hip dysplasia. Radiographic examination is one of the best methods of diagnosing joint disease of this type.

capsule, and (4) focal degenerative articular cartilage lesions. Any factor that influences the proper fit of bones can, singly or in concert with other factors such as rapid body growth, cause development of a secondary osteoarthrosis.

Joint dysplasia might be considered to be the result of an imbalance between weight-bearing forces and the maturation of cartilage to bone. If the cartilage can convert to bone forming normal shaped articular surfaces prior to abnormal stresses being placed on the hip joint, dysplasia can be avoided. However, if the cartilage model becomes malformed prior to the final conversion to bone, the joint will be dysplastic. The severity of each form of dysplasia varies, creating disease with differing clinical significance.

## Definition of osteoarthrosis (OA)

While this monograph discusses developmental lesions in the dog, it also describes in detail the resulting joint disease referred to as osteoarthrosis, or more simply, arthrosis. Osteoarthrosis is one of the most common disorders in both man and animals causing pain, suffering, and disability to millions, with great economic losses to society (Reiland 1978 b). Although the effect of osteochondrosis or joint dysplasia in the young dog may result in a painful lameness, it is the resulting arthrosis that is the permanent cause of discomfort to the dog and concern to the owner. Having to witness the long-term effects of the painful, disabling osteoarthrosis is what drives us in a search for prevention, or at least control, of the original inherited diseases. The osteoarthrosis associated with developmental bone disease in dogs is a non-inflammatory joint disease and is differentiated from inflammatory arthritis that is so common in man and is better referred to as rheumatoid arthritis.

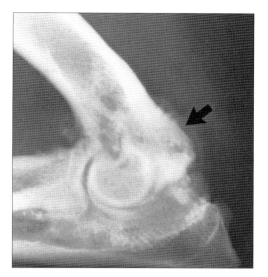
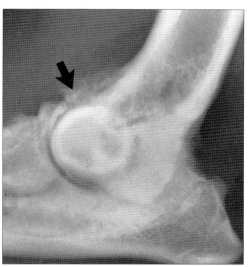
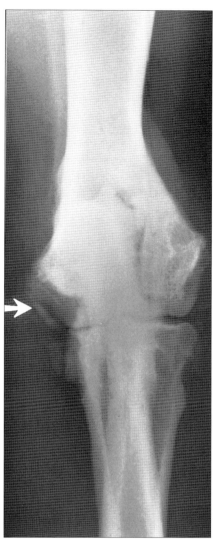

**Figure 1-9**
Radiographs of the elbow joint of an older German Shepherd Dog with severe joint disease. The radiographic changes are characterized by: (1) new bone formation (black arrows), (2) an unequal width of the joint space, and (3) by soft tissue calcification within the joint capsule and periarticular soft tissues (white arrow). The pattern of change seen with an osteoarthrosis is similar whether the cause is trauma, developmental joint disease, or, uncommonly, following infection. Thus, in this older dog, the cause of the arthrosis is more difficult to determine.

By affecting the ends of the growing bones (epiphyses), abnormal development directly influences the ultimate shape and contour of the articular surfaces (Figure 1-8). Failure to develop a perfectly formed articular surface that fits exactly or is congruent with the opposing articular surface leads to the development of osteoarthrosis that progresses as the dog ages (Figure 1-9). Progression of the arthrosis is influenced by many factors, such as inappropriate or excessive physical activity and increased body weight (Kealy, et al 1997). While relatively uncommon, trauma in the form of intra-articular fracture or luxation or infection within a joint may also produce a similar osteoarthrosis that is of a non-hereditary nature.

In the early stages, osteoarthrosis is particularly characterized by articular cartilage breakdown with an increase in production of synovial fluid that results in joint capsule distention. In addition, an increased production of lysosomal hydrolases causes exacerbation of the cartilage damage. Articular cartilage lacks blood vessels, lymphatics, and nerves, and is dependent on diffusion from the synovial fluid for nutrition. Lesions of the synovial membrane and joint capsule compromise the nutritional supply to the cartilage, limiting the range and extent of repair mechanisms. The lack of nerve endings is actually a major factor in the progression of articular disease because potentially irreversible damage may develop before clinical signs indicate joint injury. If the cartilage injury is severe enough, a network of fibrovascular stroma may extend over the articular cartilage defect. This apparent repair mechanism further compromises the nutritional supply to the damaged cartilage.

These changes are accompanied by thickening of the joint capsule and interarticular ligaments. Although it is possible that these changes may help to stabilize the joint and, thus, decrease pain, deleterious effects such as decreased joint mobility or increased pain because of increased synovial pressure are noted. Other reactions include formation of villous synovitis. Because the synovial membrane contains numerous nerves, excessive proliferation of synovial villi or increased synovial fluid pressure results in pain. The pathology of OA has been described (Pedersen and Pool 1978, Morgan 1992, 1997).

Soft tissue changes characterize the early stages of osteoarthrosis and are followed by bony changes affecting the attachments of the muscle tendons, ligaments, and joint capsule. These sites of new bone production are called entheses and the bone produced is referred to as enthesophytes. They differ from new bone that develops at the articular margins and it is known as periarticular lipping or spurring. With chronicity, the ends of the bones may become severely deformed and completely denuded of the articular cartilage. At this point, the production of synovial fluid may cease resulting in a "dry" joint.

Although dogs with advanced osteoarthrosis should receive adequate rest and avoid strenuous exercise, they should not be allowed to become invalids. Properly administered and controlled exercise is important in maintaining muscle tone and keeping joints freely movable. Controlled exercise can consist of defined periods of walking with the owner interspersed with short period of rest or other controlled periods of play, swimming, or similar activities (Millis and Levine 1997).

Others feel that CHD and OA may both be manifestations of a more generalized abnormality affecting several joints in dogs (Lust 1997). The increase in fibronectin content in cartilage from grossly normal appearing joints in dogs with a high risk for developing hip dysplasia indicates that normal appearing joints in these dogs are in fact not entirely normal (Farquhar, et al 1997). This places OA in a primary position equal to CHD. In this monograph, OA is described as secondary to a primary dysplasia or osteochondrosis since this is the manner in which the conditions are noted clinically.

## Influence of diet and growth rate

Osteochondrosis and the joint dysplasias have been studied more thoroughly in other species of animals than the dog, and these studies must be utilized in an effort to assist us in the determination of the cause of similar appearing lesions in the dog. While it may be somewhat difficult for the reader to transfer information from the pig to the dog, Grøndalen's (1974 a, b, c) and Reiland's studies in the pig (1978 a, e) are basic to a complete understanding of the role of nutrition and growth rate in the disease. They reported a high frequency of lesions with a symmetrical occurrence in certain sites in joints and in many metaphyseal plates. Examination of feeding methods answered the questions of the high frequency and location. By intensive selection for achieving fast market size, the pig has become one of the most rapidly growing of our domestic animals. Swine used for commercial purposes often reach an adult weight of more than 275 kg at 2 years of age. In contrast, swine of wild hog ancestry (Yucatan swine), in which the frequency of both osteochondrosis and clinical lameness is essentially zero, reach an adult weight of approximately 75 kg at the same age (Farnum and Wilson 1986). Reiland (1978 a) compared Swedish Landrace and Yorkshire pigs with the wild European hog and demonstrated experimentally that the incidence and severity of osteochondrosis was directly related to rapid growth (ie, weight gain) of the animal, and that the disease was not noted in slower growing animals of a more wild nature and thus, more normal variety. Reiland (1978 e) fed a diet restricted to 50% to 60% of the ration given to commercially breed controls and found that those pigs had a lower growth rate and showed no, or only mild, morphological signs of osteochondrosis. This was in agreement with studies by Grøndalen and Vangen (1974) that stated that a line of pigs selected for low growth rate had a lower incidence of osteochondrosis compared to normal pigs used for marketing. Animals with a low weight gain, nutritionally or genetically induced, had an incidence of osteochondrosis which was close to zero.

Additional important information can be gained from studies in calves. In an examination for osteochondrosis of growing bull calves, an entire group of 23 calves placed on intensive feeding were found to have lesions of osteochondrosis in the epiphyseal cartilage and within the metaphyseal growth plates. Specific locations were involved, such as the dorsocranial and central part of the humeral head, articular surface of the distal radius, lateral femoral trochlear ridge, lateral femoral condyle, tibial plateau, patella, cranial apex of the intermediate trochlear ridge of the tibia, and distal talus. Lesions were also noted within metaphyseal growth plates. However, only 13 of 25 bull calves on a lower intensity diet developed lesions of osteochondrosis. Additionally, the lesions in animals of the low intensity fed groups were less severe than those noted in the high intensity fed groups. Healing of the lesions in the low intensity fed groups was more active than healing in the corresponding lesions in the calves of the high intensity fed groups. The frequency and severity of osteochondrosis were correlated with rapid growth. The lesions histologically were similar to those seen in pigs and horses (Reiland, et al 1978 b). It has also been shown experimentally in enzygotic (same fertilized ovum) bull twins that over-nutrition induces pathologic lesions in both growth plates and joints (Andreae and Dämmrich 1972).

Studies in horses provide us with additional information concerning the appearance of osteochondrosis; the condition was positively correlated to body size in a study of 674 progeny of 20 Swedish Standardbred trotter stallions (Carlsten, et al 1993). Foals that developed osteochondrosis in the tarsus had a higher birth weight and continued to be heavier and have a higher daily weight gain than non-affected foals. They had a greater height at the withers and the croup and were bigger boned as determined from measurements made of the limb at the carpus and metacarpus. The incidence of osteochondrosis was significantly different between progeny groups. A high heritability for size of horses was demonstrated and a correlation between size and occurrence of OCD was suggested (Strömberg and Rejnö 1978). A subsequent study of OCD in the tarsus of Standardbred trotters and Swedish warm-bloods concluded that genetic factors, in addition to size, seem to contribute to the predisposition of OCD (Hoppe and Philipsson 1985). The heritability of a specific form of osteochondrosis that occurs in the tibiotarsal joint and another form of osteochondrosis characterized by formation of bony fragments in the palmar/plantar portion of the metacarpophalangeal and metatarsophalangeal joints of Norwegian Standardbred trotters was estimated to be 0.52 and 0.21. This heritability was made in both anatomical regions without reference to size or growth rate (Grøndahl and Dolvik 1993). These studies confirm the importance of both the genetic background of the animal as well as the growth rate influenced by diet.

Recently, local ischemia secondary to defects in cartilage canal blood supply is thought to be the key factor in the initiation of lesions of osteochondrosis in horses (Carlson, et al 1995). Insulin-like growth factor-I (IGF-I) and transforming growth factor-beta (TGF-ß) were found to be deficient in chondrocytes at sites of osteochondrosis. It is presumed that both of these factors are involved with chondrocyte function during endochondral ossification (Weiss and Loeffler 1996; Thorp, et al 1995).

Osteochondrosis has been noted commonly in medium or larger sized dogs and only rarely in smaller dogs. It occurs almost exclusively in individual animals with an adult weight exceeding 20 kg (Olsson 1987). It was noted that twice as many of the rapidly growing males were affected as the slower-growing females (Olsson 1976). This anecdotal information has not been treated with the importance that it deserves in an effort to understand the causes and etiology of the bone dysplasias.

Dogs with a genetic capacity for fast growth that were being overfed during their most active growth period stood the greatest chance of developing osteochondrosis in all locations. Hedhammer, et al (1974) concluded from a feeding study of Great Danes that the excessive intake of a high-energy diet, rich in protein, could induce the changes of osteochondrosis. In a study of another type of developmental bone disease, "hip dysplasia was more frequent, occurred earlier, and became more severe in dogs with rapid weight gain caused by increased caloric intake than in the dogs that had a low weight gain because of restricted feeding" (Kasström 1975).

The levels of certain vitamins, calcium, and protein that are commonly fed as supplements to animals have frequently been suggested to be a factor of importance in stimulating the occurrence of osteochondrosis. One study in dogs demonstrated experimentally that over supplementation of calcium and phosphorus can lead to skeletal changes very similar to those seen in spontaneous osteochondrosis, but a high energy diet was required as well (Hedhammer, et al 1974). Reiland's (1978 d) nutritional study in pigs suggested that high or low calcium feeding did not change the incidence of osteochondrosis. However, others have felt that the calcium content of the food played an important etiological role in the development of osteochondrosis, more so than the amount of food intake (Hazewinkel, et al 1985).

Moderate changes in protein levels in the diet were reported to not be of etiologic importance in osteochondrosis in pigs (Grøndalen 1974 c). Instead, high caloric intake was again found to be the main nutritional factor in the etiology of osteochondrosis (Reiland 1978 e).

A diet with a deficiency of vitamin D was fed to pigs and no appreciable difference in incidence and severity of osteochondrosis was noted on comparison with the control group. It was decided that lack of that vitamin was not an etiologic factor in osteochondrosis. Levels of vitamin A were also tested to evaluate the theory that hyper- or hypovitaminosis A was of any etiologic importance (Reiland 1978 d). The experimental findings did not support those theories.

It should be stressed that the majority of studies strongly support the concept that the high caloric intake rather than the specific intake of protein, minerals, or vitamins influences the frequency and severity of osteochondrosis and hip dysplasia. The causes of elbow dysplasia have not been studied as thoroughly and, therefore, are less clear.

# Heritability of hip dysplasia, elbow dysplasia, and osteochondroses in the dog

What is the genetic transmission of osteochondroses and dysplasias in the dog from parent to offspring? Between 1955 to 1959, hip dysplasia was first reported to be a disease in which there was statistically significant evidence of an hereditary nature (Grounds, et al 1955; Schales 1956, 1957; Berg 1957; McClave 1957; Henricson and Olsson 1959). Many studies since that time have confirmed these early findings. Relative to osteochondrosis, Olsson (1976) stated that there is "probably a hereditary predisposition for osteochondrosis in the dog" because of detection of a high incidence of the disease in offspring of certain dogs and detection of the disease in litters in which all or nearly all of the puppies were affected. This observation was continuously made in subsequent years by many clinicians, although while commonly accepted, it has not been well documented in the literature. Exceptions are reports of osteochondrosis in the shoulders and stifles of three of five Border Collie littermates (Knecht, et al 1977) and osteochondrosis in the shoulders in a litter of Bull Terriers (Woodard 1979). The greatest argument for the hereditary predisposition for OC, elbow dysplasia, and hip dysplasia is the fact that they occur at high frequencies in certain breeds.

Ununited anconeal process has been reported as inherited in German Shepherd Dogs (Carlson and Severin 1961; Corley, et al 1968; Hayes, et al 1979). Olsson (1976) reported this condition to have "a genetic trait because the lesion frequently is found in littermates." Lavelle and Studdert (1990) felt that there is an inherited basis for elbow disease in the Labrador Retriever with the dam contributing significantly more variation from normal than the sire. Padgett, et al (1995) considered osteochondrosis of the humeral condyle and medial coronoid disease to be inherited, but, independently.

The strongest support for heritability in these diseases is found in a recent study of elbow dysplasia diagnosed radiographically by the presence of osteoarthrosis (Swenson, et al 1997). In this study medium to high estimates of heritability were found in Bernese Mountain dog and Rottweiler breeds. The recognition of elbow dysplasia as a multifactorial polygenic threshold trait means that selection of sire and dam to be used for breeding affects the prevalence of the lesions. The term threshold suggests that the product of the gene must build up to a certain point before it can affect the development of the trait. Family records that indicate the status of full- and half-siblings as well as parents and perhaps grandparents plus progeny testing of sires all serve to further improve a breeding program.

There is strong evidence of the inheritance of these diseases in which the genes for a rapid growth may play an important role in determining expression of whether any of these developmental diseases are to be present. In

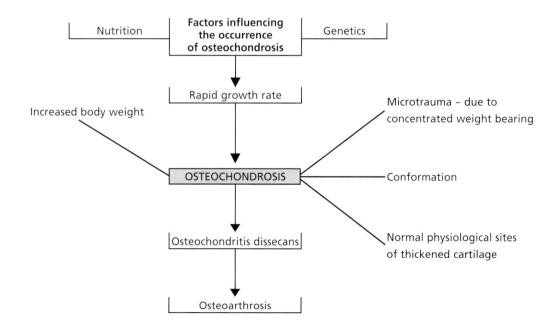

**Figure 1-10**
A model suggesting factors that influence the occurrence of osteochondrosis.

addition, environmental factors such as over-nutrition may influence the severity of the disease. Based on studies of the occurrence of osteochondrosis in pigs, horses, cattle, poultry, and turkeys, Olsson and Reiland (1978) showed conclusively "that the two interrelated factors, nutrition and the genetic trait which determine growth rate, are of importance for the frequency of osteochondrosis in animals." This permits us to develop a model suggesting factors that influence the occurrence of osteochondrosis (Figure 1-10).

Examination of genetic studies in the horse adds information of value in our understanding of osteochondrosis in the dog. Nutritional as well as genetic and biomechanical factors are suggested to contribute to the development of this condition in the horse. Large, rapidly growing individuals are thought to be more affected with osteochondrosis. While ponies are seldom found with osteochondrosis, 10% to 15% of Standardbred trotters and Warmblood riding horses commonly have osteochondrosis (Hoppe and Philisson 1985). Knowing whether certain stallions give a significantly higher incidence of osteochondrosis in their progeny than do other stallions is valuable in understanding the genetic role. Five studies from the Scandinavian countries reveal highly significant differences in the incidence of disease among progeny group (Strömberg and Rejnö 1978; Hoppe and Philisson 1985; Schougaard, et al 1990; Grøndahlen and Dolvik 1993; Philipsson, et al 1993). Most of these studies were based on radiographic findings in yearlings. The studies showed that the occurrence of osteochondrosis was nearly three times as high among the progeny of stallions affected with osteochondrosis as among those from non-affected stallions. This is strong proof of the importance of hereditary factors in contributing to the development of osteochondrosis and suggests that the inheritance has a polygenic nature. A recent review of the occurrence of osteochondrosis in different joints of the horse indicates a multifactorial background in which genetic factors have been shown to be quite important (Philipsson 1996). Progeny testing of Swedish Landrace and Yorkshire boars showed heritability estimates ranging from 0.14 to 0.30 for osteochondrosis lesions at three sites (Reiland, et al 1978 a).

Heritability is a parameter used in both the estimation of breeding values for quantitative characteristics and for predicting the response expected from various selective schemes. It is of value in discussing the possibility of altering the frequency of a trait noted within a population. Heritability in the broad sense is defined as the ratio of the genetic variance to the phenotypic variance and describes what proportion of the total variation is due to differences among genotypes of individuals in the population. Heritability is specific to the population and trait under consideration. If either the genetic or environmental variance for the same trait in two populations differs, heritability will also be different (van Vleck, et al 1987).

The level of heritability often reported for osteochondrosis (0.25 to 0.35) is of the same magnitude as that of important traits such as milk yield and growth rate in cattle, traits that are subject to successful selection programs. This level of heritability indicates that good progress in decreasing the incidence of osteochondrosis could be expected from the elimination of affected animals from breeding. A higher demand of accuracy in the determination of osteochondrosis within a breeding animal must not only be based on a negative radiographic finding but also must be based on progeny-testing results.

## Sites of disease predilection in the dog

If osteochondrosis is a disease affecting skeletal maturation, why are there certain sites of predilection? Osteochondrosis of the shoulder joint is almost exclusively located in the centrocaudal portion of the humeral head where the cartilage remains thicker than in the other parts of the humeral head until the age of 4 to 5 months. The reason for this may be that the center of ossification of the humeral epiphysis is located eccentrically with the caudal portion delayed in development. Thus, the blood supply is further from the maturing cartilage of the caudal epiphyseal growth plate (Carrig and Morgan 1974). This tendency is accentuated in the large and giant breeds offering an explanation for the increased frequency of osteochondrosis of the humeral head in those breeds. Osteochondrosis of the elbow joint is exclusively located in the medial condyle of the humerus where a thickened joint cartilage is retained for a longer period than in the lateral condyle. In the distal femur, osteochondrosis occurs in the condyles, both of which can be late in their ossification. Obviously, a critical time in the development of osteochondrosis in the dog appears to be the age of 4 to 5 months when these sites of predilection remain cartilaginous (Olsson 1976).

Many lesions of osteochondrosis never proceed to the clinical disease of OCD. What causes an osteochondrosis lesion to change to an OCD? Are weight bearing stresses important? Examination of anatomic sites frequently affected by clinically significant lesions indicates that in these joints all of the stress of weight bearing is borne on a relatively small area of the articular surface. This is particularly suggested in lesions of the femoral condyles and the trochlear ridges of the talus. Less obvious is the mechanistic explanation of the lesions of the humeral head. Osteochondrosis of the distal ulnar metaphyseal growth plate is unique and probably is caused by an interference of blood supply leading to cessation of cartilage maturation.

## Diagnosis

Diagnosis of osteochondrosis or osteochondritis dissecans is based on clinical signs and symptoms and radiographic studies. Since the joints are frequently involved bilaterally and many of the predisposed breeds have combinations of osteochondrosis, elbow dysplasia, and hip dysplasia, it is advisable to determine the status of all of the most likely affected joints before recommending treatment of a single pain-producing lesion (Olsewski, et al 1983; Morgan, et al 1998). Be aware that severe pain in one joint may camouflage pain caused by the presence of disease in other joints. While pain may be detected within a joint, diagnostic radiology is the only non-invasive technique readily available at this time that can be used to support the clinical findings.

Early diagnosis is paramount to the successful treatment of a single patient if we are to have a positive influence on the outcome of the disease. Accurate diagnosis is also important if we are to have an impact on selection of dogs to be used for breeding or training.

Because of the high incidence of bilateral involvement of a specific lesion, it is strongly suggested following detection of a single lesion that the opposite joint should be examined radiographically. This is important since often only one joint is painful. Because osteochondroses and elbow and hip dysplasia are diseases that can be present concurrently, skeletal survey radiographs should be considered in predisposed breeds when it is economically feasible (Poulos 1982; Olsson 1987; Morgan, et al 1998). The need for a limited or general skeletal survey may be determined by considering the confidence of the examining clinician as well as the wishes of the owner. Use of a radiographic skeletal survey is especially advisable prior to treatment so that a decision relative to surgical treatment and determination of the prognosis can be based on the most complete knowledge of the orthopedic status of the patient. In dogs without clinical signs that are to be placed in working programs or to be used as breeding stock, a survey radiographic study is most certainly indicated to determine most accurately the orthopedic status of this special patient.

While any combination of affected joints within a single dog can be found in survey studies, in our experience, the most common combination is that of elbow and hip dysplasia. However, these combinations are breed dependent and the reader is directed to the discussion of disease in the chapter concerning the study on Labrador Retrievers (see Chapter 9).

## Treatment and prognosis

The treatment of an individual patient must take into account many factors, among which are the expected use of the dog or the specific wishes of the owner. In some instances, conservative treatment (weight and exercise control) or medical treatment may be recommended, while in other cases, surgical treatment should be strongly considered. In cases of lesions with advanced osteoarthrosis, surgery is often not an option and conservative and medical treatment may be all that remains. However, this limitation may change with the increased use of prosthetic implants. The prognosis cannot easily be predicted because of the individual differences and circumstances of each patient. Still, an effort will be made to describe the prognosis in general in the following chapters so that the reader can have some knowledge of what to expect following treatment of a particular disease.

## Significance of osteochondrosis and dysplasia

It seems appropriate to spend a few minutes and again consider the status of osteochondrosis in the pig, since it has been so thoroughly studied, to learn if there are some warning signs for those breeding large dogs. Reiland (1978 a) found that the modern pig is the product of genetic selection for fast growth and for specific qualities such as increased lean meat and less fat. The modern pig weighs about 100 kg at 6 months of age, a weight that a wild hog does not reach until it is about 12 months of age. The modern boar at maturity weighs about 350 kg at an age of 3.5 years while the adult wild boar at that age weighs about 200 to 250 kg. What have been the consequences of breeding the modern pig to this stage? Almost 100% of the modern pigs under 18 months of age have osteochondrosis. These findings by Reiland are in agreement with figures reported by Grøndalen (1974 b). It is important to recognize that growth can be influenced both by genetic and nutritional factors. This scenario suggests that we need to look carefully at our selection of dogs used for breeding and also the way in which we feed them. It is not totally impossible that we could breed and raise dogs in a manner that is similar to what has been used in pigs and have to face the painful consequences.

# Goals of this monograph

The goal of this monograph is to describe in detail the osteochondroses as well as elbow and hip dysplasia and lumbosacral lesions from the standpoint of the individual dog. This includes: (1) clinical signs, (2) physical diagnosis, (3) radiographic diagnosis, (4) treatment, and (5) prognosis. Particular attention has been given to the working or performance dog since much time and effort can go into their training with little reward when these skeletal diseases are unexpectedly discovered. The heritability of the conditions is stressed because breeders must come to understand the responsibility they shoulder in selection of breeding stock. The limited sensitivity of diagnostic methods that can detect only phenotype has been stressed, as has the importance of knowing the status of littermates and offspring that more clearly reflects the genotype. The consequences of using a dog with a normal phenotype and an affected genotype for breeding must be understood as we look at the persistence of the diseases.

The authors have written in such a manner that hopefully both the owner/breeder and clinician can gain an understanding of these diseases, methods of diagnosis, and schemes that are in effect that attempt to control the frequency of OC and the dysplasias. The role of the rapidly growing dog and how this has influenced the frequency of skeletal disease has been stressed. It is our hope that from this work, a better understanding can be gain of how to reach our goal in control of inherited skeletal disease (Figure 1-11).

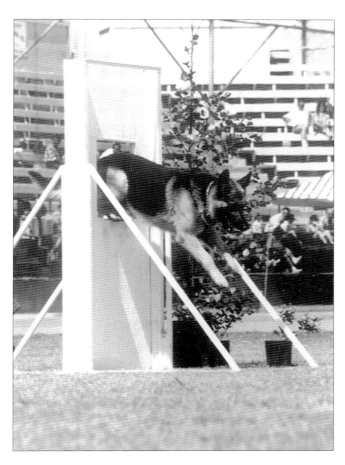

**Figure 1-11**
The type of healthy, active, physically strong dog that can be the result of careful selection of breeding stock and management of growth.

# References

ANDREAE U, Dämmrich K. Über die Beeinflussung der Skelettentwicklung durch energetisch unterschiedliche Fütterung bei eineiigen Zwillingsbullen. Berl Münch Tierärztl Wsch 85:261-265,1972.

BERG E. Die angeborene Hüftgelenksdysplasie beim Hund. Deutsche tierärztl Wsch 64:509-511,1957.

CARLSON CS, CULLINS LD, MEUTEN DJ. Osteochondrosis of the articular-epiphyseal cartilage complex in young horses: evidence for a defect in cartilage canal blood supply. Vet Path 32:641-647,1995.

CARLSON WD, SEVERIN GA. Elbow dysplasia in the dog: A preliminary report. JAVMA 138:295-301,1961.

CARLSTEN J, SANDGREN B, DALIN G. Osteochondrosis in the tarsocrural joint in young Standardbreds. Early development and epidemiology. 2nd EAVDI Annual Congress,1993.

CARRIG CB, MORGAN JP. Microcirculation of the humeral head in the immature dog. JAVRS 15:28-33,1974.

CORLEY EA, SUTHERLAND TM, CARLSON WD. Genetic aspects of canine elbow dysplasia. JAVMA 153:543-547,1968.

CRAIG PH, RISER WH. Osteochondritis dissecans in the proximal humerus of the dog. JAVRS 6:40-49,1965.

DUPRUIS J, BRETON L, DROLET R. Bilateral epiphysiolysis of the femoral heads in two dogs. JAVMA 210:1162-1165,1997.

DUTHIE IF, LANCASTER MC. Polyarthritis and epiphyseolysis of pigs in England. Vet Rec 76:263-272,1964.

EKMAN S, CARLSON CS. The pathophysiology of osteochondrosis. Vet Clinics of NA/SAP:28:17-32,1998.

FARNUM CE, WILSMAN NJ. Ultrastructural histochemical evaluation of growth plate cartilage matrix from healthy and osteochondritic swine. Am J Vet Res 47:1105-1115,1986.

FARQUHAR T, BERTRAM J, TODHUNTER RJ, BURTON-WURSTER N, LUST G. Variations in composition of cartilage from the shoulder joints of young adult dogs at risk for developing canine hip dysplasia. JAVMA 210:1483-1485,1997.

GOLDMAN AB, LANE JM, SALVATI E. Slipped capital femoral epiphyses complicating renal osteodystrophy: A report of three cases. Radiology 126:333-339,1978.

GROUNDS OV, HAGEROORN Al, HOFFMAN RA. Hereditary subluxation. J. Canine Genetics January 1955.

GRONDAHL AM, DOLVIK NI. Heritability estimations of osteochondrosis in the tibiotarsal joint and of bony fragments in the palmar/plantar portion of the metacarpo- and metatarsophalangeal joints of horses. JAVMA 203:101-104,1993.

GRONDALEN T. Osteochondrosis and arthrosis in pigs. I. Incidence in animals up to 120 kg live weight. Acta vet scand 15:1-25,1974a.

GRONDALEN T. Osteochondrosis and arthrosis in pigs. II. Incidence in breeding animals. Acta vet scand 15:26-42,1974b.

GRONDALEN T. Osteochondrosis and arthrosis in pigs. VI. Relationship to feed level and calcium, phosphorus and protein levels in the ration. Acta vet scand 15:147-169,1974c.

GRONDALEN T, VANGEN O. Osteochondrosis and arthrosis in pigs. V. A comparison of the incidence in three different lines of the Norwegian Landrace breed. Acta vet scand 15:61-79,1974.

HAYES HM, SELBY LA, WILSON GP, HOHN RB. Epidemiologic observations of canine elbow disease (Emphasis on dysplasia). JAAHA 14:449-453,1979.

HAZEWINKEL HAW, GOEDEGEBUURE SA, POULOS PW, WOLVEKAMP WThC. Influences of chronic calcium excess on the skeletal development of growing Great Danes. JAAHA 3:377-391,1985.

HEDHAMMER Å, WU F-M, KROOK L, SCHRYVER HR, DELAHUNTA A, WHALEN JP, KALLFELZ FA, NUNEZ EA, HINTZ HF, SHEFFY BE, RYAN GD. Overnutrition and skeletal disease. An experimental study in growing Great Dane Dogs. Cornell Vet 64:(Suppl) 5,1-160,1974.

HENRICSON B, OLSSON S-E. Hereditary acetabular dysplasia in German Shepherd Dogs. JAVMA 135:207-210,1959.

HOPPE F, PHILIPSSON J. A, genetic study of osteochondrosis dissecans in Swedish horses. Eq Pract 7:7-15,1985.

KASSTRÖM H. Nutrition, weight gain and development of hip dysplasia. An experimental investigation in growing dogs with special reference to the effect of feeding intensity. Acta Radiol (Suppl) (Stockh) 344:136-178,1975.

KEALY RD, LAWLER DF, BALLAM JM, LUST G, SMITH GK, BIERY DN, OLSSON S-E. Five-year longitudinal study on limited food consumption and development of osteoarthritis in coxofemoral joints of dogs. JAVMA 210,222-225,1997.

KINCAID SA, ALLHANDS RV, PIJANOWSKi GJ. Chondrolysis associated with cartilage canals of the the distal humerus of growing pigs. Am J Vet Res 46:726-732,1985.

KNECHT CD, VAN SICKLE DC, BLEVINS WE, AVOLT MD, HUGHES RB, CANTWELL HD. Osteochondrosis of the shoulder and stifle in 3 of 5 Border Collie littermates. JAVMA 170:58-60,1977.

LAVELLE RB, STUDDERT VP. Elbow dysplasia (osteochondrosis) A report. 2nd Internat Elbow Working Group Meeting, San Francisco March 1990.

LEE R. Proximal femoral epiphyseal separation in the dog. J small Anim Pract 17:669-679,1976.

LUST G. An overview of the pathogenesis of canine hip dysplasia. JAVMA 210:1443-1445,1997.

McCLAVE PL. Elimination of coxofemoral dysplasia from a breeding kennel. Vet Med 52:241-243,1957.

MILLIS DL, LEVINE D. The role of exercise and physical modalities in the treatment of osteoarthritis. Vet Clinics of NA/SAP 27:913-930,1997.

MORGAN JP, WIND A, DAVIDSON AP. Bone dysplasias in the Labrador Retriever: A radiographic study. JAAHA in press,1999.

MORGAN SJ. The pathology of canine hip dysplasia. Vet Clin North Amer/ SAC 22:541-550,1992.

MORGAN SJ. Pathologic alterations in canine hip dysplasia. JAVMA 210:1446-1450,1997.

OLSEWSKI JM, LUST G, RANDANO VT, SUMMERS BA. Degenerative joint disease: Multiple joint involvement in young and mature dogs. AJVR 44:1300-1308,1983.

OLSSON S-E. Osteochondrosis dissecans in the dog. A study of pathogenesis, clinical signs, pathologic changes, natural course and sequelae. Abstract JAVRS 14, 4,1973.

OLSSON S-E. Osteochondritis dissecans in the dog. Proc AAHA 42 Ann Meeting p360.1975a.

OLSSON S-E. Lameness in the dog. A review of lesions causing osteoarthrosis of the shoulder, elbow, hip stifle and hock joints. Proc AAHA 42 Ann Meeting p363.1975b.

OLSSON S-E. Osteochondrosis- A growing problem to dog breeders. Gaines Progress, Summer 1976 p.1-11.

OLSSON S-E. Osteochondros hos hund. Symposium om ärftligt betingade sjukdomar hos hund. Svensk Veterinärtidning Supplement 11:78-90,1986.

OLSSON S-E. General and local aetiologic factors in canine osteochondrosis. Vet Quart 9:268-278,1987.

OLSSON S-E, REILAND S. The nature of osteochondrosis in animals. Summary and conclusions with comparative aspects on osteochondritis dessicans in man. Acta Radiol (Suppl) (Stockh) 358:299-306,1978.

PADGETT GA, MOSTOSKY UV, PROBST CW, THOMAS MW, KREKE CF. The inheritance of osteochondritis dissecans and fragmented coronoid process of the elbow joint in Labrador Retrievers. JAAHA 31:327-330,1995.

PAATSAMA S, ROKKANEN P, JUSSILA J, SITTNIKOW K. A study of osteochondritis dissecans of the canine humeral head using histological, OTC bone labelling, microradiographic and microangiographic methods. J Sm Anim Pract 12:603-611,1971.

PEDERSEN NC, POOL RR. Canine joint disease (so called osteochondritis dissecans) Vet Clinics of NA 8:465-493,1978.

PHILIPSSON J. Pathogenesis of osteochondrosis - Genetic implications. in Joint Disease in the Horse. C. Wayne McIlwrath and Gayle W. Trotter. Saunders, Philadelphia 1996.

PHILIPSSON J, ANDREASSON E, SANDGREN B. Osteochondrosis in the tarsocrural joint and osteochondral fragments in the fetlock joints in Standardbred trotters : II. Heritability. Eq Vet J 16(suppl):38-41,1993.

POULOS PW Jr. Canine osteochondrosis. Vet Clinics of NA SAP 12:313-328,1982.

REILAND S. Growth and skeletal development of the pig. Acta Radiol (Suppl) (Stockh) 358:15-22,1978a.

REILAND S. Pathology of so-called leg weakness in the pig. Acta Radiol (Suppl) (Stockh) 358:23-44,1978b.

REILAND S. Morphology of osteochondrosis and and sequelae in the pig. Acta Radiol (Suppl) (Stockh) 358:45-90,1978c.

REILAND S. Effects of Vitamin D and A, calcium, phosphorus, and protein on frequency and severity of osteochondrosis in pigs. Acta Radiol (Suppl) (Stockh) 358:91-105,1978d.

REILAND S. The effect of decreased growth rate on frequency and severity of osteochondrosis in pigs. Acta Radiol (Suppl) (Stockh) 358:107-122,1978e.

REILAND S, ORDELL N, LUNDEHEIM N, OLSSON S-E. Heredity of osteochondrosis, body consititution and leg weakness in the pig. A correlative investigation using progency testing. Acta Radiol (Suppl) (Stockh) 358:123-137,1978a.

REILAND S, STRÖMBERG B, OLSSON S-E, DREIMANIS I, OLSSON IG. Osteochondrosis in growing bulls. Pathology, frequency and severity on different feedings. Acta Radiol (Suppl) (Stockh) 358:179-196,1978b.

REJNÖ S, STRÖMBERG B. Osteochondrosis in the horse. II Pathology. Acta Radiol (Suppl) (Stockh) 358:153-178,1978.

RISER WH. The dog. His varied biological makeup and its relationship to orthopaedic diseases. AAHA 1-24, 1985.

SALMERI KR, BLOOMBERG MS, SCRUGGS SL, SHILLE V. Gonadectomy in immature dogs: Effects on skeletal, physical, and behavioral development. JAVMA 198:1193-1203,1991.

SCHALES O. Genetic aspects of dysplasia of the hip joint. North Am Vet 37:476-478,1956.

SCHALES O. Hereditary pattern in dysplasia of the hip. North Am Vet 38:152-159,1957.

SCHOUGAARD H, FALK-RONNE J, PHILIPSSON J. A radiographic survey of tibiotarsal osteochondrosis in a selected population of trotting horses in Denmark and its possible genetic signficane. Eq Vet J 22:288-289,1990.

SILVERMAN CL, THOMAS PRM, McALISTER WH, WALKER S, WHITESIDE LA. Slipped femoral capital epiphyses in irradiated children: Dose, volume, and age relationships. Int J Radiation Oncology 7:1357-1363,1981.

STRÖMBERG B, REJNÖ S. Osteochondrosis in the horse. I. A clinical and radiologic investigation of osteochondritis dissecans on the knee and hock joint. Acta Radiol (Suppl) (Stockh) 358:139-152,1978.

SWENSON L, AUDELL L, HEDHAMMER A. Prevalence and inheritance of and selection for elbow arthrosis in Bernese Mountain Dogs and Rottweilers in Sweden and benefit:cost analysis of a screening and control program. JAVMA 210:215-221,1997.

THORP BH, EKMAN S, JAKOWLEW SB, GODDARD C. Porcine osteochondrosis: deficiencies in transforming growth factor-beta and insulin-like growth factor-I. Cal Tissue Inter 56:376-381,1995.

VAN BREE H. Evaluation of subchondral lesion size in osteochondrosis of the scapulohumeral joint in dogs. JAVMA 294:1472,1994.

VAN BREE H, VAN RYSSEN B. Positive contrast shoulder arthrography with Iopromide and Diatrizoate in dogs with osteochondrosis. Vet Rad & Ultra 36:203-206,1995.

VAN VLECK LD, POLLAK EJ, OLTENACU EAB. Genetics for the Animal Sciences. W.H. Freeman and Company, New York,1987.

WEISS S, LOEFFLER K. Histological study of cartilage channels in the epiphyseal cartilage of young dogs and their relationship to that of osteochondrosis dissecans in the most frequently affected locations. Dtw. Deutsche Tierärzt Wochenschrift 103:164-169,1996.

WOODARD DC. Osteochondritis dissecans in a family of bull terriers. Vet Med SAC 74:936,1979.

YAMASAKI K, IKEDA J, ITAKURA C, Bone lesions in pigs with locomotor dysfunction of hind legs. J Comp Path 100:313-322,1989.

# Chapter 2

# Osteochondrosis of the humeral head

## Introduction

Osteochondrosis (OC) of the humeral head is a hereditary developmental disease resulting from a disturbance in endochondral ossification in which cartilage cells are not resorbed and replaced by bone as occurs normally (Olsson 193, 1975, 1976, 1977). This is one location at which osteochondrosis may occur in the dog. The hereditary nature is suggested because of its high frequency in certain breeds of dogs and within certain bloodlines. With fissure formation between the thickened cartilage and the subchondral bone, the previously non-painful OC progresses to a clinically painful osteochondritis dissecans (OCD). The resulting defect causes an incongruity within the articular surface of the humeral head that leads to the development of an osteoarthrosis. The lesion is often bilateral. The terms osteochondrosis and osteochondritis dissecans are used separately when reference is made to a specific form of the disease. However, in some instances, "osteochondrosis" within quotation marks is used as a general term making reference to both forms of the disease.

## History

Osteochondrosis was first described in the humeral head in the dog in the 1950s (Schnelle 1954, Brass 1956). It was thought for a long time to exist at that anatomical location exclusively. In the early literature, confusion existed between the meaning of osteochondrosis and osteochondritis dissecans and as a result the terms were used interchangeably. The abbreviation OCD was used for either form but was usually reserved for osteochondritis dissecans.

Schnelle's report from the Angell Memorial Animal Hospital in Boston (1954) was primarily concerned with hip dysplasia, but he included a discussion of osteochondritis of the humeral head and referred to it as "Perthes" syndrome. Brass, from the school in Hannover, discussed six cases and his was probably the first thorough report of the condition. Wamberg (1966) included in his book examples of bilateral osteoarthrosis deformans of the shoulder that were likely secondary to OCD. Since that time a large number of papers have reported the general appearance of shoulder "osteochondrosis." A recent search of old records at the Veterinary Medical Teaching Hospital, University of California, Davis brought forth radiographs made in 1954 of the shoulder of a 6 months old dog with a lesion typical of osteochondrosis of the humeral head. First reported as an aseptic necrosis of bone from the school in Vienna (Pobish 1952), it was later considered more correctly to be a developmental bone disease (Cordy and Wind 1969).

An early paper in the United States by Mostosky (1964) reported nine cases and was particularly valuable because a sire and son, in addition to male littermates from another litter, were included. Unfortunately, this was not widely circulated because it was contained within in a proceedings report. The 16 cases described by Craig and Riser (1965) received much wider attention. The familial nature of the disease was again reported in littermates of Border Collies (Knecht, et al 1977) and in a litter of bull terriers (Woodard 1979). Eventually, the disease was uniformly recognized as especially affecting large and giant breeds such as the Great Dane and the Saint Bernard (Craig and Riser 1965; Vaughan and Clayton-Jones 1968; Griffiths 1968; Paatsama, et al 1971; Ticer 1973; Smith and Stowater 1975). But, as is often found within descriptions of diseases, exceptions began to appear and somewhat questionable reports of the disease were made in a 6 kg Miniature Poodle (Dingwall, et al 1973) and a 13 kg Beagle (Johnson and Dennis, 1978). In our experience, the Great Pyrenees, Newfoundland, Labrador Retriever, Bernese Mountain dog, and Old English Sheepdog are predisposed breeds. Also, OCD has been reported in the racing greyhound (Milton, et al 1980).

The male has always been reported to be over-represented when compared with the female, usually in a ratio of 4:1 (Pobish 1962; Craig and Riser 1965; Vaughan and Clayton-Jones 1968; Griffiths 1968; Paatsama, et al 1971; Olsson 1977; Smith and Stowater 1975). This overrepresentation of males continues to hold in a review of 50 recent cases including various breeds from the University of California.

The bilateral occurrence of the lesions was eventually appreciated, with approximately 65% of the cases involving both shoulders (Griffiths 1968; Clayton-Jones and Vaughan 1970; Robins, et al 1978; Berzon 1979; Whitehair and Rudd 1990). We recently noted over 60% bilateral involvement in the 50 cases studied. Bilateral involvement is probably under-detected because of the unfortunate practice of radiographing only the shoulder with the most severe clinical signs. This is partially explained because of the failure to detect the problem in the less involved shoulder clinically since dogs with bilateral lesions are rarely equally symptomatic in both shoulders at the same time (Whitehair and Rudd 1990). Thus, the owner and/or clinician notice only unilateral lameness. Pain may be detected on the less-symptomatic shoulder only with careful examination.

## Course of the disease

Following cartilage necrosis, the overlying cartilage may separate from the underlying bone possibly from traumatic forces, perhaps the result of normal activities. With extension of the cleft from the depth of the lesion, a fissure forms which may reach the articular cartilage surface permitting synovial fluid to flow into this opening, causing further injury to the cartilage cells. Beneath the cleft, an intense mesenchymal reaction occurs with granulation tissue, active fibrogenesis, fiberbone formation, and osteoclastic activity. Cartilage necrosis is seen at the depth of the lesion. Surrounding the lesion, the cancellous spicules of bone thicken. At this time, the first signs of lameness may be detected and the lesion may be called an osteochondritis dissecans. As the fissure increases in size, the cartilaginous fragment loosens to the degree that it maintains only a partial attachment and may be referred to as a "flap." This attachment may persist or the "flap" may become unattached.

The size of the subchondral defect influences the character of the overlying cartilage. The larger the size of the lesion, the greater is the chance that the cartilage has formed a flap, while the smaller lesions often have an intact cartilage covering the osteochondrosis. This has a direct affect on clinical signs; the larger sized lesions being associated with clinical signs while the smaller lesions often have none (van Bree 1994).

The natural course of the disease consists of the gradual release of the cartilage flap leaving a defect within the epiphysis. After the flap detaches, it may fall into the caudal pouch and (1) totally disintegrate, (2) break into smaller pieces that persist, or (3) remain an intact fragment. The future appearance of the fragment(s) depends to a great extent on whether they gain a synovial attachment. Loose remnants that are not absorbed may become nour-ished by the joint fluid and become larger loose cartilaginous bodies (joint mice or osteochondromas) (Schawalder 1980). The fragments are not identified on the non-contrast radiograph if they remain cartilaginous, but may become attached to the synovium where they can become vascularized and may ossify becoming osteochondromas that increase in size (Lincoln and Potter 1976; LaHue, et al 1988; Muir, et al 1992). Thus, fragments may increase in size gaining nourishment from the synovial fluid within the joint and remaining cartilaginous, or may become attached to the synovial lining and, upon invasion by blood vessels, undergo endochondral ossification, becoming visible radiographically. Cartilage bodies in the caudal pocket of the joint capsule may remain quiescent but may through a shifting of position also serve as a stimulus for development of an acute tenosynovitis at a later date. These joint bodies may or may not play an active role in the degree of clinical signs dependent on their location within the joint. The appearance of the primary OCD lesion radiographically may not satisfactorily explain the degree of clinical signs and lameness. This may be due to the presence of cartilaginous joint bodies that are not calcified and thus are not identified radiographically but cause a severe synovitis. Since they cannot be identified radiographically, the nature of the lesion as seen on the non-contrast films may not correlate well with the clinical signs (Morgan 1972). In this instance, contrast arthrography is required for their identification in which they appear as filling defects within a positive contrast pool (van Bree 1985, 1990).

Because the bicipital tendon sheath is a continuation of the shoulder joint capsule, fragments may migrate to this location and produce a severe tenosynovitis. In many cases, the tenosynovitis produces adhesions between the tendon and surrounding sheath and the resulting condition is very painful necessitating transposition of the origin of the biceps tendon from the scapular tubercle to the proximal humerus. In other cases, the inflammation may extend to the surrounding tissues where inflammation and even ossification of the intertrabecular ligament can occur. This ligament confines the bicipital tendon between the greater and lesser tubercles. The possibility of a tenosynovitis is a severe complication of OCD of the humeral head especially in dogs with an early and large lesion and is a reason for early surgical treatment. The most severe pattern of complications of an OCD lesion occurs with development of a persistent, progressive osteoarthrosis of the joint plus the development of a bicipital tenosynovitis.

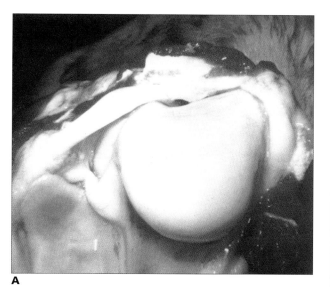 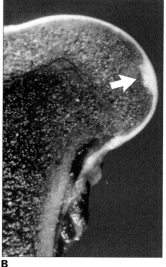 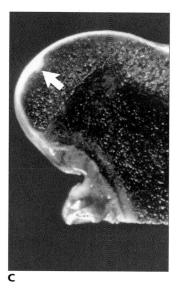

**Figure 2-1**
Photographs of the humeral head of a 5-month-old female Saint Bernard showing (A) the surface of what appears to be normal articular cartilage. However, on sectioning of the humeral head (B, C), areas of cartilage thickening are identified that are characteristic of an early osteochondrosis (arrows). It is possible for this lesion to progress to an osteochondritis dissecans or, more likely, for it to heal with formation of a near-normal articular surface. This error is skeletal maturation is one cause of false radiographic diagnosis of humeral head osteochondrosis in the immature puppy.

The flap can become free through normal use of the limb or as a result of surgical treatment. The resulting cartilage defect, if relatively small, can more or less fill in with granulation tissue, which can, through joint movement, change into a form of functional hyaline cartilage. The contour of the joint is thus partially re-established. In the young dog with early surgical removal of the flap, the chance for development of a grossly normal contour of the humeral head is good. Once a normal contour is re-established, the degree of osteoarthrosis is mild or non-existent clinically. These dogs have normal limb function. Some surgeons advise curettage of the defect in order to achieve the earliest vascular ingrowth and healing of the defect.

As long as the cartilage flap remains in position, degenerative products from the flap and free cartilage fragments result in perpetuation of a chronic synovitis and a delay in healing of the cartilage defect. Filling of the defect is markedly delayed, because the movement of the flap prevents capillaries from growing into the defect, thus discouraging formation of healing connective tissue. Because of a failure to understand this process of healing, disagreement exists among clinicians regarding treatment (Fox and Walker 1993). The longer the delay of healing of the cartilage defect, the more severe is the resulting osteoarthrosis.

In the dog in which the flap has spontaneously become detached, surgical removal of the cartilage fragments is indicated to reduce the chronic synovitis. If the flap is removed surgically, joint lavage is critical to accomplish removal of the irritating cartilage products and joint mice. This policy of cleansing of the joint capsule probably plays a small role in the healing of the cartilage defect, but is important in reducing the pain.

## Gross lesion

Grossly the earliest lesions of osteochondrosis have overlying cartilage that is normal in appearance (Figure 2-1). Normal cartilage appears at the time of surgery as a slightly bluish shiny covering over the epiphysis. The bluish color is due to the proximity of the underlying blood supply. Early lesions of osteochondrosis have the normal shiny surface but have lost the bluish color. In OCD with the flap in situ, the flap appears extremely white and can be "bounced" against the underlying bone. The surface of the humeral head acquires the character of a loose floor tile that has a "hollow" sound and feel upon tapping with a surgical instrument. With separation of the cartilage flap from the underlying bone, its surface acquires a "wrinkled" appearance, although the cartilage remains shiny (Figure 2-2).

Frequently, the flap remains attached cranially and medially with a ragged appearance to the free margin. Thickened fibrous joint capsule and excessive and hyperemic synovium are noted. With complete separation of

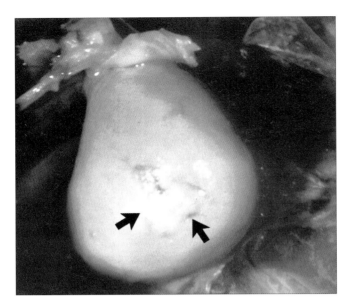

**Figure 2-2**
Photograph of the humeral head in a young adult dog with an early lesion of OCD with "wrinkling" of the articular surface (arrows). The cartilage cap is beginning to separate from the underlying cancellous bone.

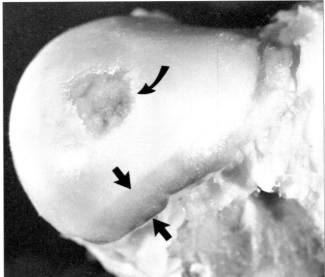

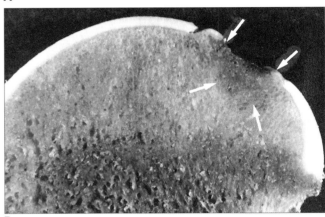

**Figure 2-3**
Photograph of (A) a humeral head with a lesion of osteochondritis dissecans (curved arrow) following separation of the cartilaginous cap. Note the extent of the secondary periarticular lipping (straight arrows). Photograph of (B) a sagittal section made through the center of the lesion shows its depth (white arrows) more clearly.

the flap, a shallow cavity in the contour of the humeral head is evident (Figure 2-3). Eventually, the underlying bone begins to repair, but in the larger lesions, it fails to form a normal articular contour. The formation of fibrocartilage that later converts to a hyaline cartilage will partially fills the defect.

On direct visual examination, the typical secondary changes of osteoarthrosis are noted in addition to the primary lesion. These changes include: (1) generalized thinning of the articular cartilage, (2) eburnation (shiny bone surface), indicative of subchondral bone sclerosis (hardening), (3) periarticular lipping, and (4) enthesophyte formation at the sites of soft tissue attachments (Figure 2-3). The pattern of change is principally dependent on the size of the original OCD lesion. With the absence of a portion of the cartilage contour of the humeral head due to an OCD, the opposing cartilage on the glenoid cavity fails to be properly nourished and dies, creating a "kissing" lesion (Figure 2-4). A thickened capsule and hypertrophic, hyperemic synovium is usually evident. Some, but not all, of these changes are clearly observed at the time of surgical exploration.

On histological examination, a cross section of the humeral head reveals hyperemic, sclerotic bone around the lesion that is more prominent in an OCD than in an OC. If the flap has completely separated, the defect varies in depth from a few mm to rarely as much as 5mm. Raw cancellous bone, scar tissue, or cartilaginous remnants may be apparent. Color of the underlying bone varies from red to white suggesting the degree of vascularity.

## Clinical signs

The clinical signs of a shoulder OCD are a rather nonspecific forelimb lameness, which usually can be first detected between the ages of 4 to 8 months. At this time, the lameness is caused by a painful synovitis precipitated by the cartilaginous debris within the joint. The age of first presentation of most patients was originally reported to be in young dogs between 6 to 8 months (Craig and Riser 1965), 5 to 10 months (Griffiths 1968), and 4 to 14 months (Paatsama, et al 1971). Most owners recognize clinical signs prior to 1 year of age. While many patients are presented at an early age, some are not recognized to have shoulder lameness until later. This delay is especially understandable in dogs with bilateral lesions in which the lameness remains unnoticed because both shoulders are equally sore and the dog displays an altered forelimb gait rather than an obvious lameness in one limb. Of the 50 patients surveyed at UCD, 20% were not presented for diagnosis and treatment until after 12 months of age, and some were not seen for the first time until 36 months of age.

The lameness can be unilateral if only one humeral head is involved, however, the lameness can also be seen in only one limb if both humeral heads are involved but with different degrees of severity and resultant pain. The shoulder with the largest lesion usually has the most obvious clinical signs. If the degree of pain is equal in both shoulders, an altered, restricted gait can be present, rather than obvious forelimb lameness. The restricted gait is due to a decreased range of motion because of the painful shoulder and the dog's effort to limit the discomfort.

Dependent on the duration of these clinical signs, muscle atrophy can be noted on physical examination, especially in the supraspinatus, infraspinatus, and deltoid muscles, due to diminished use of the limb. The muscle atrophy may be recognized by palpating the shoulder region and noting the prominence of the spine of the scapula. Asymmetry in muscle mass may be an indication of disuse atrophy due either to unilateral involvement or unequal involvement in dogs with bilateral disease. However, disuse muscle atrophy is not pathognomonic for this disease and may be secondary to other causes of disuse, both orthopedic and neurological.

Early in the course of OCD in the untreated young dog, the lameness increases with exercise and decreases with rest. The dog often is hesitant to rise. Sometimes a clinician advises prolonged rest in an apparent effort to provide a chance for the cartilage lesion to heal. However, this is an unrealistic expectation and the dog will evidence lameness again when physical activity is resumed. The pain is persistent because of the synovitis associated with the presence of a partially attached cartilage "flap."

In the 7 to 8 months old affected dog of the lighter breeds, the size of the cartilage defect is usually small and natural shoulder motion causes the cartilage flap to breakdown spontaneously. Filling of the defect occurs and only a mild or moderate amount of osteoarthrosis follows. This dog often appears to be clinically sound to the owner

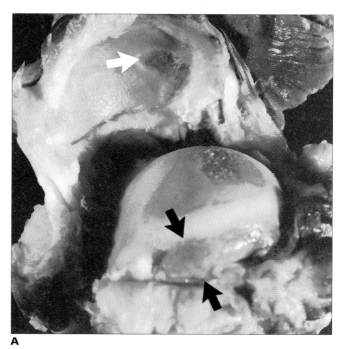

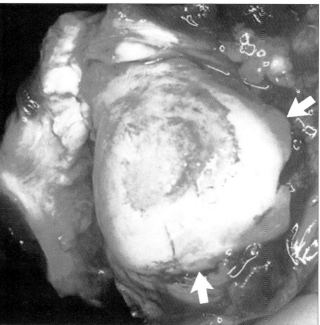

**Figure 2-4**
Photographs of the shoulder joints in two older dogs. (A) The shoulder joint has a large OCD lesion in the humeral head and a "kissing" lesion on the glenoid cavity (white arrow). Note the size of the periarticular new bone formed around the articular margin of the humeral head (black arrows) as the secondary osteoarthrosis progresses. (B) A large OCD lesion is seen in a malformed, flattened humeral head with secondary periarticular new bone (arrows) indicating chronicity.

throughout the course of the OCD or evidences only a brief period of mild lameness.

In contrast, in the untreated older dog of the larger breeds, clinical signs are already present at the age of 4 to 5 months. The pain in the acute phase, which was the result of synovitis, becomes complicated by the development of a painful osteoarthrosis. The degree of pain may vary dependent on the severity of the osteoarthrosis. In these dogs, marked stiffness may be noted upon rising in the morning; sleeping in a cold room or on a cold floor exacerbates this. However, the signs tend to moderate with exercise, the dog "warms out" of the lameness, and often this dog can eventually undergo physical activity later in the day without apparent discomfort. If exercise is excessive however, the dog can again become acutely lame and refuse to use the forelimb.

Not infrequently, forelimb lameness due to elbow dysplasia has been misinterpreted as shoulder lameness because of the prominence given to the diagnosis of OCD of the shoulder and the relatively late recognition of elbow dysplasia as a cause of forelimb lameness. In other dogs, the clinical signs of forelimb lameness can become less obvious in the presence of painful hind limb lameness due to hip dysplasia, for example. Often these dogs are described by their owner as being particularly "well behaved", probably the result of pain in all four limbs that effectively controls the dog's activity and prevents it from wanting to jump up on people or play actively.

In summary, in the lighter breeds, the lesion of OCD is small, the onset of clinical signs is usually late, and the possibility of spontaneous recovery is good. In contrast, if the breed is large, the lesion is probably large, the onset of clinical signs is early (van Bree 1990), and healing of the defect is possible but with a high likelihood of development of severe osteoarthrosis.

## Physical examination

Shoulder muscle atrophy develops rather quickly in patients with marked disuse due to pain and is a valuable finding noted visually or on physical examination. The range of motion of the forelimb usually appears to be normal to the casual observer, even if somewhat restricted. However, hyperflexion and hyperextension of the shoulder joint often elicits a pain response. A number of patients with lameness have been identified with unilateral or bilateral lesions that fail to show pain on physical examination. This may be due to the stoic character of the dog. Cases have also been described in which the

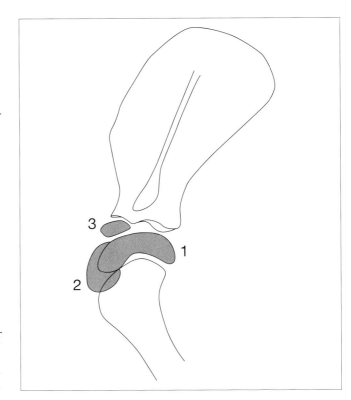

**Figure 2-5**
Drawing of a lateral radiograph of the shoulder joint in a 3-month-old dog with shading of: (1) the proximal epiphysis of the humerus, (2) the tubercles of the humerus, (3) and the supraglenoid tubercle of the scapula.

functional disorder was thought to be unilateral, while the necropsy examination revealed the existence of a clinically silent lesion on the opposite shoulder (Craig and Riser, 1965). An inadequate physical or radiographic examination most likely explains this problem.

Pieces from the cartilage defect can drift into the synovial pouch surrounding the bicipital tendon, causing an acute tenosynovitis and a somewhat unique pattern of clinical signs. As a result of the inflammatory lesion, severe pain can be elicited on direct pressure on the tendon in the bicipital groove, cranial to the shoulder joint. In addition, pain can be detected in these dogs on hyperflexion of the shoulder joint, which results in a painful stretching of the tendon. Either of these findings can indicate this particular complication of shoulder OCD. The bicipital tendon sheath can become affected as early as 6 to 12 months of age. If the acute condition is present, it can convert to a chronic one with adhesions between the tendon and tendon sheath. The physical findings mimic those seen in the more acute phase of an OCD. However, a bicipital tenosynovitis may be secondary to trauma in the absence of an osteochondrosis. Bicipital tenosynovitis was early described as a complication of OCD of the humeral head (Suter and Carb 1969).

While breed, age, history, clinical signs, and physical examination may lead one toward a tentative diagnosis of OCD, shoulder radiographs are necessary to confirm the diagnosis and determine its severity.

False results from physical examination may be obtained in: (1) the presence of panosteitis of the humerus, radius, or ulna or in (2) the presence of elbow dysplasia. Therefore, one should not grasp the above mentioned bones tightly or flex and extend the elbow joint unduly while examining the shoulder. Other differential diagnoses may include traumatic injuries to the shoulder region or infectious lesions in either bone or joint. As the dog ages, neoplastic lesions need to be included in the differential diagnosis.

Also, the clinical signs can be complicated by the presence of lesions in the hind limbs associated with skeletal development (Clayton-Jones and Vaughan, 1970), particularly hip dysplasia, cranial cruciate ligament disease, osteochondrosis of the femoral condyle, or hind limb panosteitis.

## Anatomy and development of the shoulder joint

The shoulder joint is a very loose ball-in-socket joint consisting of the glenoid cavity of the scapula proximally and the humeral head distally. The proximal end of the humerus has 2 ossification centers, the proximal epiphysis and the greater tubercle. The scapula has a separate growth center in the supraglenoid tubercle (Figure 2-5). The major growth of the humerus is obtained through the proximal metaphyseal growth plate (Figure 2-6). Only the proximal epiphysis is influenced by the osteochondrosis originally. The glenoid cavity articulates with the humeral head and becomes affected secondarily because of development of an osteoarthrosis.

The main movements of the joint are flexion, extension, and rotation with both adduction and abduction being possible. Medial stability of the joint is achieved through the articular capsule as well as from the medial glenohumeral ligament and the tendons of the biceps brachii, subscapularis, and coracobrachialis muscles. Laterally, the lateral glenohumeral ligament and the tendons of the infraspinatus muscle support the joint. The radiographic anatomy of the normal shoulder joint is well studied by arthrography with detection of the transchondral fissures beneath the cartilage flap described in the disease shoul-

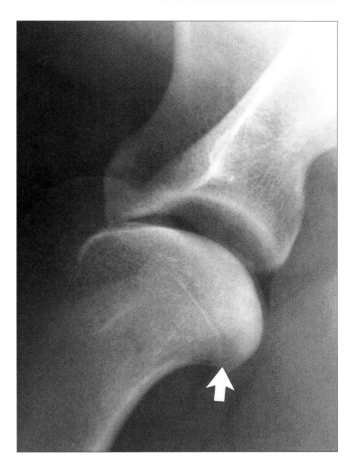

**Figure 2-6**
Lateral radiograph of a normal shoulder joint in a young adult dog in which the proximal humeral metaphyseal growth plate has closed leaving a radiopaque scar (arrow). The width of the joint space varies because of normal joint laxity. The glenoid cavity forms a "cap" that sits over the humeral head.

der (Suter and Carb 1969, van Bree and Van Ryssen 1991).

## Radiographic diagnosis

The definitive diagnosis of humeral head "osteochondrosis" is made by radiographic examination. The dog is positioned on top of the cassette and tabletop radiographic technique is used. The lateral view is made with the limb to be radiographed next to the table top and extended in a craniodistal direction, so the shoulder joint is not superimposed over the air-filled trachea or the manubrium (Figure 2-7). The opposite limb is pulled caudally so that the upper shoulder is beyond the well-collimated x-ray beam. The caudocranial view is used rarely and is made with the dog in dorsal recumbency and the limb pulled cranially (Figure 2-7). This is one of the few le-

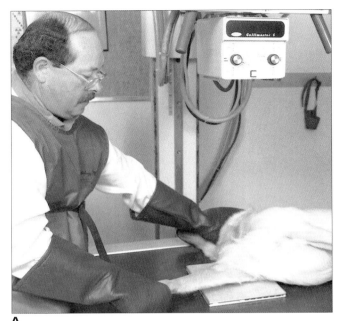
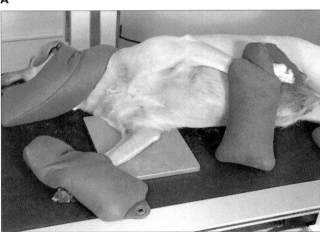
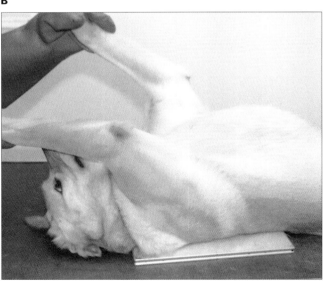

**Figure 2-7**
Photographs of a dog showing various positions used for radiographic evaluation of the shoulder joint. The lateral view (A, B) is made with the dog recumbent with the affected limb next to the cassette and extended cranially. The unaffected limb is displaced caudally. The patient may be positioned by use of gloved hands or held in position by sandbags. The caudocranial view (C) is used uncommonly and is made with the dog on its back with the affected limb pulled cranially. Tabletop technique is used for both views.

sions in the dog that can be studied effectively from lateral radiographs only, however, it is imperative that the radiographs be of good quality. Sedation or anesthesia is not necessary as a rule to obtain the necessary radiographic positioning (Morgan 1990).

In a joint under tension from distraction of opposing articular surfaces, nitrogen gas collects within the joint space creating a shadow resembling that seen with an arthrogram performed with air. This vacuum sign has been reported in 20% of non-contrast studies of the shoulder (van Bree 1992) (Figure 2-8). Theoretically, when opposing articular surfaces are separated, a negative pressure is created within the joint space and nitrogen from the surrounding extracellular fluid is attracted to the joint space. When the articular surfaces are re-opposed, the pressure within the joint returns to normal and the nitrogen is re-absorbed. Because of the positioning required for the lateral view of the shoulder joint in the dog, as well as the general laxity of this joint, the vacuum phenomenon is seen frequently. It can be of diagnostic value because the gas outlines the margin of the articular cartilage which otherwise can not be seen on a routine diagnostic radiograph. Since osteochondrosis first causes change in thickness of the cartilage, the presence of intracapsular gas serves as a contrast agent and can aid in its diagnosis.

Arthrography is used to help show the existence of the cartilaginous flap and its location (Story 1978, van Bree 1985, 1990). Both negative and positive arthrography have been used (Muhumuza, et al 1988; van Bree, et al 1989). Negative arthrography is performed with injection of air or $CO_2$ while positive arthrography is performed with injection of a sterile iodine-containing contrast agent. The use of low-osmolar, non-ionic iodine containing contrast media definitely produces more diagnostic studies (van Bree and van Ryseen 1995). The diagnosis is made by the identification of the contrast agent located between the flap and the underlying bony defect (Figure 2-9). If the flap has broken free, the positive contrast agent can identify the fragment(s) within the caudal joint pouch or within the bicipital tendon sheath as a filling defect within the contrast pool as well as outlining the defect in the contour of the humeral head. Arthrography may be of value in attempting to relate the clinical signs with the nature of the lesion, since, contrast medium that reaches beneath the cartilage flap usually correlates positively with signs of pain and lameness (van Bree 1990, 1993).

The relevant sign of osteochondrosis as seen on a mediolateral radiograph of the extended shoulder joint is a defect in the contour of the subchondral bone of the caudocentral aspect of the humeral head. In mild or early cases, only a small area of flattening of the contour of the humeral head is seen (Figure 2-8). Olsson (1967) and Callahan and Ackerman (1985) described lesions that were more lateral, rather than central, in location. In addition, the authors have seen lesions located medially. In these dogs, a radiograph made in a true lateral projection does not project the lesion as a defect in the contour of the bone, and only the area of altered bone density within the caudal part of the head is seen. By making radiographs of the limb in internal or external rotation, these unusually located lesions are placed in a location where they are projected in a tangential manner and thus are more easily identified. If tension is placed in the joint, a resulting "vacuum sign" is helpful in diagnosis (Morgan 1992).

In the very young patient, the defect within the humeral head and the change in the surrounding bone may not be seen radiographically and the thickened cartilage covering or underlying fissures can only be seen following use of arthrography (Figure 2-8) (van Bree 1985). In this patient as well as in the shoulder with a more advanced lesion, the arthrogram offers the possibility to evaluate the: (1) thickness of the articular cartilage, (2) presence of a dissecting fissure, and (3) presence of joint mice (LaHue, et al 1988) (Figure 2-9). It is also possible to withdraw synovial fluid for examination at the time of needle placement. However, the combination of clinical signs plus the radiographic appearance of the lesion on non-contrast radiographs may permit the diagnosis of osteochondritis dissecans to be made with assurance without use of arthrography. However, if a distinction cannot be made between an OC and an OCD lesion, the use of arthrography should be strongly considered. Some clinicians will not choose to do this because of a fear of secondary sepsis. Cases of septic arthritis following arthrography in man are extremely rare, probably due in part to the anti-bacteriocidal action of the contrast media (Dory and Wautelet 1985). The most common complication seen by the authors when using a positive contract study is a painful, sterile, chemical synovitis.

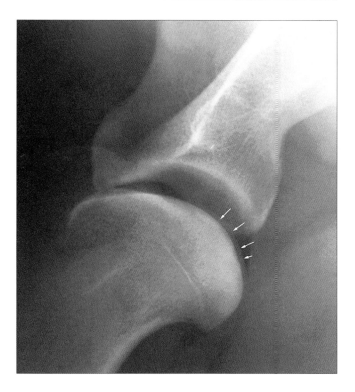

**Figure 2-8**
Lateral radiograph of a shoulder of a 2-year-old Giant Schnauzer lame on both forelimbs. The osteochondrosis is characterized by only minimal alteration in the contour of the humeral head plus a sclerotic pattern of new bone surrounding the lesion. By placing tension on the limb, a "vacuum sign" is created and the resulting gas within the joint permits identification of the thickness of the articular cartilage (arrows). The increased thickness of the cartilage over the lesion assists in confirming the diagnosis of osteochondrosis. Note that secondary bony changes are not present suggesting the minimal nature of the lesion. A similarly appearing lesion was seen on radiographs of the opposite shoulder. Because the cartilage flap has not separated, the humeral head lesion may not be the cause of the clinical signs and the elbow joints should be carefully examined as another cause of forelimb lameness.

As the patient ages, a zone of increased density that surrounds the defect creates a halo that usually has the shape of an inverted cone (Figures 2-8, 2-9, 2-10). This pattern of increased bone density is helpful in directing a search for a lesion. In addition, with chronicity, secondary changes begin to develop and bony spurs are seen on the caudal aspect of the glenoid cavity and surrounding the humeral head.

## Radiographic grading of lesions

Grading of the lesions of "osteochondrosis" is helpful in understanding the sequence of change noted in the disease (Craig and Riser 1965, Vaughan and Clayton-Jones 1968).

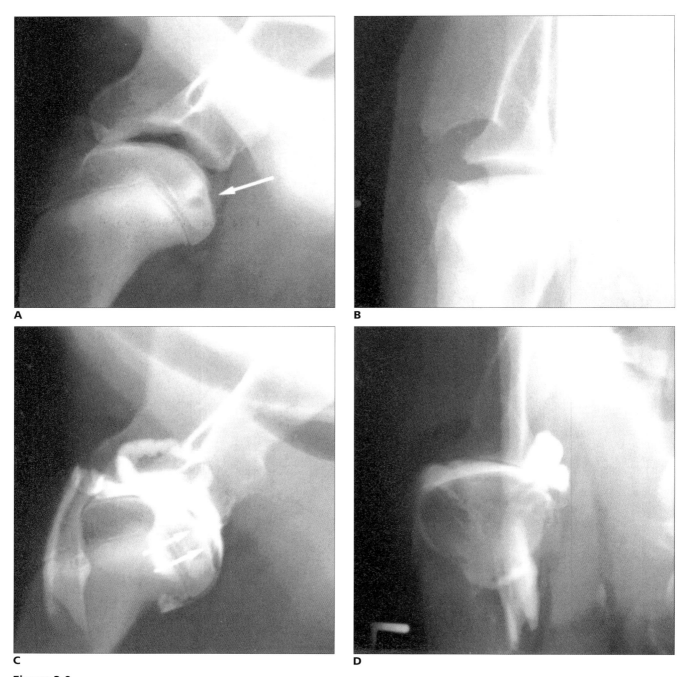

**Figure 2-9**
Survey radiographs (A, B) and arthrography (C, D) of the left shoulder of a 6-month-old male Great Dane with lameness and pain due to an OCD lesion of the humeral head. On the lateral view of the non-contrast study (A), changes within the subchondral bone consist of flattening of the humeral head, sclerosis, or hardening, of the subchondral bone, and a large subchondral cyst (arrow). On the caudocranial view (B), the lesion is not identified. On the lateral view of the arthrogram (C), the contrast agent flows beneath the cartilage flap that remains in situ (arrows). The contrast agent also flows around the normally appearing bicipital tendon (D). The round smooth filling defect adjacent to the tendon is an air bubble.

Grade 1 is assigned to a lesion found in a dog that is 3 to 5 months of age and is characterized by a defect in the bony contour of the caudocentral half of the ossification center (Figures 2-1, 2-2). This may be diagnostic of an osteochondrosis that may develop into an OCD or it may only be indicative of a simple delay in ossification with an anticipated normal, but delayed, development of the humeral head. In this stage, since the lesion is covered by grossly normal articular cartilage, it has, as yet, no clinical significance. Vaughan and Clayton-Jones (1968) have in particular warned against the possibility of over diagnosis of lesions of this type in the young dog. Olsson (1976) also described many similar cases in which he reported spontaneous healing. A defect of this type in the bony epiphysis after the age of 6 months is more likely to become an OCD lesion that will not spontaneously repair and therefore has clinical significance.

A grade II lesion is characterized by an increase in the size of the defect in the bony epiphysis. The surrounding radiodense zone of bone has a mottled appearance and often assumes the form of an inverted cone with the apex at the physis (Figure 2-8). Vaughan and Clayton-Jones (1968) recognized that some patients had adjacent areas of rarefaction or cyst formation (Figure 2-9a) within the adjacent epiphyseal bone that were identified on the early radiographs. These lucent lesions tend to coalesce with time. This is typical for an early OCD lesion.

Grade III is assigned to lesions characterized by flattening of a large segment of the bony contour of the humeral head. Formation of further cavities occurs within the bony epiphysis. Mottled or granular elements of calcified cartilage are noted within the gap beneath the cartilage defect (Figure 2-10). The sclerotic cone remains surrounding the lesion. This suggests a more progressive lesion in an older dog, but can also be found in a young, heavy dog. This lesion is clinical and should be referred to as an OCD.

Grade IV lesions represent a continuation of the above changes, with the addition that a free fragment of cartilage may be identified over the articular defect. Usually this is identified by calcification within the depth of the cartilage cap, but a cartilage flap without mineralization can be identified by use of arthrography (Figure 2-9c) (Vaughan and Clayton-Jones 1968). This represents an older lesion since time is needed for the cartilaginous flap to mineralize.

Grade V is reserved for lesions that are progressive and the cartilaginous flap has become free and shifted in position (Figure 2-11). The free fragments are usually identified on the radiograph because of calcification or subsequent ossification and have thus become radiopaque (Vaughan and Clayton-Jones 1968). The fragments can also be identified by use of arthrography as they create a filling defect within the positive contrast pool (van Bree 1985). After the flap becomes free, it drops first into the caudal pouch of the joint capsule where it usually divides into several fragments of varying sizes. Later, fragments may shift into the region of the bicipital tendon and become trapped in this location causing a clinically significant tenosynovitis. Following displacement of the cartilage flap, the underlying bony lesion within the epiphysis

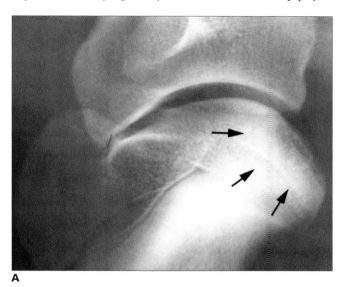

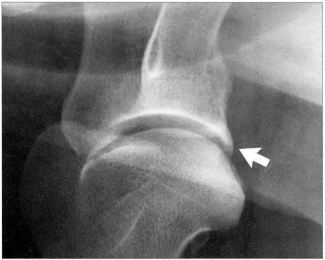

**Figure 2-10**
Lateral radiographs of affected shoulders in an immature dog and mature dog. In a younger dog (A), the lesion is limited to the defect within the humeral head with an increase in density in the surrounding bone (arrows). In an older dog (B), the lesion is more chronic and the subchondral bone is more clearly identified beneath the lesion. Periarticular bony spurs have formed on the caudal aspect of the glenoid cavity (arrow). Note the early mineralization of the cartilage flap. Both of these dogs should be considered to have formed flaps and the lesions are typical of pain-producing lesions of osteochondritis disecans.

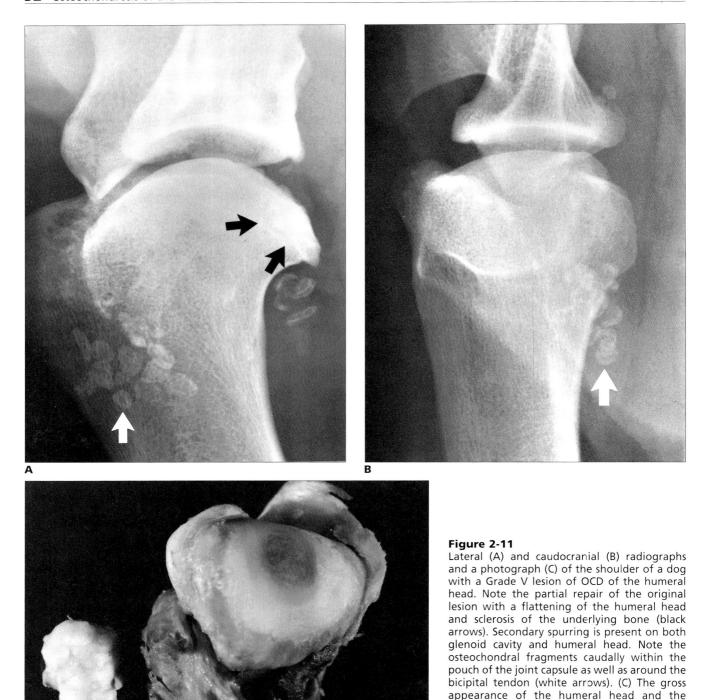

**Figure 2-11**
Lateral (A) and caudocranial (B) radiographs and a photograph (C) of the shoulder of a dog with a Grade V lesion of OCD of the humeral head. Note the partial repair of the original lesion with a flattening of the humeral head and sclerosis of the underlying bone (black arrows). Secondary spurring is present on both glenoid cavity and humeral head. Note the osteochondral fragments caudally within the pouch of the joint capsule as well as around the bicipital tendon (white arrows). (C) The gross appearance of the humeral head and the largest osteochondral fragment is seen following dissection. The "polishing" of the articular surface (eburnation) can be appreciated easily.

usually begins to fill in with a fibrocartilaginous material, but the bony defect remains visible. Arthrography is required to identify the extent of the repair. Some improvement in uniformity in bone density begins to occur within the epiphysis indicating bony healing due to restored weight bearing on the limb.

Grade VI lesions are found in older patients and are limited to shoulders in which secondary osteoarthrosis is prominent (Figure 2-12). These may occur in either the non-treated or surgically treated patient. The osteoarthrosis is characterized in the older patient by capsular thickening, eburnation and subchondral sclerosis, generalized disappearance of articular cartilage, periarticular lipping and enthesophyte formation. Periarticular bony lipping is recognized around the margin of the humeral head, around the margin of the glenoid cavity, and near the bicipital groove with ossification of the intertubercular ligament (Vaughan and Clayton-Jones, 1968). The degree of osteoarthrosis is dependent on the size of the original lesion, the age of the dog at the time of any surgical intervention, and the age at the time of radiography.

Closure of the metaphyseal growth plate of the proximal humerus may occur earlier than expected in the dog with OCD. This feature has not been used to influence a grade assignment. In a dog with bilateral OCD, the radiographic appearance of physeal closure in one shoulder can mimic that of the contralateral shoulder or they can differ remarkably. Usually the resulting length of the humerus is not affected.

In later stages of the disease with calcification of the base of the cartilage flap, radiographic diagnosis can be made positively without the use of arthrography. When the flap is calcified and falls free into the caudal pouch, or around the bicipital tendon in the form of fragments, it can be identified on the radiograph (Figure 2-11). In cases where the flap is not identified because of a lack of calcification, arthrography may be necessary to locate it in

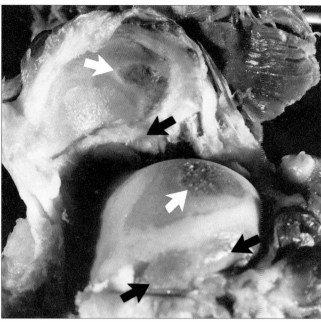

**Figure 2-12**
Photograph of the shoulder of an older dog with severe secondary osteoarthrosis characterized by wearing of the articular cartilage with visible subchondral bone (eburnation) (white arrows) on both articular surfaces. Periarticular new bone is seen on both sides of the joint (black arrows). The etiology of the osteoarthrosis is difficult to ascertain in the older dog even at the time of surgery or necropsy.

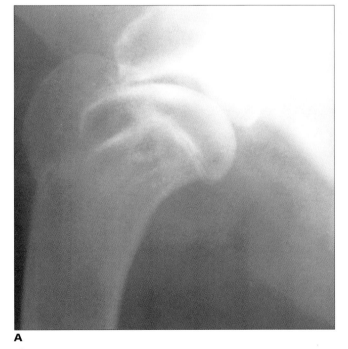

A

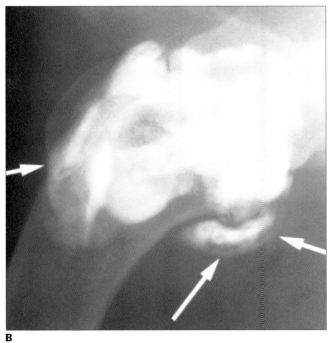

B

**Figure 2-13**
Lateral radiographs of the shoulder of a 1-year-old Sheepdog with lameness in the right shoulder. The non-contrast radiograph (A) is unremarkable while the arthrogram (B) reveals filling defects within the caudal pouch (arrows) and around the bicipital tendon sheath (arrow) indicative of cartilage fragments. Cartilage fragments or osteochondral fragments may be secondary to an OCD lesion or may be secondary to a chronic synovitis.

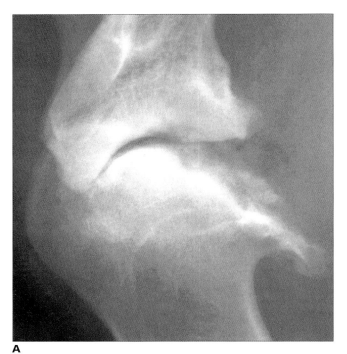 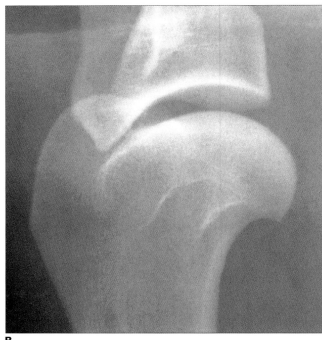

**Figure 2-14**
Lateral radiographs of the shoulders of an 8-year-old female Malamute with a developmental disease within one humeral head. (A) Severe change are present in the shoulder joint in the affected limb with a partial absence of the caudal portion of the ossification center of the humeral head with flattening and secondary osteoarthrosis. The caudal portion of the glenoid cavity has failed to form normally. (B) The normal unaffected shoulder joint is shown. This lesion might better be referred to as an epiphyseal dysplasia affecting a specific portion of the humeral head.

situ, or to locate cartilage fragments in the caudal pouch or around the bicipital tendon (Figures 2-9, 2-13) (van Bree 1985). Experience has shown that the identification of these fragments is critical to enable cleansing of the joint by curettage and lavage to ensure the most favorable prognosis.

## Differential radiographic diagnosis

Consideration of a differential diagnosis is important because OCD is often the only lesion considered in event of shoulder lameness especially in a member of a large breed. Another developmental disease involving the humeral head occurs when the caudal portion of the ossification center of the humeral head fails to form. In this dog, the collapse of the caudal portion of the shoulder joint is present shortly after birth. Because of the lack of a caudal articular support, a secondary bowing of the humerus results with concavity directed caudally. The caudal aspect of the glenoid cavity also fails to form because of the absence of a normal apposing articular surface. The condition is relatively easy to differentiate from a humeral head osteochondrosis at a young age; however, in the older dog the changes of osteoarthrosis confuse the diagnosis although the humeral bowing remains (Figure 2-14). This lesion might be referred to more accurately as an epiphyseal dysplasia affecting a specific portion of the humeral head.

In the older dog, a severe secondary osteoarthrosis in the shoulder may be characterized by such prominent periarticular spurring and modeling that the etiology of the original lesion may not be determined (Figure 2-12). However, OCD should be considered the most likely cause of osteoarthrosis in the older dog, especially if the lesion is bilateral and in a predisposed breed. This diagnosis should be entertained even if the original bony lesion is difficult to ascertain.

The diagnosis is difficult in a mature dog with minimal osteoarthrosis without evidence of an OC lesion, even if it was the original disease. Because, with repair, the articular surfaces becomes nearly normal and the stimulus for the development of a secondary osteoarthrosis is minimal. The genotype of these dogs should be considered suspect. However, it is possible for this osteoarthrosis to have followed another type of injurious lesion.

Older dogs of the heavier breeds may have tenosynovitis of the bicipital tendon. Radiographically this is characterized by soft tissue mineralization within the bicipital

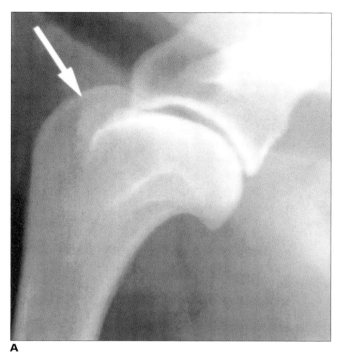 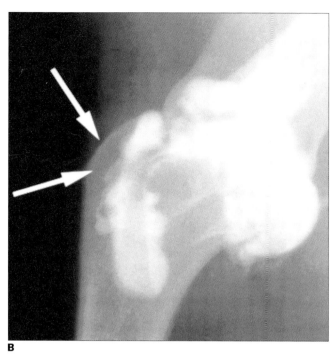

**Figure 2-15**
Lateral radiographs of the shoulder of a 9-year-old male Brittany. (A) On the non-contrast study, a pattern of calcified tissue is identified (arrow). (B) On the contrast study, the distention of the bicipital tendon sheath is limited by the calcified mass located cranial to the sheath (arrows). The humeral head is normal in appearance without evidence of an OCD. The diagnosis was that of a tenosynovitis of unknown etiology.

groove and sclerosis within the surrounding bone (Figure 2-15) or the lesion may not be evident until arthrography is performed (Figure 2-16). This tenosynovitis may be a consequence to traumatic rupture of the bicipital tendon or may be a complication of OCD in which cartilaginous fragments have drifted into the tendon sheath. In either case, focal mineralization of the synovium may be present. The osteochondromas have their origin in detached cartilage fragments or may have originated in the chronically inflamed synovium. Differentiation between osteochondromas associated with trauma and fragments secondary to OCD that have re-attached and mineralized is difficult. The use of arthrography is helpful in determination of the: (1) presence of non-mineralized cartilage fragments, (2) status of the tendon, and (3) presence of adhesions within the sheath. Determination of these clinically important lesions is important (Barthez and Morgan 1993).

## Treatment

In general, surgical removal of the "flap" is highly advisable in the young members of heavy breeds with large lesions. Conservative or medical treatment is indicated in light breeds with a small lesion, in which the clinical signs are first noted at 7 to 8 months, and natural breakdown and absorption of the flap is likely with a natural filling of the bony defect. However, conservative or medical treatment is better reserved for the older dog with pain due to chronic osteoarthrosis secondary to OCD.

## Conservative treatment

Conservative treatment in the form of analgesics and moderate exercise can be satisfactory if the lesion and the cartilage flap are small and the clinical signs are not noted until the age of 7 to 8 months. However, Olsson (1976) felt that a dog with osteochondritis dissecans of the humeral head should be allowed to move the shoulder joint as much as possible; the chance is greater that the flap is dislodged and subsequent healing of the bone at the depth of the lesion can occur. Therefore, moderate exercise can be advised to assist in the dislodging of the flap, allowing the cartilage defect to fill. It is difficult to ascertain the pain associated with this type of treatment. Even if the flap becomes dislodged, surgical removal of the fragment is recommend to minimize the secondary synovitis and osteoarthrosis. To rest the dog is a waste of time because the flap does not re-attach and no repair of the defect occurs with the flap in its original position. Steroid

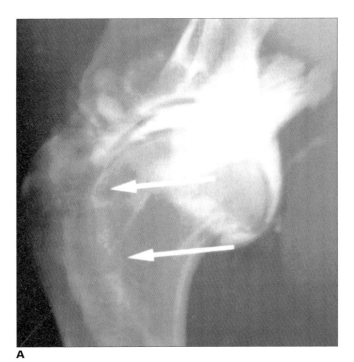 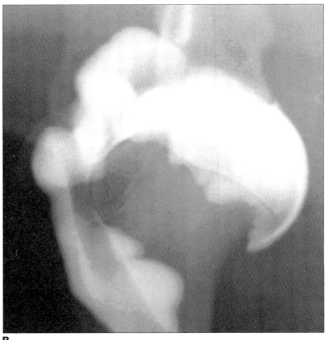

**Figure 2-16**
Lateral radiographs of the shoulders of two adult Labrador Retrievers following positive contrast arthrography. (A) On the affected limb, the bicipital tendon sheath is incompletely filled, has an irregular surface, and contains filling defects (arrows). (B) On the unaffected limb, the bicipital tendon sheath is normally distended and filled with the contrast agent. In the absence of changes typical of an OCD lesion, the diagnosis was that of a tenosynovitis of unknown etiology.

therapy delays healing and is contraindicated. Weight reduction and control of exercise are important in control of clinical signs of osteoarthrosis found in any orthopedic problem and should be included in any treatment regimen (Vaughan and Clayton-Jones 1968, Siemerina 1979).

## Surgical treatment

The authors feel that if the OCD lesion is large and/or has occurred at an early age, or if a month of conservative treatment has not produced clinical improvement, surgical treatment should be considered. This may hasten the filling in of the defect and remove the detrimental effect of the degenerated cartilage. In addition, surgical treatment shortens the time of discomfort, prevents the formation of large joint bodies, minimizes the degree of osteoarthrosis that develops, and makes the development of bicipital tenosynovitis less likely. The important indication for surgical intervention is the persistence of the cartilage flap in situ, since it delays or prevents repair of the lesion. The size of the lesion has been reported to not affect the outcome of cases treated surgically (Rudd, et al 1990). This is in agreement with early reports (Griffiths 1968, Clayton-Jones and Vaughan 1970, Leighton 1971).

Birkeland (1967) was the first to suggest that conservative treatment of rest and analgesics or intra-articular injections of steroids was not entirely satisfactory in the control of clinical signs and that surgical removal of the flap was indicated to achieve soundness in the patient. Later, it was suggested that following surgical removal of a partially loosened cartilage cap, the underlying bone should be scarified. It was thought that surgical removal of the flap with or without curettage would permit more rapid healing of the bony lesion and the results would be better than more conservative treatment (Griffiths 1968, Olsson 1976, Clayton-Jones and Vaughan 1970, Vaughan and Clayton-Jones 1970).

If the flap has dislodged at the time of examination, it often drops in the caudoventral pouch of the joint cavity and the value of surgery has been questioned. Some have suggested that the presence of the cartilage flap as a joint body does not cause clinical signs (Olsson 1976) while others feel strongly concerning its removal to prevent the perpetuation of a clinically important sterile chronic synovitis. Clinical signs may be used to decide the appropriateness of surgery in these cases. However, in rare instances, a clinically silent healed OCD lesion with fragments in the caudal pocket may suddenly become acutely lame because of fragment movement into the bicipital sheath.

If the flap has fallen free spontaneously, some feel that the edges of the original cartilage defect need to be trimmed surgically, however, deep curettage of the lesion is not recommended, although opinions are divided (Rudd, et al 1990). Extensive lavage of the joint helps to remove the small fragments of cartilage and debris that would otherwise perpetuate the chronic synovitis.

The surgery can be performed through an arthrotomy in which the joint capsule is opened widely or with the aid of arthroscopy which utilizes a small opening in the capsule (Person 1989; Van Ryssen, et al 1993; van Bree and Van Ryssen 1998). However, the surgical opening of the bicipital tendon sheath remains the method of choice to remove joint mice from this location since this area in inaccessible for arthroscopic viewing (van Bree and Van Ryssen 1991). Regardless of technique used, the surgery should include extensive lavage to flush free the cartilage debris, especially from sites around the bicipital tendon.

## Prognosis

In a dog of a lighter breed (less than 20 kg) with a small lesion evidenced at 7 to 8 months, it is expected that the flap will disintegrate spontaneously without surgical removal. The prognosis in this case is good with or without use of analgesics and controlled exercise, and the owner can expect a clinically sound dog. However, if the dog remains painful for more than 1 month after conservative treatment, surgical intervention should be considered with projection of a good prognosis. Our experience in treatment of this type of case is limited because of their infrequent occurrence.

In the dog of a heavier breed (more than 20 kg) with a large lesion first noted at 4 to 5 months, the prognosis following conservative treatment is poor because the flap often remains in position for some time. If this patient is operated early with flap removal and joint lavage, the prognosis is good. If this patient is managed conservatively and operated later with flap removal and joint lavage, the prognosis is only fair because of the chronic synovitis and development of an osteoarthrosis.

In the dog in which the flap has become dislodged due to physical activity and the defect undergoes spontaneous repair, there is the possibility that the cartilaginous fragment will perpetuate a chronic synovitis. Thus, it is highly likely that the clinical signs will persist with additional development of a progressive osteoarthrosis and the prognosis is guarded. Without surgery, the prognosis is only fair because of the continued inflammatory disease and surgical lavage of the joint is highly recommended. Following surgery, the prognosis is thought to be good.

If a combination of OCD and bicipital tendon synovitis is present simultaneously, clinical signs should be used to determine which site is most clinically important in determining the prognosis. In some cases, two surgical approaches need to be used in treatment. Whatever the circumstances, the flap should be removed surgically.

In the heavy breed dog with a large lesion that is not presented for treatment until 2 years of age or older, it is probable that conservative treatment has been attempted first with only a temporary and incomplete improvement. The presence of tenosynovitis, in addition to the developing osteoarthrosis, greatly affects the prognosis in a case such as this. Surgical treatment of the OCD lesion may be attempted following the use of conservative treatment, but there is little chance of improvement because of a co-existing tenosynovitis, which is the major cause of pain. This aspect of the disease may be treated successfully by surgery.

## Heritability

An early report suggested incorrectly that the lesion was an aseptic necrosis of the bone (Pobisch 1962). Later, Craig and Riser 1965, recognized the lesion was due to an error in bone formation and was either: (1) trauma induced, (2) due to late skeletal development, (3) due to excessive weight of the patient, or (4) any combination of these. Trauma was suspected because the position of the humeral head relative to the glenoid cavity might result in excessive forces on the caudal aspect of the humeral head. A widely accepted proposal relative to the etiology of osteochondrosis suggested that the shoulder joint in full extension allowed the caudal rim of the glenoid cavity of the scapula to contact the susceptible area within the humeral head (Craig and Riser 1965). This idea has continued through the years despite the fact that the humeral head rolls within the glenoid cavity and does not, even in full extension, ride in a manner that the edge of the glenoid cavity contacts the susceptible area on the humeral head (Morgan 1972).

Weakening in subchondral support structures was thought possible due to late development within the caudocentral epiphysis. This could create a susceptibility to injury, due to an increase in pressure at this site due to increasing levels of physical activity in the growing dog. Microcirculation of the developing humeral head determined by filling of the capillaries in specimens, showed that delayed ossification occurs in the medial half of the humeral head when compared with the lateral half. Thus, the caudomedial aspect is exposed to the effects of trauma for longer periods of time (Carrig and Morgan 1984).

The late development of the caudocentral epiphysis seems to create an "anatomic susceptibility" to indentation of the bone by the articular surface of the glenoid cavity.

Hormonal disturbances have been suggested as a cause of the disease (Paatsama, et al 1971). Later, an effort to prove the lesion heritable was not successful and it was thought, instead, that any imbalance of calcium, phosphorus, or vitamin D in conjunction with minimal trauma might be the cause of the lesions (Palmer 1970). This was perhaps a first attempt to determine causation by observation and test breeding of a large group of suitable animals. The discovery of lesions within littermates may be supportive of the possibility of nutritional errors, but also continues to suggest the possibility of an inheritable disease (Knecht, et al 1977). The frequent identification of lesions within certain breeds strongly suggests a hereditary disease.

Dietary studies using a variation in energy levels in Great Danes have shown a failure of maturation of the epiphyseal cartilage in dogs fed free-choice with inconsistent development of OCD lesions within the humeral head. The lesions were located in a similar location and had the same histological appearance as those seen in spontaneous cases. It was thought that the experimental feeding demonstrated that excessive intake of food rich in energy, protein, calcium and phosphorus accelerated growth and induced the anatomical changes of osteochondrosis dissecans of the humeral head (Hedhammer, et al 1973). The occurrence of this condition in heavier breeds and in specific bloodlines certainly provides for a strong suspicion that this condition is the result of genetic predisposition on the part of the parents and that rapid skeletal growth is a contributing factor.

# References

BARTHEZ PY, MORGAN JP. Bicipital tenosynovitis in the dog: evaluation with positive contrast arthrography. Vet Radiol Ultrasound. 1993;34:325-330.

BERZON JL. Osteochondritis dissecans in the dog: Diagnosis and therapy. JAVMA.175:796-799,1979.

BIRKELAND R. Osteochondritis dissecans in the humeral head of the dog. Comparison of results achieved with conservative and surgical treatment. Nord Vet Med. 1967;19:294-306.

BRASS W. Über die Osteochondrosis des Hundes. Tierärztl Umsch. 1956;11:200-204.

CALLAHAN TF, ACKERMAN N. The suspinated mediolateral radiograph for detection of humeral head osteochondrosis in the dog. Vet Radidol. 1985;26:144-148.

CARRIG CB, MORGAN JP. Microcirculation of the humeral head in the immature dog. JAVRS.15:28-33,1974.

CLAYTON-JONES DG, VAUGHAN LC. The surgical treatment of osteochondritis dissecans of the humeral head in dogs. J Sm An Pract.11:803-812,1970.

CORDY DR, WIND AP. Transverse fracture of the proximal articular cartilage in dogs (so-called osteochondritis dissecans). Path Vet. 1969;6:424-436.

CRAIG PH, RISER WH. Osteochondritis dissecans in the proximal humerus of the dog. JAVRS. 6:40-49,1965.

DINGWALL JS, STAPLES JW, PENNOCK PW. Osteochondritis dissecans in a miniature poodle. Mod Vet Prac 53:47,1973.

DORY MA, WAUTELET MJ. Arthroscopy in septic arthritis: Lidocaine- and iodine-containing costrast media are bacteriostatic. Arthritis and Rheumatism. 1985;98:198-203.

FOX SM, WALKER AM. OCD of the humeral head: Its diagnosis and treatment. Vet Med February 1993:123-131.

GRIFFITHS RC. Osteochondritis dissecans of the canine shoulder. JAVMA.153:1733-1735. 1968.

HARRISON JW. Osteochondritis dissecans. Proc AAHA Meet.:423,1975.

HEDHAMMER Å, WU FM, KROOK L, SCHRYVER HF, et al. Over nutrition and skeletal disease: An experimental study in growing Great Dane dogs. Cornell Vet. 1974;5 (suppl):1-160.

JOHNSON KA, DENNIS KA. Osteochondritis dissecans in a beagle. Aust Vet J. 1978;54:364.

KNECHT CD, VANSICKLE DC, BLEVINS WE, AVOLT MD, HUGHES RB, CANTWELL HD. Osteochondrosis of the shoulder and stifle in 3 of 5 Border Collie littermates. JAVMA.170:58-60,1977.

LAHUE TR, BROWN SG, ROUSH JC, TICER JW. Entrapment of joint mice in the bicipital tendon sheath as a sequela to osteochondritis dissecans of the proximal humerus in dogs: A report of six cases. JAAHA.24:99-105,1988.

LEIGHTON RL. Osteoochondritis dissecans of the shoulder joint of the dog. Vet Clinics of NA (SAP). 1971;1:391-401.

LINCOLN J, POTTER K. Tenosynovitis of the biceps brachii tendon in dogs. JAAHA.12:475-480,1976.

MOSTOSKY UV. Osteochondritis dissecans of the canine shoulder. Proceed 13th Gaines Vet Sym, 1964:16-19.

MILTON JL, RUMPH PF, REED AD. Osteochondritis dissecans of the shoulder in the racing greyhound: A report of two cases and a survey of 109 greyhound anatomy specimens. JAAHA.17:617-622,1981.

MORGAN JP. Osteochondritis in the proximal humerus of the dog. In: Morgan JP, Radiology in veterinary orthopedics, Philadephia: Lea & Febiger. 1972:341-345.

MORGAN JP, ed. Techniques of Veterinary Radiography. 5th ed. Ames, Iowa: Iowa State University Press;1990.

MOSTOSKY UV. Osteochondritis dissecans and synovial fluid analysis. Gaines Progress. Spring,1964.

MUHUMUZA L, MORGAN JP, MIYABAYASHI T. Positive-contrast arthrography: A study of the humeral joints in normal Beagle Dogs. Vet Radiol. 1988;29:157-161.

MUIR P, GOLDSMID SE, ROTHWELL TL, BELLENGER CR. Calcifying tendinopathy of the biceps brachii in a dog. JAVMA.201:1747-1749,1992.

OLSSON S-E. Osteochondritis dissecans in dogs: A study of pathogenesis, clinical signs, pathologic changes, natural course and sequelae. Abstracts of Third International Conference of Veterinary Radiologists. JAVRS.14:8,1973.

OLSSON S-E. Lameness in the dog. A review of lesions causing osteoarthrosis of the shoulder, elbow, hip, stifle and hock joints, in Proc AAHA Meet.:363-370,1975.

OLSSON S-E. Osteochondrosis- A growing problem to dog breeders. Gaines Progress. Summer, 1976:1-11.

OLSSON S-E. Osteochondrosis in the dog. In: Kirk RW, ed. Current veterinary therapy VI. Philadplphia, PA: WB Saunders; 1977:881-886.

PAATSAMA S, ROKKANEN P, JUSSILA J, SITTNIKOW K. A study of osteochondritis dissecans of the canine humeral head using histological, OTC bone labeling, microradiographic and microangiographic methods. J Sm Anim Pract.12:603-611,1971.

PALMER CS,. Osteochondritis dissecans in Great Danes. Vet Med/SAC. 1970;65:994-1002.

PERSON MW. Arthroscopic treatment of osteochondritis dissecans in the canine shoulder. Vet Surg. 1989;18:175-189.

POBISCH R. Aseptische Nekrose des Humeruskopfes eine Lahmheitsursache bei Junghunden. Wien Tierärzlt Mschr. 1962;49:571-587.

ROBINS GM. Osteochondritis dissecans in the dog. Aust Vet J.54:272-279,1978.

RUDD RG, et al. Results of management of osteochondritis dissecans of humeral head in dogs: 44 cases (1982 to 1987). JAAHA.26:173-178,1990.

SCHAWALDER P. Die Synoviale Osteochondromatose (Synoviale Chondrometaplasie) beim Hund. Schweiz Arch Tierheilk. 1980;122:673-678.

SCHNELLE GB. Congenital dysplasia of the hip (canine) and sequelae. Proc. 91st Annual Meet. AVMA.253-258,1954.

SIEMERING B. A review of the diagnosis and treatment of common forelimb lameness in immature dogs. Compend Cont Ed. 1979;5:357-365.

SMITH CW, STOWATER JL. Osteochondritis dissecans of the canine shoulder joint: A review of 35 cases. JAAHA. 11:658-662,1975.

STORY EC. Prognostic value of arthrography in canine shoulder osteochondrosis (osteochondritis) dissecans. Vet Clinics N A Sm Anim Pract.8:301-308,1978.

SUTER PF, CARB AV. Shoulder arthrography in dogs - Radiographic anatomy and clinical application. J Sm Anim Pract.10:407-413,1969.

TICER JW. Radiographic interpretation. Mod Vet Pract.53:38-42,1973.

VAN BREE H. OCD and shoulder arthrography in dogs. Proceedings 7th International Veterinary Radiology Conference:30,1985.

VAN BREE H. Evaluation of the prognostic value of positive-contrast shoulder arthrography for bilateral osteochondrosis lesions in dogs. Am J Vet Res.51;1121-1125,1990.

VAN BREE H. Vacuum phenomenon associated with osteochondrosis of the scapulohumeral joint in dogs: 100 cases (1985-1991). JAVMA. 201: 1916-1917,1992.

VAN BREE H. Comparison of diagnostic accuracy of positive-contrast arthrography and arthrotomy in evaluation of ostechondrosis lesions in the scapulohumeral joint in dogs. JAVMA.203: 84-88,1993.

VAN BREE H. Evaluation of subchondral lesion size in osteochondrosis of the scapulohumeral joint in dogs. JAVMA.204:1472-1474,1994.

VAN BREE H, VAN RYSSEN B. Arthrography of the dog's shoulder. The Veterinary Annual 1991;31:213-220.

VAN BREE H, VAN RYSSEN B. Positive contrast shoulder arthrography with Iopromide and Diatrizoate in dogs with osteochondrosis. Vet Rad Ultrasound. 1995;36:203-206.

VAN BREE H, VAN RYSSEN B. Diagnostic and surgical arthroscopy in osteochondrosis lesions. Vet Clinic of NA/SAP. 1998;28:161-189.

VAN BREE H, VAN RYSSEN B, DESMIDT M. Osteochondrosis lesions of the canine shoulder: Correlation of positive contrast arthrography and arthroscopy. Vet Radiol. 1992;33:342-347.

VAN BREE H, VERHAEGHE B, MAENHOUT D. Positive contrast arthrography of the dog's shoulder with meglumine-sodium diatrizoate. J.Vet Med.36:421-430,1989.

VAN RYSSEN B, VAN BREE H, VYT Ph. Arthroscopy of the shoulder joint in the dog. JAAHA.29:101-105,1993.

VAUGHAN LC, CLAYTON-JONES DG. Osteochondritis dissecans of the head of the humerus in dogs. J Sm Anim Pract.9:283-294,1968.

WAMBERG K. Atlas Radiologica, Copenhagen:The Medical Book Company; 1966:71.

WHITEHAIR JG, RUDD RB. Osteochondritis dissecans of the humeral head in dogs. Compend Cont Ed. 1990;12;195-203.

WOODARD DC. Osteochondritis dissecans in a family of bull terriers. Vet Med Sac. 1979;74:936.

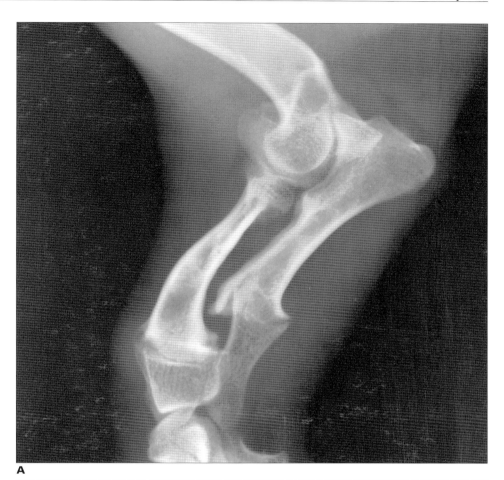

**Figure 3-2**
Radiographs of a 6-month-old Welsh Corgi showing joint morphology as seen in chondrodystrophic breeds. The lateral radiograph of the elbow illustrates the malformed trochlear notch of the ulna and radial head (A). Joint incongruity is severe. Note the alteration in appearance of the distal ulnar and distal radial physes. Joint morphology of this nature when seen in non-chondrodystrophic breeds is not a form of elbow dysplasia. The ventrodorsal radiograph of the pelvis shows the malformed hip joints characterized by poorly fitting femoral heads (B). Joint morphology of this nature when seen in non-chondrodystrophic breeds is not a form of hip dysplasia.

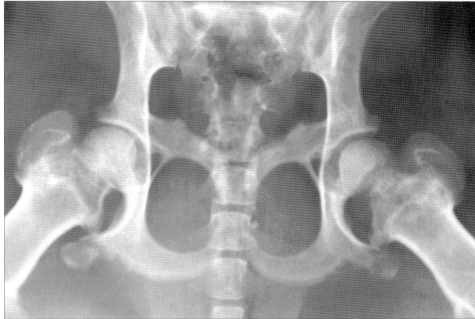

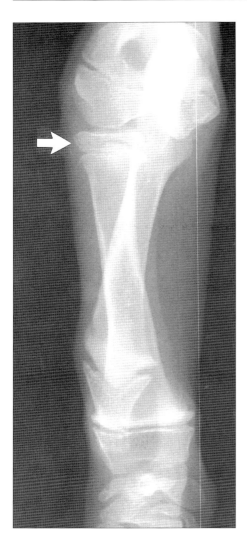 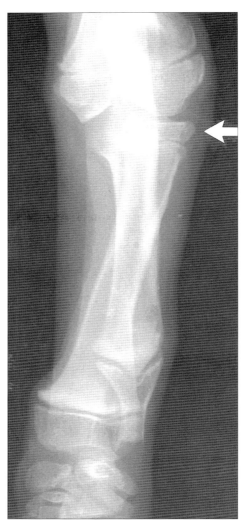

**Figure 3-3**
Craniocaudal radiographs of the antebrachii of a 15-week-old male Doberman Pinscher with an abnormal gait and shortened limbs. The comparative overgrowth of the radii had resulted in lateral subluxation of the radial heads (arrows) and hypoplastic development of the medial portion of the humeral condyle (trochlea). With the unequal growth of the radius and ulna, the bones form an "X" as seen on this projection rather than the near parallel appearance that would be seen in the normal dog. The resulting elbow sub-luxation is associated with chondrodysplasia occurring sporadically in this non-chondrodystrophic breed.

unfractured) elbow of Cocker Spaniels that had suffered a fracture of the opposite elbow. A secondary osteoarthrosis often developed in the normal elbow that could cause a problem in diagnosis of elbow dysplasia (Marcellin-Little, et al 1994).

## Proposed etiologies

Olsson (1974) proposed that all three forms of elbow dysplasia are manifestations of osteochondrosis. However, the primary role of osteochondrosis has been somewhat discounted because of the additional finding of joint incongruity and thus, joint instability. Because the incongruity exists in the different forms of elbow dysplasia, a common etiology has remained attractive. The finding of all forms of elbow dysplasia within both elbows of a single dog plus the finding of various forms of elbow dysplasia within the same elbow suggests a common etiology. Joint incongruity has been suggested as a result of underdevelopment of the ulnar trochlear notch and is strongly suggested as a cause of elbow dysplasia (Wind 1986, Weiss 1983, Bienz 1985)

The incongruity observed between the distal edge of the ulnar trochlear notch (medial coronoid process) and the radius suggests either asynchronous growth of the radius and ulna, or insufficient development of the ulnar trochlear notch. Measurements of radial and ulnar length have indicated a statistically significant relative increase in length of the proximal ulna in breeds with elbow dysplasia. Length ratios (proximal ulna to radius) in rarely affected sight hounds ranged from 0.17 to 0.19 and in commonly affected breeds from 0.19 to 0.23 (Wind 1986).

The "step" between the distal edge of the ulnar trochlear notch and the articular surface of the radius is at most 5mm (Figures 3-5, 3-6, 3-7). This degree of incongruity is compatible with a lagging radial growth although this, in itself, is insufficient to explain the relative increase in

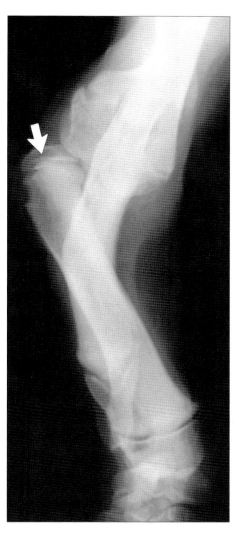
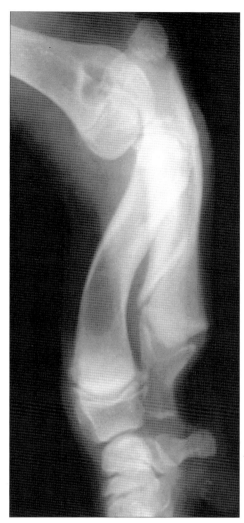

**Figure 3-4**
Craniocaudal and lateral radiographs of the forelimb showing congenital elbow luxation with lateral displacement of the hypoplastic radial head (arrow) in a nonchondrodystrophic breed. Note the destruction of the elbow joint. This is thought to be a further stage of the lesion shown in Figure 3-3.

the length of the proximal ulna. It is possible that a lagging radial growth may contribute to the relative increase in size of the proximal ulna, however, comparison of relative proximal ulnar measurements of affected animals with those of non-affected animals within the same breed did not show a consistent increase in the affected animals. Another contradictory finding is the radiographic appearance. Instead of an increase in the joint space between the anconeal process and humerus, as is seen with traumatic premature closure of either of the radial physes, this joint space usually appears narrower.

An alternative explanation is underdevelopment of the ulnar trochlear notch, resulting in a notch with too small a curvature to encompass the humeral trochlea. The increase in the relative size of the proximal ulna in affected (heavier) breeds most likely represents an adaptation to accommodate an ulnar trochlear notch of sufficient size to encompass a larger humeral trochlea. Because the ulnar trochlear notch surrounds to a considerable extent the humeral trochlea, the rate of bone production by the articular epiphyseal growth plate of the ulnar trochlear notch needs to be a great deal more rapid than the growth rate of the humeral trochlea. Failure to keep pace with the growth of the humeral trochlea may be the underlying cause for the observed incongruity.

The presumed underdevelopment of the ulnar trochlear notch and the resulting incongruity becomes evident between the age of 4 and 6 months. The skeleton at that time is as yet incompletely ossified and a separate center of ossification for the anconeal process may still be present in some breeds. Depending upon the degree of underdevelopment, and also upon the breed involved, the ultimate effect may be only an osteoarthrosis. This is observed in cases of very mild incongruity as seen in the Brittany with little clinical affect. However, the level of athletic performance may be decreased in these dogs and it is recommended that breeding stock should be radiographed for evaluation of this level of disease. In cases of

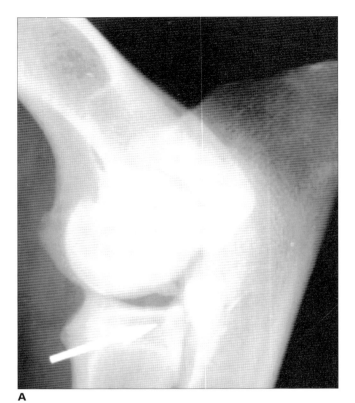 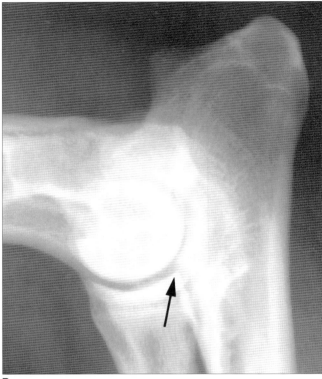

**Figure 3-5**
Lateral radiographs of an elbow joint of an 11-month-old male Bernese Mountain Dog (A) and a 1-year-old male Shar Pei (B) that illustrate the "step" between the ulnar trochlear notch and the articular surface of the radius (arrows). The joint space between the humeral condyle and the anconeal process is narrowed. The distal humerus is displaced cranially as evidenced by the humeroradial joint space that is narrowed cranially and widened caudally in a manner that the condyle is shifted cranially to the cranial margin of the radial head.

more severe incongruity; fracture, fragmentation, or fissure of the medial coronoid process (and perhaps the distal end of the ulnar trochlear notch) may occur due to increased weight-bearing forces on the too-high lying parts of the ulna.

Another possibility of disease occurs in development of a UAP in dogs in which a separate center of ossification within the anconeal process is still present after the onset of incongruity. This non-union is most likely due to micro-movement of the cartilage bridge between the separate center of ossification and the olecranon. This movement is caused by too tight a fit between the anconeal process and the humerus, the result of the too small curvature of the trochlear notch.

A final form of disease is seen in the development of an OCD lesion of the medial aspect of the humeral condyle in which interference with endochondral ossification of the epiphyseal growth plate is caused by excessive pressure generated by the too high lying medial coronoid process. Combinations of any of the above may be found within one elbow or between both elbows of a single dog.

## Clinical signs

Initial clinical signs of elbow dysplasia occur at the age of 4 to 6 months and are generally irrespective of the form of the disease or the breed involved and include frequent episodes of lameness, a "paddling" gait, and a wide forelimb stance that may possibly be an effort to minimize painful weight bearing (Table 3-3). In addition, the animal may stand with the elbows either out or in with the feet rotated outward. However, dogs affected by other elbow diseases also adduct the elbows. The clinical signs are in particular influenced by whether the disease is unilateral or bilateral. The abnormal "paddling" gait is especially noted when both elbows are involved and additionally, may be characterized by excessive supination of the front paws during extension of the limb. This observation is not pathognomonic however, because many apparently normal dogs of the affected breeds also supinate the paw on extension of the limb. Because of pain and especially with bilateral involvement, exercise endurance may be limited, affecting the personality of the dog causing it to appear quieter than expected (often to the pleasure of the owner). Usually, the specific form of elbow dysplasia cannot be distinguished by signalment, history, or clinical signs, and this determination, if made at all, may be only by radiographic examination or at the time of surgery.

**Table 3-3: Acute clinical signs of elbow dysplasia due to early onset of osteoarthrosis in dogs 6 months of age (authors' observations)**

- Episodes of lameness
- Elbows may be abducted or adducted on standing
- "Paddling" forelimb gait with supination during forward motion
- Outward rotation of the forefeet on standing
- Reluctance to flexion and extension of the elbow joint
- Stiff, stilted forelimb gait (in more severely affected dog)

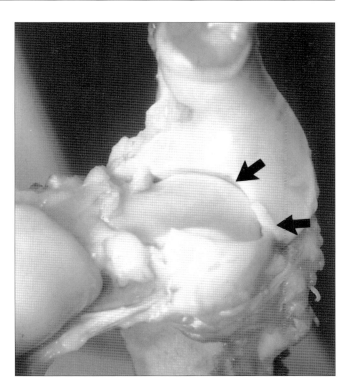

**Figure 3-6**
A photograph of a specimen of an elbow of a 11-month-old male Bernese Mountain Dog with dysplasia showing the "step" between the surface of the trochlear notch and the surface of the radial head (arrow). Note the fragmented medial coronoid process (arrow).

**Figure 3-7**
Lateral radiographs of specimens from the elbow joints of a 6-month-old female German Shepherd Dog following removal of the humeri which show the "step" between the distal surface of the ulnar trochlear notch and the articular surface of the radius (arrows). Note the malformed curvature of the trochlear notch more obvious on the more severely affected joint. Also note the pattern of new bone that creates a sclerotic appearance in the adjacent proximal ulna (arrows).

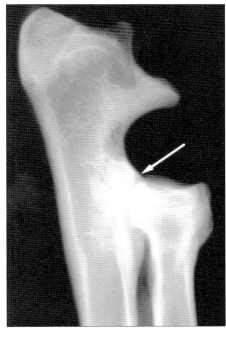 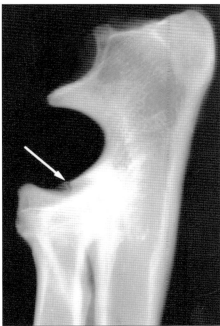

These early clinical signs are most likely due to the early stages of osteoarthrosis especially that of a sterile synovitis. Not all cases of elbow dysplasia have clinically observable signs especially if the condition is bilateral and symmetrical. Minimal joint incongruity fails to cause clinical signs of lameness or discomfort.

With time, osteoarthrosis progresses and a more chronic pattern of clinical signs develops. The dog now sits or lies down much of the time and plays for shorter periods of time than other dogs of a comparable age. Some severely affected dogs can barely walk around the block with their owner. It is at this stage that the lameness becomes more mechanical in nature due to a limitation of movement of the joint because of thickening of the joint capsule and new bone production.

It is interesting that the clinical degree of lameness often fails to have a positive correlation with radiographic changes of osteoarthrosis. Also, determination of a score obtained by evaluation of the radiographic changes of osteoarthrosis does not make it possible to predict the extent of the lesion to be found at surgery (Guthrie 1989 a). This inconsistency can be partially explained by the fact that surgical exploration used to confirm the status of the joint disease may provide an incomplete comparison and the results are therefore questionable. In particular, surgical exploration often does not permit evaluation of the degree of incongruity, thus missing this important aspect of elbow dysplasia. A similar inconsistency between radiographic changes and clinical signs is found in other forms of joint disease, especially in the osteoarthrosis associated with hip dysplasia, in which, many of the most severely affected dogs as determined radiographically are often without observable clinical signs according to the owners. However, the authors have noted that frequently the clinical signs do correlate positively with the radiographic changes; in general, the authors feel that the radiographic changes reflect the degree of the lesion more objectively while the clinical signs are more likely to be influenced by the personality of the dog. Ideally, the findings from the history, clinical observations, physical examination and radiographic examination should lead to a quite accurate prediction of the nature of the joint disease.

The variation in impact of elbow dysplasia on a dog's behavior can be seen from a study in which the elbows were examined following death. The dogs in one group were presented for diagnosis and treatment and were ultimately euthanized because of lameness on one or both forelimbs caused by elbow lesions diagnosed in one or both forelimbs. Over 93% of this group had lesions of elbow dysplasia. The average age of these dogs was 25 months and larger breeds were over-represented. However, this only partially tells the story of the clinical impact of elbow dysplasia. A second smaller group of dogs with unknown clinical history regarding lameness of the forelimbs and a third group of dogs that had never revealed lameness of the forelimbs were presented for clinical examination. The average age at the time of examination of these last two groups was 83 and 70 months, respectively. In these groups, the owners were not cognizant of an elbow disease and the dogs had continued to live what was thought to be a pain-free life until they were presented for clinical examination for another reason. Over 87% and 83% of these groups respectively had lesions of elbow dysplasia at necropsy with a rather severe degree of osteoarthrosis. This means that elbow dysplasia and the resulting osteoarthrosis exerts its affect on dogs differently. Dogs in group I were of larger breeds with recognizable clinical signs, and were euthanized because of the lameness. The other two groups were dogs of smaller breeds with clinical signs undetected by the owners or clinicians, and dysplasia was evident in the majority and must have influenced the quality of life or certainly the working ability of the dogs (Grøndalen 1982 a).

In another study, a group of 207 Rottweilers over 12 months of age was divided into one group of 66 dogs suffering from elbow lameness and a second group of 141 dogs that had never revealed forelimb lameness. New bone formation (osteophytes) was noted in 89.4% of lame dogs (group I) and 68.1% of dogs free from lameness (group II). Consequently it was noted that a large number of dogs had secondary osteoarthrosis characterized by extensive new bone formation in the elbow joints and were without sufficient pain to cause them to have a clinically obvious lameness. The obvious conclusion is that the number of dogs with elbow lesions far exceeds the number of dogs showing detectable lameness recognized by owners (Grøndalen 1982 b). It suggests in addition, that a large number of dogs are being used for breeding without the knowledge that they have an inheritable joint disease and illustrates the need to perform radiographic examination of the elbow joints prior to breeding in breeds commonly affected.

It is reported in the literature that the type of elbow dysplasia influences the time of appearance for clinical examination. However, the owner often does not recognize lameness or fails to present the dog for examination even if minimal lameness is noted. Reports often describe the age at which the dogs were presented for treatment to a referral clinic and not the age of first lameness. These problems complicate determination of the age at which dogs are first expected to show signs of lameness. Generally, it is reported that dogs with OCD seem to have clinical signs at a younger age than seen in other forms of dysplasia. Dogs with coronoid disease range from 6 to 20 months at the time of presentation, while dogs with a loose anconeal process are older and range from 14 to 46 months. In one report of 77 Bernese Mountain Dogs, lameness was first noted in dogs between the ages of 5 months and 8 years (Bienz 1985). The authors' experience suggests detection of all forms of the disease at a younger age than generally reported, probably reflecting a higher interest in this form of lameness (Table 3-4).

**Table 3-4: Age of first clinical signs due to specific lesions (authors' experience)**

| | |
|---|---|
| Ununited anconeal process: | 6 to 12 months |
| Coronoid process disease: | 5 to 12 months |
| Osteochondrosis: | 5 to 6 months |
| Minor joint incongruity: | non-clinical |

## Physical examination

On physical examination at approximately 6 months of age, manipulation of the diseased elbow joint may be resented with pain demonstrated on both flexion and extension of the elbow joint. The presence of crepitation can be misleading because it may be detected in many normal elbows at this age. In more severe cases, joint effusion may be palpable beneath the anconeal and extensor muscles, and this may become more pronounced after physical activity. At a later age when the disease has become more chronic, thickening of the joint capsule is noted along with increased prominence of the medial humeral epicondyle. Muscle atrophy may be associated with loss of physical activity. Exercise endurance may be limited because of pain, especially with bilateral involvement. This affects the personality of the dog and causes it to appear quiet.

With time, secondary joint disease in the form of osteoarthrosis progresses and it is at this stage that the lameness becomes more mechanical in nature because of development of heavy bony enthesophytes and marked thickness of the joint capsule. These changes result in a limitation of motion within the joint causing this different form of lameness. The lameness is now referred to as a mechanical lameness rather than one associated with pain. The findings on physical examination are similar in elbows regardless of the specific form of the dysplasia (Table 3-5).

**Table 3-5: Physical signs identified with elbow dysplasia (authors' observations)**

**I.** Acute disease
    A. Pain on flexion and extension
    B. Joint effusion

**II.** Chronic disease
    A. Thickening of the joint capsule
    B. Increase in prominence of medial humeral epicondyle
    C. Muscle atrophy
    D. Mechanical limitation of motion

## Anatomy and development of the elbow joint

The elbow joint is a tight hinge joint consisting of the humerus proximally and the radius and ulna distally. The distal part of the humerus is called a condyle. The medial part of the condyle is called the trochlea, and consists of a depressed central area for articulation with the "keel" of the ulnar trochlear notch and a narrow downward sloping ridge for articulation with the medial coronoid process of the ulna. It also articulates with the medial aspect of the radial head. The remainder of the radial head has the principle weight bearing function and articulates with the lateral aspect of the humeral condyle, or capitulum. The main movement of the joint is flexion and extension that occurs between the trochlear notch of the olecranon portion of the ulna and the olecranon fossa of the humerus, and the head of the radius and the lateral aspect of the humeral condyle. An additional joint exists between the radius and the ulna, which permits the radius a few degrees of rotation resulting in supination and pronation of the forelimb (Figure 3-8). Coordinated growth of the articular growth plates in the three articulating bones, as well as of the metaphyseal growth plates of these bones, is required to create a perfectly fitting joint (Riser and Shirer 1965).

Several separate ossification centers are involved in the development of the elbow joint (Hare 1961) The humeral condyle is formed by two secondary ossification centers and the proximal radius by one secondary ossification center. The ulna, in most instances has only one radiographically recognizable secondary ossification center distally near the carpal bones and an apophyseal center in the olecranon. The coronoid, and anconeal processes of the ulna usually have no recognizable secondary centers of ossification, instead the entire cartilage model of the proximal ulna gradually changes into bone after birth. There are exceptions, however, especially in the German Shepherd Dog, and the Greyhound. In some dogs of

## 52 Elbow dysplasia

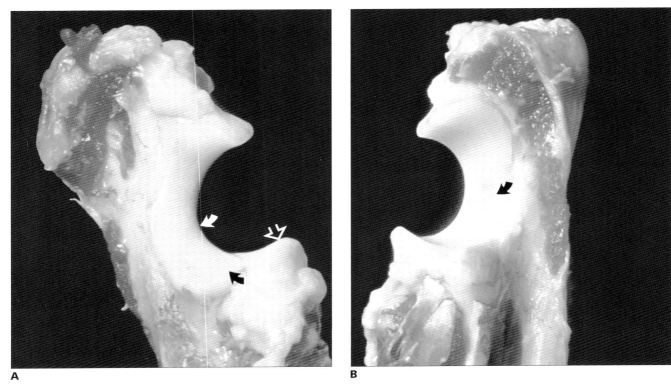

**Figure 3-8**
Photographs of specimens of the normal elbow joint of a 5-year-old Boxer showing two different views. The medial aspect of the elbow joint with the humerus removed. Note the shape of the ulnar trochlear notch and its "keel" (white arrow) (A). The medial coronoid process (black arrow) is a downward continuation of the downward sloping medial aspect of the radius. The articular cartilage has a uniform thickness. The radial head (hollow arrow) is identified. The lateral aspect of the elbow joint with the humerus removed shows the slight thinning of the articular cartilage in the central portion of the lateral flange of the ulnar trochlear notch (arrow) and the smooth transition of this notch onto the proximal radial articulation (B).

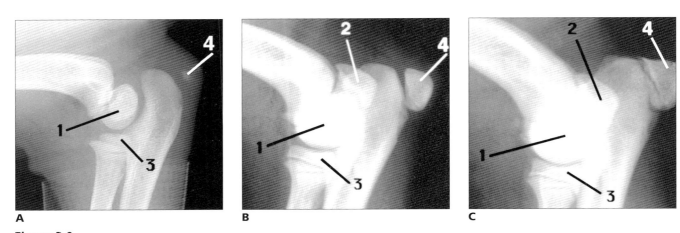

**Figure 3-9**
Lateral radiographs of the elbow joints of a Beagle at: 60 days (A), 120 days (B), and 180 days (C). The two separate centers of ossification within the humeral condyle are superimposed on these views (1). The center of ossification of the medial epicondyle is seen ossified at 120 days and remains ununited at 180 days (2). The proximal radial epiphysis is seen ununited in all three studies and consists of a horizontally directed portion and a downward slanting portion (3). This conformation separates the lateral radial eminence from the remainder of the radial head on the radiograph. The center for the olecranon process is seen ununited in all three studies (4). Ossification of the anconeal process is difficult to see because of the overlying center for the medial epicondyle. Early ossification of the medial coronoid process is superimposed by the lateral radial eminence.

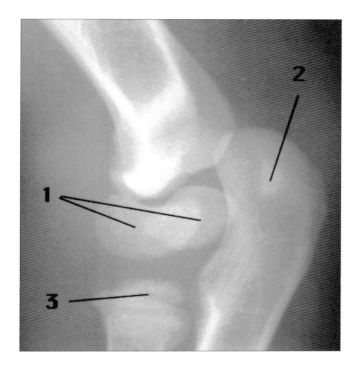
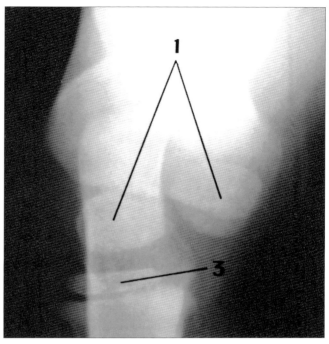

**Figure 3-10**
Craniocaudal and lateral radiographs of the elbow joint of a 6-week-old Rhodesian Ridgeback showing the major ossification centers. The two separate centers of ossification within the humeral condyle (1), the medial epicondyle (2), and the proximal radial epiphysis (3) are identified. The center for the olecranon, the anconeal process, and the medial coronoid are not ossified at this time. Because of incomplete ossification, the joint spaces appear wide caused by the presence of the radiolucent cartilage that serves both as a growth cartilage and an articular cartilage at this time.

these breeds, a separate center of ossification may be present in the anconeal process, which unites with the olecranon between the age of 4 to 6 months (Figure 3-9).

Ossification of the centers of growth occurs early (Figure 3-10). The medial and lateral condyles of the humerus are first noted to be ossified at 2 to 4 weeks of age and the head of the radius at 3 to 5 weeks of age. The medial epicondyle ossifies later at 6 to 9 weeks. The olecranon ossifies at 7 to 9 weeks. The method by which these centers unite and the approximate ages are listed (Table 3-6).

Looking inside the elbow joint after removal of the humerus, the normal radioulnar joint surface is characterized by a smooth transition from the ulnar trochlear notch onto the horizontal articular surface of the radius, and from the medial downward slope of the radius onto the medial coronoid process (Figure 3-8). The main radial articular surface is horizontal, while the ulnar articulation slopes downward. This appearance implies that the radius is the main weight-bearing bone and that the ulna serves more as a lever arm for the extensor muscles of the elbow joint. Compared to the coursing breeds, the heavier-set breeds have a relatively larger proximal ulna and appear to have a slightly larger, wider, less steeply sloping medial coronoid process. This may indicate an increase in the weight-bearing function of the ulna in these breeds (Wind and Packard 1986).

The articular cartilage of the ulnar trochlear notch extends medially and laterally to the site of attachment of the joint capsule, with only a slight thinning of this cartilage along the lateral aspect of the notch. The uninterrupted continuity of this cartilage implies that the entire ulnar trochlear notch is in close contact with the articular cartilage of the olecranon fossa and the humeral trochlea. In some dogs, a thinning of the articular cartilage occurs in the central portion of the trochlear notch. This is thought normal in some of the larger breeds, however, it is often associated with more severe forms of elbow dysplasia where the thinning of the articular cartilage involves the lateral flange of the trochlear notch. In the more severe cases the entire cartilage and underlying bone is missing (Figure 3-11). The main weight-bearing surface of the humerus in the elbow joint is the humeral trochlea, which articulates with both the radius and the ulna. Only the cranially sloping lateral part of the radial head articulates with the capitulum humeri.

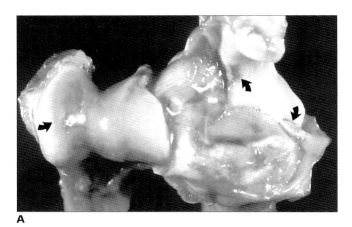 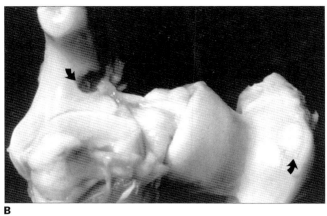

**Figure 3-11**
Photographs of specimens of dysplastic elbow joints from two different dogs show the character of injury to the articular cartilage of the trochlear notch. A 7-month-old male Golden Retriever has marked thinning of the articular cartilage (arrow) of the lateral flange of the ulnar trochlear notch (A). A fragmented MCP (arrow) is seen with abrasion of the articular cartilage on the opposite medial aspect of the humeral condyle (arrow). Also note the "step" (arrow) between the ulnar trochlear notch and the radial head. A 6-month-old female Rottweiler has disappearance of the cartilage and underlying bone (arrow) of the lateral flange of the ulnar trochlear notch (B). An abrasion of the cartilage of the MCP is seen and the process lies slightly above the level of the radial head. An OCD lesion is on the opposing articular cartilage of the medial aspect of the humeral condyle (arrow).

## Radiographic diagnosis

### Radiographic views

In young dogs between 5 and 7 months of age, the diagnosis of all forms of elbow dysplasia is primarily based on clinical signs, physical examination, and radiographic evaluation. The radiographic study should include views of each elbow because of the high frequency of bilateral elbow dysplasia. Correct radiographic technique as well as a high quality of film processing is critical in the production of diagnostic radiographs. The most diagnostic radiographs are made with a tabletop technique using a slow speed film-screen combination and a relatively low kVp setting (50 to 60). The central beam is directed on

**Table 3-6: Radiographic appearance of ossification centers in the normal elbow**

| Ossification centers | Earliest visualization | Fusion |
| --- | --- | --- |
| Distal humerus | | |
|     Capitulum | 2 to 3 weeks | |
|     Trochlea | 2 to 3 weeks | |
|         Capitulum joins trochlea | | 6 weeks |
|         Combined trochlea joins | | 6 months |
|         Distal epiphysis | | |
|     Medial epicondyle | 6 to 8 weeks | |
|         Epicondyle joins distal humerus | | 5 to 7 months |
| Radius | | |
|     Proximal epiphysis | 3 to 5 weeks | |
|         Epiphysis joins proximal radius | | 10 months |
|     Radial sesamoid bone | inconsistent | |
| Ulna | | |
|     Olecranon apophysis | 7 to 9 weeks | |
|         Joins the proximal ulna | | 8 months |
| Ossification of the | | |
|     Anconeal process | 3 to 4 months | |
|     Medial coronoid process | 3 to 6 months | |

the elbow joint. The arrangement of the bones of the elbow joint results in some degree of superimposition of the bones in each view, which makes interpretation more difficult. Detection of the more free-lying ununited anconeal process is much easier on the lateral view because of its larger size. The non-ossified cartilage bridge can be seen on this view between the anconeal process and the main body of the ulna. A variety of radiographic views have been recommended (Webbon and Clayton-Jones 1976, Robins 1980, Henry 1984) including the use of oblique views.

The major views used in routine radiographic examination of the elbow include the craniocaudal (CrCa) view and two lateral view(s) (Figures 3-12, 3-13). The lateral views are made with the dog lying on its side with the object limb dependent and the beam centered on the elbow joint. For the extended view, the elbow is extended with an inside angle of 120° with the paw held in a relaxed position of 15° supination causing a positioning of the limb that results in the best evaluation of the joint. Moderate supination of the paw places the medial coronoid process parallel to the tabletop for optimum visualization. A flexed lateral view of the elbow joint with an inside angle of less than 90° may also be advisable since it permits a more clear visualization of the anconeal process and the lateral epicondylar ridge. Another reason for use of the flexed lateral view is to permit a better evaluation of the condylar region of the distal humerus to better differentiate between a UAP and the normal growth plate of the medial epicondyle. A disadvantage of positioning of the limb in tight flexion is the resulting muscle tension that forces the elbow into an adducted position placing the lateral aspect of the humeral condyle distal to the medial condyle making evaluation of the joint spaces difficult (Figure 3-14).

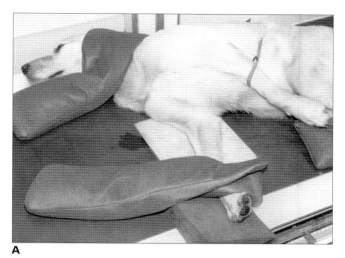

A

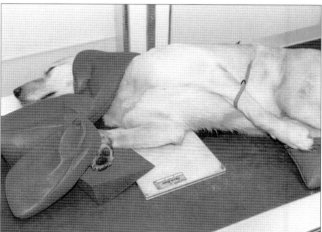

B

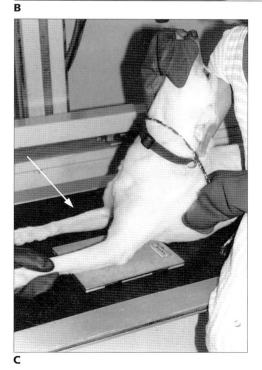

C

**Figure 3-12**
Photographs illustrate the positioning used in radiographic examination of the elbow joint. The lateral views are made with the dog lying on its side with the object limb dependent. For the extended lateral view, the limb is positioned with the joint at an angle of 120° with the foot held in a relaxed position of minimal supination (A). For the flexed lateral view, the elbow is positioned with an angle of less than 90° (B). Positioning for this view often causes the lateral head of the triceps and anconeus muscles to "bulge" resulting in elevation of the distal humerus. This results in adduction of the elbow joint and the resulting radiograph shows the articular margin of the lateral part of the condyle to appear distal to the medial part of the condyle. For the craniocaudal view, the animal is positioned on its sternum with the object limb in maximum extension and mild supination (C). The x-ray beam is angled distoproximally 10° to 20° (arrow). Note that the limb cannot be fully extended because of the position of the dog.

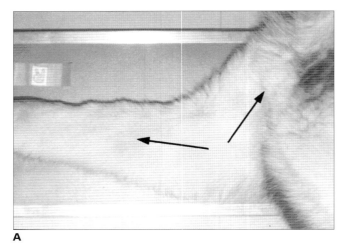

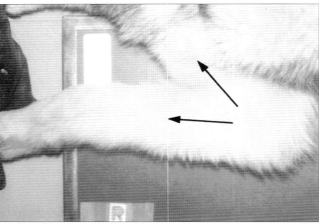

**Figure 3-13**
Photographs made from the location of the x-ray tube clearly show the exact positioning of the bones (arrows) within the fore limb in making the extended (>120°) (A) and flexed (<90°) (B) lateral views of the elbow joint.

For the craniocaudal view, the animal is positioned on its sternum with the object limb in maximum extension and mild supination (Figure 3-12). Because the dog is positioned on its sternum, the actual angle of limb extension is probably limited to approximately 120°. The x-ray beam should be centered on the olecranon and the x-ray beam angled distoproximally 10° to 20°. Thus, the beam is directed so it is nearly perpendicular to the long axis of the humerus. Greater angulation of the beam is required in the severely diseased elbow joint because of increased limitation of limb extension. Angulation of the beam projects the caudal portion of the humeral condyle, which is the common location for an OCD lesion. Regardless of the degree of flexion and the angle of the x-ray beam, the CrCa view allows comparison of the width of the medial and lateral aspects of the joint space. In the authors' experience, little information is added by the use of medial or lateral oblique views to that available on the conventional views.

Screening of elbow joints for registries is allowed at an age of 1 year or older. The screening must be performed in a practical manner, which means that the cost must be low and the study made in a short time. For these reasons, the use of lateral view(s) alone is suggested. Protocol recommendations made by the IEWG (Anomymous 1994) include a listing of minimal guidelines for radiographic diagnosis recommended for use by elbow screening registries and stresses use of both an extended and flexed lateral view.

## Purpose of study

The sequence of views used for examination of the elbow joint is dependent on the age of the patient and the presence of clinical signs and whether the study is used for diagnosis of clinical lameness or used for screening (Table 3-7).

In radiographic examination of the young (6 months old) clinically lame dog that is suspected to have elbow dysplasia, the extended lateral and craniocaudal views should be utilized. The presence of joint incongruity is best evaluated on the relaxed lateral view. The CrCa view is of value in the recognition of joint incongruity and in differentiation between coronoid disease and OCD of the humeral condyle. The flexed lateral view can be of value to confirm the presence of a UAP or new bone (enthesophytes) on the anconeal process and/or the lateral condylar ridge.

In the radiographic examination of an older clinically lame dog suspected of having elbow dysplasia, the signs of incongruity may be less conspicuous and the diagnosis of elbow dysplasia is made much easier than in the young dog because of the presence of the advancing osteoarthrosis. However, the exact form of the dysplasia may be hidden by the secondary pattern of bony changes. Both extended lateral and CrCa views clearly demonstrate the new bone production associated with osteoarthrosis.

In the screening of the younger dog for dysplasia (6 to 12 months), flexed and extended lateral views are usually sufficient for a survey, use patient positioning that is easier to obtain, and require less time for examination. The CrCa view adds information in the detection of joint incongruity.

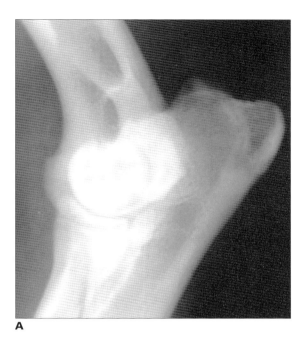 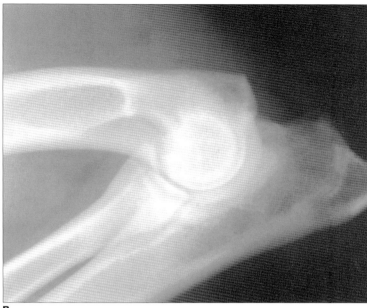

**Figure 3-14**
Lateral radiographs of the elbow joint of a 1-year-old male Labrador Retriever made with the joint extended (A) and tightly flexed (B). The proximal margin of the anconeal process is more clearly identified when the limb is flexed.

**Table 3-7: Views used in radiographic examination of the elbow joint(s)**

I. Young clinically lame dog - extended and flexed lateral and craniocaudal views

II. Older clinically lame dog - extended lateral and craniocaudal views

III. Young clinically sound dog (screening study) - extended and flexed lateral views and craniocaudal views

## Techniques for evaluation

In this monograph, diagnostic radiology is the recommended technique for evaluation for the presence of elbow dysplasia because it is most readily available and least expensive. Other imaging techniques have been recommended for use in the diagnosis of elbow dysplasia in certain diagnostic centers. These include: (1) xerography (Carpenter, et al 1993, (2) linear tomography (Voorhout and Hazewinkel 1987; Fox and Roberts 1987; Carpenter, et al 1993), (3) arthrography (Carpenter, et al 1993; Lowry, et al 1993), (4) computed tomography (Carpenter, et al 1993), and (5) microfocal radiography (Guthrie, et al 1991). The authors feel that with a consideration of the history of the dog, a good clinical and physical examination, and routine radiography, in most instances an accurate diagnosis, including determination of the specific form of elbow dysplasia, can be made and proper treatment instituted.

## Radiographic appearance of the normal elbow joint

The elbow or cubital joint forms from the articulation of the distal humerus, proximal radius, and proximal ulna. The articular surface of the distal humerus has two ossification centers, the laterally located capitulum and the medially located trochlea, that join to form the distal condyle. The capitulum articulates with the radial head and the trochlea articulates with the radius and ulna. The medial condyle maintains a thicker joint cartilage than the lateral condyle. A third ossification center of the distal humerus is nonarticular and forms the medial epicondyle. These centers are usually joined to the distal humerus prior to radiography for elbow dysplasia (Figure 3-15). The proximal radius has a single ossification center that often remains ununited at the time of first examination of many patients (Figures 3-9, 3-10) (Table 3-6)

The persistent appearance of a sesamoid bone craniolateral to the radius has been reported to be associated with the tendon of origin of the supinator muscle in 31% of dogs studied (Wood, et al 1985). It has been identified at about the same frequency in lame dogs as compared with those free from lameness. Consequently the presence of this bone does not seem to affect the function of the joint (Väänänen and Skutnabb 1978, Berzon and Quick 1980, Grøndalen 1982 a, b).

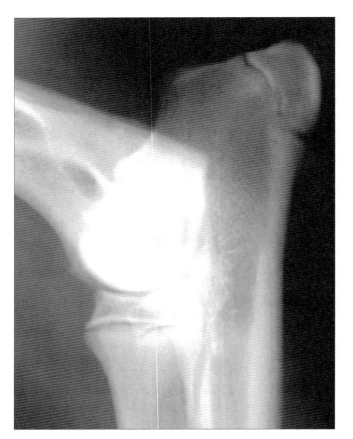 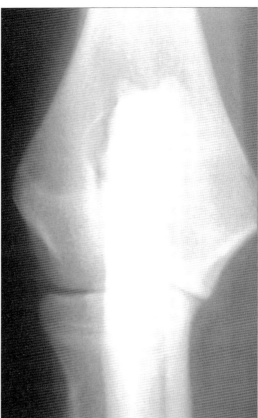

**Figure 3-15**
Lateral and craniocaudal radiographs of a normal elbow joint of a 7-month-old male Collie. The congruity of the joint is characterized by a deeply seated humeral condyle with equal width of the surrounding joint space. The shape of the trochlear notch of the ulna is full and it accepts the humeral condyle. No evidence of new bone production is noted.

The ossification center for the anconeal process of the ulna is inconstant in its appearance and develops from a separate center of ossification in some German Shepherd Dogs; it is first seen radiographically at 93.7 days (±11.25) and unites with the ulnar diaphysis at 124.5 days (±17.1) (van Sickle 1965). The age of fusion differs between breeds. The larger size of the cartilaginous anconeal process of the German Shepherd Dog may account for its slower ossification when compared to that of the Greyhound (van Sickle 1966). In the Beagle, this center of ossification is not identified radiographically (Corley and Carlson 1965). Because of the early age of ossification of the anconeal process, a separate center of ossification may not have been recognized in other breeds. If it is identified as a separate center of ossification on a radiograph of a dog greater than 4 months of age with clinical signs of lameness, this can be the source of the clinical signs.

The normal elbow joint in the dog over 6 months of age is characterized by congruity, with thin even joint spaces between the humerus, radius, and ulna (Figures 3-9, 3-15). On the lateral view, the sagittally placed ridge of the ulnar trochlear notch and the head of the radius appear to lie on a continuous arc. The ridge is an important radiographic feature and is described as the "keel" of the trochlear notch. The important medial and lateral flanges extend from the "keel" and are not identified on the lateral radiograph. The medial coronoid process is well ossified by the age of 6 months, and its radiographic outline is clearly defined (Figure 3-15).

## Radiographic appearance of the dysplastic elbow joint

The radiographic appearance of the dysplastic elbow joint is characterized by incongruity and sequential osteoarthrosis. The specific radiographic appearances of the different forms of elbow dysplasia are described later when each form is discussed in detail. Regardless of the type of dysplasia, the pattern of osteoarthrosis is similar. New bone appears in two patterns: in the periarticular region where

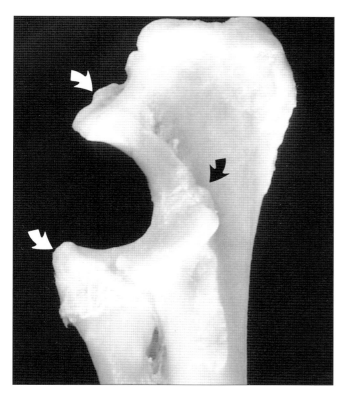

**Figure 3-16**
Photograph of the medial aspect of a specimen of the proximal radius and ulna from a dog with osteoarthrosis secondary to elbow dysplasia. Enthesophytes have formed on the dorsal surface of the anconeal process (arrow) (1), adjacent to the medial flange of the trochlear notch (arrow) (2), caudal to the medial coronoid process (3), and on the cranial aspect of the radial head (arrow) (4). Note the shape of the trochlear notch is less spherical than normal.

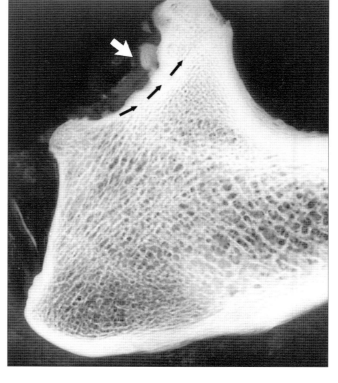

**Figure 3-17**
Radiograph of a section taken from the proximal ulna from an elbow with osteoarthrosis due to elbow dysplasia. Enthesophytes have begun to form on the proximal surface of the anconeal process (arrows). Note the line indicating the original cortex (small arrows).

it attempts to increase the size of the articular surface and as enthesophytes resulting from abnormal tension placed on the soft tissue attachments near the joint (Table 3-8).

**Table 3-8: Location of new bone production in all forms of elbow dysplasia as seen radiographically**

### Lateral view
I. Dorsal surface of the anconeal process (Figures 3-16, 3-17)
II. Ulna adjacent to the trochlear notch (Figure 3-16)
III. Caudal to the medial coronoid process (Figure 3-16)
IV. Cranial aspect of the radial head (Figure 3-16)
V. Caudal surface of the lateral condylar ridge (Figure 3-18)
VI. Cranial aspect of the distal humerus

### Craniocaudal view
I. Medial coronoid process
II. Surface of the medial epicondyle

The radiographic changes noted with osteoarthrosis in the case of elbow dysplasia are influenced by the incongruity, which leads to joint instability and secondary changes in the articular cartilage and bone. Subchondral bone becomes sclerotic and may contain small cystic lesions. The margins of the articulations may enlarge with expansion of the articular cartilage and development of underlying bone that has the appearance on the radiograph of periarticular bony spurs or lips. In addition, bony changes may occur prematurely because of unusual tension due to joint instability that is placed on the attachments of tendons, ligaments, and joint capsules to bone. These sites of attachment are referred to as entheses and the new bone that results from the "tearing" of the soft tissue attachments is referred to as an enthesophyte. While a degree of enthesophyte formation is expected with increasing age, greater than usual athletic activity, and heavy body weight, the formation of enthesophytes seen in association with elbow dysplasia is more rapidly accelerated and therefore uncharacteristic.

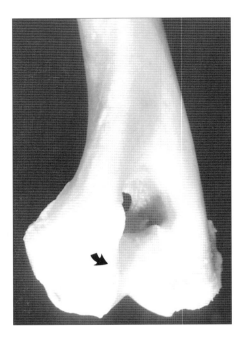 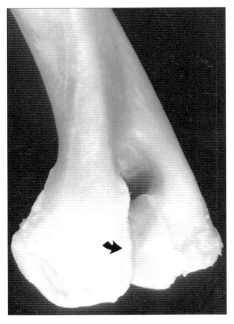

**Figure 3-18**
Photographs of the caudal aspect of the distal humerus from a dog with osteoarthrosis due to elbow dysplasia. Enthesophytes have formed on the caudal margin of the lateral condylar crest (arrows).

The appearance of the new bone is similar to that of periarticular new bone also associated with osteoarthrosis and varies only with its location. Since many of the soft tissue attachments are located at or near the articular rim, the new bone from periarticular expansion may be combined with the new bone resulting from enthesophyte formation due to tearing of the soft tissue attachments. A scoring technique for the assessment of dogs with elbow disease was undertaken using the two standard views (Guthrie 1989). It is interesting that often the score indicating the degree of osteoarthrosis was higher in the more clinically sound limb than in the more severely affected limb. Also, the severity of lameness did not always reflect the score that was assigned by evaluation of the radiograph. In this study, it was noted that the form of the dysplasia was breed dependent and influenced the pattern of osteoarthrosis that developed (Guthrie 1989 a).

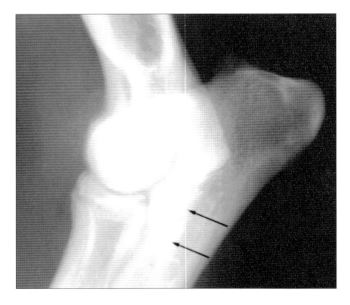 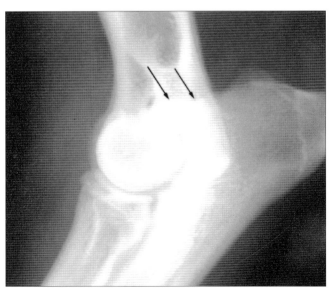

**Figure 3-19**
Lateral radiographs of both elbows of a 2-year-old male Collie-cross with minimal osteoarthrosis (grade I) as indicated by osteophyte formation on the proximal edge of the anconeal process (arrows) and sclerosis adjacent to the distal end of the ulnar trochlear notch (arrows). The humeral condyle is displaced cranially. The humeroradial joint space is narrower cranially and wider caudally. The medial coronoid processes are not identified suggesting MCPD. Note the narrow joint space between the humeral condyle and the anconeal process.

## Differential radiographic diagnosis

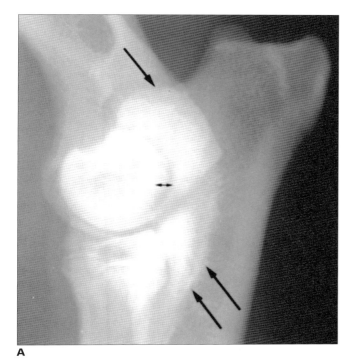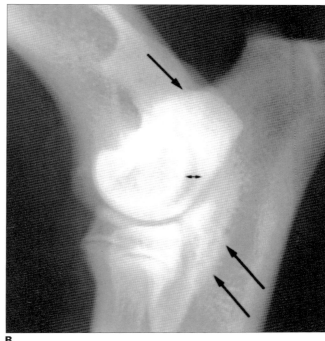

**Figure 3-20**
Lateral radiographs of both elbows of an 8-month-old male Rottweiler with moderate osteoarthrosis (grade II) on the right (A) and minimal osteoarthrosis (grade I) on the left (B). Changes are similar on both joints but more severe on the right. Osteophyte formation is seen on the proximal edge of the anconeal process (arrows) and prominent sclerosis is adjacent to the distal end of the ulnar trochlear notch (arrows). The humeral condyles are displaced cranially (double-headed arrows). Narrowing of the joint spaces is noted between the anconeal process and the humeral condyle adding to the impression of joint incongruity.

The IEWG felt that a grade of arthrosis should be determined and recorded for the use of the owner and veterinarian and that knowledge of the grade may be of future value in the determination of the heritability of the disease. This was based on the system classification used for elbow dysplasia used in Sweden (Audell 1993). Borderline arthrosis was classified as increased radiographic density in the ulna caudal to the trochlear notch and/or the presence of lipping on the head of the radius. These borderline cases should be re-examined in a minimum of 6 months to evaluate progression of the changes.

Minimal arthrosis (grade I) is diagnosed when one or more of the following is found:
- Less than 2 mm high osteophyte formation on the dorsal edge of the anconeal process;
- Minimal osteophyte formation (less than 2 mm in any direction) on the dorsal proximal edge of the radius or the lateral palmar part of the humeral trochlea; or
- Obvious sclerosis in the area caudal to the distal end of the ulnar trochlear notch and proximal portion of the radius (Figure 3-19).

Moderate arthrosis (grade II) is diagnosed when osteophytes are 2 mm to 5 mm high on the anconeal process and/or moderate osteophyte formation (2 mm to 5 mm in any direction) can be seen on the radial head, medial margin of the medial coronoid process, or lateral condylar ridge of the humerus (Figure 3-20).

Severe arthrosis (grade III) is diagnosed when the osteophyte formation on the anconeal process is more than 5 mm high and/or severe osteophyte formation (more than 5 mm in any direction) can be seen on the radial head, medial margin of the medial coronoid process, or lateral condylar ridge of the humerus (Figure 3-21).

## Differential radiographic diagnosis

Many additional conditions within the developing elbow joint have been identified and may be confused as elbow dysplasia as defined in this chapter. Generally, these can be separated from elbow dysplasia by consideration of the clinical signs, physical examination, and radiographic examination. Some of these cause clinical signs early and include congenital elbow luxation with lateral displacement of the radial head (Campbell 1969; Pass and Ferguson 1971; Grøndalen 1973; Stevens and Sande 1974; Bingel and Riser 1977; Carrig, et al 1977) (Figure

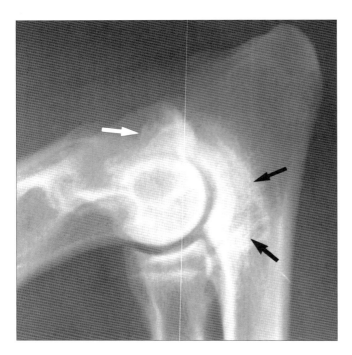 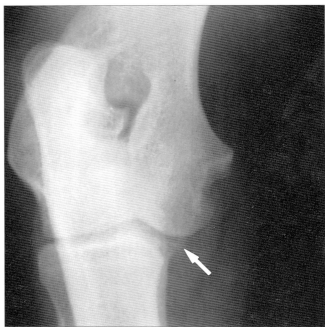

**Figure 3-21**
Lateral and craniocaudal radiographs of one elbow of a mature Shar Pei with severe osteoarthrosis (grade III) as indicated by prominent osteophyte formation on the proximal edge of the anconeal process (white arrow) and the tip of the medial coronoid process (white arrow) and by extensive sclerosis adjacent to the distal end of the ulnar trochlear notch (black arrows). The MCP is not outlined. Joint incongruity remains evident as indicated by the narrowing of the joint space between the anconeal process and the humeral condyle, the wider joint space between the ulnar trochlear notch and the humeral condyle, the "step" between the distal edge of the ulnar trochlear notch and the radial head, and by the cranial displacement of the humeral condyle.

3-3). A more difficult diagnostic problem is found in a young dog during skeletal maturation as a result of premature closure or delayed growth in the distal radial physis. This causes a shortened radius, a high-lying coronoid process, and a badly deformed elbow joint. However, a major difference exists as the shortened radius displaces the humeral condyle distally causing a marked increase in the width of the joint space between the condyle and the anconeal process. Examination of the distal antebrachium along with comparison studies of the opposite forelimb confirms the etiology of the elbow disease (Figure 3-22).

Joint morphology in members of chondrodystrophic breeds varies markedly from that seen in the more normal appearing long-limbed dogs. Radiographs of the elbow joint often have features similar to those used in diagnosis of elbow dysplasia. This included the malformation of the medial coronoid process and a poorly fitting humeral condyle within the trochlear notch. Usually the elbows in these breeds are characterized by shortening of the ulna with overgrowth of the radial head being the cause of the malformed elbow joint (Figure 3-2).

In a middle or larger breed dog with bilateral arthrosis in both elbows, elbow dysplasia is the first etiology to be considered. However, the arthrosis noted following the developmental disease of elbow dysplasia is similar to that caused by a traumatic or chronic inflammatory event or senile joint disease. Thus, it may be difficult in the older dog to determine the specific cause of the joint disease radiographically. Thus, the clinician and owner need to understand that there are limitations in the accuracy of evaluation of the older patient (Figure 3-23).

However, in the event of a healed articular fracture, the old fracture line and resulting fragment malunion are often identified making it possible to determine the exact etiology of the secondary osteoarthrosis. Also, destructive changes within the subchondral bone commonly associated with an infectious arthritis are not present in osteoarthrosis secondary to elbow dysplasia and they serve as a method of differentiation of this uncommon cause of elbow arthrosis. The bone destruction associated with tumors can be of value in making their diagnosis; however, it is possible for any of these lesions to be superimposed over the changes previously related to dysplasia (Figure 3-24).

While rather easy to differentiate radiographically, panosteitis needs to be considered in the differential diagnosis of forelimb lameness in the young dog because of the

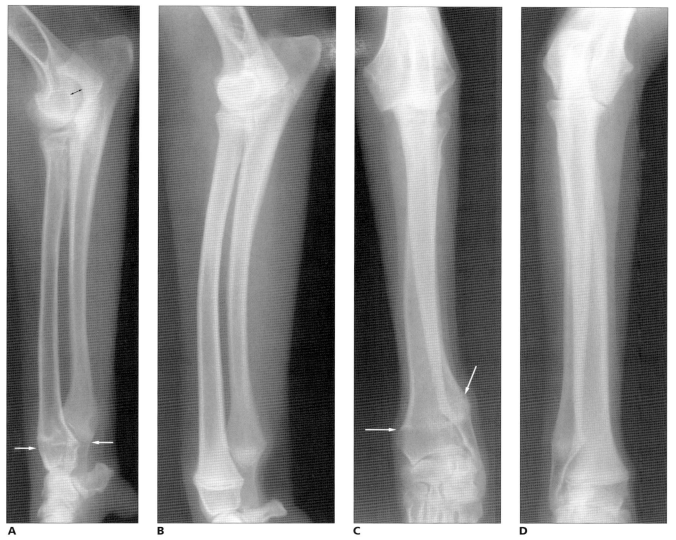

**Figure 3-22**
Craniocaudal and lateral radiographs of both forelimbs of a 9-month-old male German Shorthair Pointer made after 3 months' lameness on the left. On the affected limb, the high-lying distal edge of the trochlear notch, subluxation, and the failure of formation of the medial coronoid process suggest the possibility of elbow dysplasia (A, C). However, the distal displacement of the humeral condyle suggested by the increased width of the joint space between the condyle and the anconeal process (double-headed arrow) indicates instead a delay in bone growth resulting in a shortened radius. Examination of the distal antebrachii shows the premature closure of the growth plates of both bones (arrows). The owner had not noticed the injury that caused the premature closure. The right limb is normal by comparison (B, D).

similar ages and breeds affected and the similarity in clinical signs (Figure 3-25).

## Treatment

Therapy is dependent on the character of the original lesion, the severity and rate of progression of the secondary osteoarthrosis, and the degree of pain (Houlton 1984). Joint incongruity of itself leads to cartilage damage and osteoarthrosis with the level of joint disease dependent on the degree of incongruity. In general, when the incongruity is minor, secondary lesions (OCD, FCP, and UAP) are not present and the osteoarthrosis is often of no clinical significance. With greater incongruity, the secondary forms of the dysplasia are commonly seen and both the incongruity and the secondary lesion contribute to the severity of the osteoarthrosis and possibly the clinical signs.

Regardless of the age at which the dog is presented for treatment, common therapy for any orthopedic disease includes weight control, intelligent nutrition, and a wise

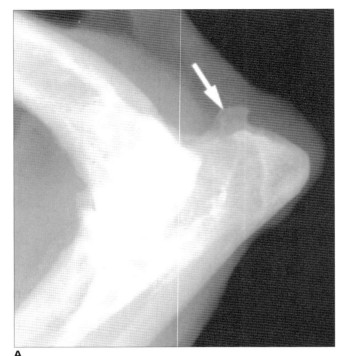

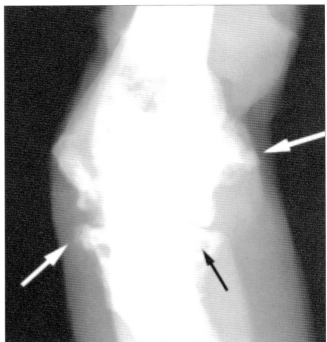

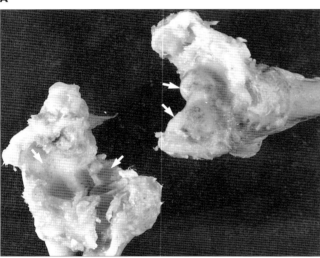

**Figure 3-23**
Radiographs of the elbow joint (A) and photograph of the gross specimen of this elbow joint (B) from an aged Beagle dog with severe osteoarthrosis. The cause of the joint disease cannot be determined after secondary changes have become so extensive. In addition to the extensive enthesophyte formation (white arrows), note the subchondral cyst formation (black arrow). The osteoarthrosis was not evident on radiographs made earlier in the life of the dog and did not begin until later in life. Because of this and because elbow dysplasia is not seen frequently in this breed, it is rather certain that the cause of the osteoarthrosis is not elbow dysplasia. Both joints were similarly affected.

selection of the exercise program. All of these diminish or at least control progression of the secondary arthrosis that might otherwise be seen in a dysplastic elbow.

Standards (FCI) applied to exterior conformation in the most affected breeds, ie, Rottweiler and the retrievers, encourage heavy, massive dogs, which may easily lead to obesity (Sundgren 1980). This rapidly growing heavy dog tends to potentiate the lesions and cause more rapid development of the osteoarthrosis. By decreasing the standard measurements of dogs presented at shows, a less heavy and more functional dog may be bred. While owners should not be misled into feeding puppies excessively to attain standards of adult dogs, they should also not be misled into believing that by limiting the feeding of puppies they can control or eliminate dysplasia. They can only influence the severity of the disease in that dog. In addition to conservative treatment, therapy of the affected dog may be medical or surgical. The selection is influenced by the age and the desired use of the dog. Understandably, the cost of the treatment, the nursing care required, plus the pain to the dog during surgical treatment that is perceived by the owner often influence treatment decisions. Intermittent use of analgesics may be required, depending on the severity of the condition. Long-term medical treatment is useful if the osteoarthrosis is the main cause of the discomfort as would be in a case characterized by minimal joint instability. In younger dogs with a sudden onset of lameness, intermittent use of analgesics may be indicated with an observation of the effects, while waiting to make a more definitive decision of whether to perform surgery on the elbow. If surgery is considered and advisable, medical management of the lesions should not be prolonged unduly because the "window" of opportunity during which best results from surgery can be expected is relatively short and is measured in weeks not months or years. The types of analgesics recommended are discussed thoroughly in the chapter on hip dysplasia (see Chapter 5).

## Conservative treatment

Mildly affected dogs that are treated conservatively using weight control and limited exercise along with analgesics when the dog is obviously in pain manage to cope with the problem quite adequately. However, the osteoarthrosis is most likely progressive because of the combined effect of the joint incongruity and the presence of a UCP, an MCPD, or an OCD and the need for analgesics can increase. Working dogs frequently show increased limitation in their athletic performance. Dogs with severe degrees of any form of elbow dysplasia show a rapid progression of osteoarthrosis, which leads to a crippling disease often by an age of 3 years (Figure 3-26).

## Surgical treatment

Justification for surgical treatment requires further understanding of the pathological changes that can occur with elbow dysplasia. The early onset of acute pain between the ages of 4 and 6 months is associated with joint fluid entering exposed subchondral bone. The joint fluid may gain access to the subchondral bone via chondral fissures, due to fragmentation of the medial coronoid process, or in association with an OCD lesion. A persistent separate center of ossification of the anconeal process (UAP) can also expose subchondral bone to synovial fluid via chondral fissures within the cartilaginous bridge. Degenerative cartilage products are a constant irritant causing a chronic synovitis. Bone or cartilage fragments are a constant irritant perpetuating the chronic synovitis that adds to the discomfort. The in-situ movement of the bony or cartilaginous fragments prevents union of the anconeal process, filling in of the OCD lesion, or union of the coronoid fragment. In cases of the fragmented coronoid process, the fragment itself can do active damage to the opposing articular surface of the humeral condyle causing a "kissing" lesion. This contributes to the overall damage to the joint. Surgical removal of the gross cartilaginous fragment limits the damage caused but surgery does not correct the joint incongruity. It is interesting to

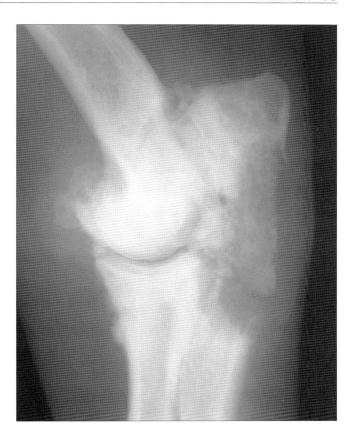

**Figure 3-24**
A lateral radiograph of an elbow of a 3-year-old male Labrador Retriever that was correctly diagnosed with elbow dysplasia 1 year earlier. Continued progression of clinical signs occurred despite conservative treatment. The repeat radiographs clearly show a pathologic fracture through a large destructive lesion within the proximal ulna that was later proven to be an undifferentiated sarcoma. The malformed anconeal process and the reactive new bone cranially on the humeral condyle and radial head are associated with the osteoarthrosis secondary to elbow dysplasia.

note that as the osteoarthrosis in the joint becomes more severe the pain is less acute, probably because of stabilization of the joint due to thickening of the joint capsule.

Thus, because of the poorly formed trochlear notch, elbow dysplasia is like the foot with a shoe that fits poorly and is painful. However, the elbow joint may be additionally affected by a separated fragment of cartilage or bone and now resembles a situation in which there is a pebble in the poorly fitting shoe. Surgical removal of the fragment(s) is therefore recommended as a way of diminishing the pain due to the ingress of the synovial fluid or the in-situ movement of the fragments, by encouraging the sealing off of the lesion through creation of a fibrocartilage covering. However, the underlying incongruity remains unaltered and the client should be made aware of the expected progressive nature of the osteoarthrosis.

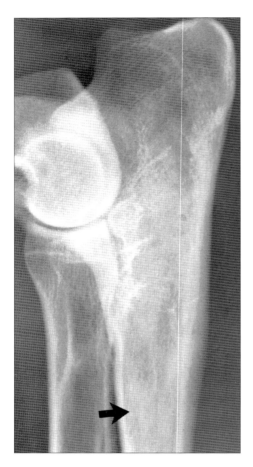 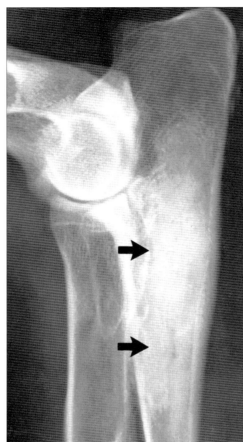

**Figure 3-25**
Lateral views of both elbow joints of a mature male German Shepherd Dog with normally formed elbow joints. The clinical signs in this dog were due to panosteitis characterized by medullary new bone (arrows) more prominent in one ulna than in the other.

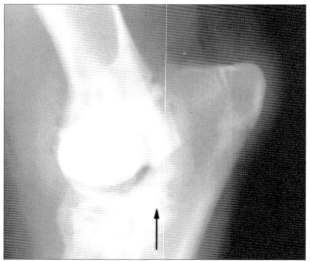 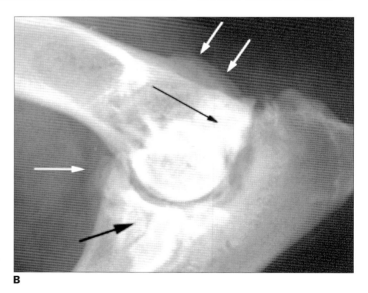

A  B

**Figure 3-26**
Lateral radiographs of the left elbow joint of a male Saint Bernard with MCPD made at 6 months of age show joint subluxation and marked joint incongruity (A). Note the increased subtrochlear sclerosis (arrow). The MCP is poorly defined. At 2 years of age, the subluxation is still evident but complicated by the severe osteoarthrosis that includes a deformed anconeal process (small black arrow), traction osteophytes on the lateral epicondylar ridge (white arrows), and radial lipping (white arrow) (B). The MCP is now ossified with apparent fragmentation of the cranial portion (large black arrow). Note in the early study that the growth plate of the apophyseal center of the medial epicondyle is partially superimposed over the anconeal process causing a radiolucent line that can be confused with an UAP (A). In the later study, the radiolucent line through the intact anconeal process is caused by different tissue densities (B).

Because of the incongruity, a decrease in discomfort, not normalcy, is the goal of the surgery.

It is advisable prior to the time surgical treatment is instituted to carefully examine the dog for the presence of other developmental bone disease, such as hip dysplasia, in order to more accurately counsel the owner relative to treatment. This examination will prevent disagreeable surprises at a later time. If, following a satisfactory recovery from a specific surgery, a new lameness is noted, it is readily apparent that an additional cause of pain is present in the same or other limb not previously expected. Owners of sporting dogs need to be advised that following surgery, their dog can be expected to be less lame, but it can not become a top performer as a result of the surgery. Also, the future of a working dog, such as a police dog, is highly dependent on the degree of severity of the lesion prior to surgery and the level of work expected.

The results of treatment of elbow disease were noted in a group of over 100 affected dogs, one half of whom were treated medically and one half of who were treated surgically. No positive correlation was noted between the two groups relative to: (1) the severity of the lameness prior to and after treatment, (2) severity of radiographic changes, and (3) the type of lesion detected at surgery. While the surgical treatment did not remove the post treatment lameness, the surgically treated dogs were more active and less severely lame after treatment. Recommendations offered in the report were that mild lameness did not appear to benefit from surgery while dogs with chronic, moderate to severe lameness had a better prognosis if surgically treated (Read, et al 1990).

## Prognosis

The prognosis of elbow dysplasia, in general, is dependent on the following:

- Degree of incongruity and the type of ensuing lesion.
- Nature of the predisposing cause for elbow disease,
- Severity of the clinical signs at first examination,
- Treatment used,
- Age at beginning of treatment,
- Form of physical therapy used by the owner, and
- Weight of the dog.

### Non-operated dogs

Dogs with severe degrees of all forms of elbow dysplasia that are not operated show rapid progression of the osteoarthrosis which leads to a crippling disease often by an age of 3 years. Dogs with minimal to moderate degree of osteoarthrosis, regardless of the type of lesion, may lead a happy, active life being managed only by selection of a good exercise regime, a wise diet, and thoughtful owners. However, it is possible that surgery might have improved the prognosis in some of these cases.

### Operated dogs

Reports of the results of surgical treatment of elbow dysplasia are confusing because of the grouping together of patients that are both immature and mature, patients with differing types of elbow dysplasia, patients with varying degrees of secondary osteoarthrosis, and patients with variation in the intended use following treatment. In addition, many follow-up evaluations are conducted through telephone calls and lack physical examination or stress-plate evaluation, both of which would be a more accurate form of evaluation. The following discussion attempts to separate the patients into groupings that allow for more accurate prediction of the treatment to be recommended and the expected prognosis.

### Immature dogs

Immature dogs with slight to moderate incongruity and minimal osteoarthrosis due to MCPD are the best surgical candidates. Similarly affected dogs, with an MCPD in association with an OCD lesion have a somewhat less optimal prognosis, probably because the OCD lesion contributes to the incongruity and causes additional damage to the articular surface of the medial coronoid process. Both groups, however, benefit from the surgical removal of the OCD flap and/or removal of the coronoid fragment with curettage of the lesion bed. An in situ fragmented coronoid process may cause mild clinical signs. However, if a similarly sized fragment is dislodged, the clinical pain may be more severe and the surgical indications become more obvious. Thus, the nature of the lesion, the size of the lesion, and range of movement of a fragment all influence the clinical signs and the decision to operate (Table 3-9).

#### Table 3-9: Prognosis following surgical treatment of immature dogs

**I.** With minimal to moderate incongruity and
1. FCP - good prognosis
2. FCP plus OCD - good to guarded prognosis
3. OCD (small lesion) - good prognosis
4. UAP - poor prognosis

**II.** With severe incongruity and
1. FCP - poor prognosis
2. OCD (large lesion) - poor prognosis
3. UAP - poor prognosis
4. UAP plus FCP - worst prognosis

Immature dogs with marked incongruity and a large displaced coronoid fragment may benefit from surgery because of the immediate decrease in pain. However, the development of the arthrosis may be severe enough by the age of 2 years to considerably decrease their exercise tolerance and to warrant the use of analgesics intermittently. Nevertheless, many of these dogs manage to cope with the problem through use of limited exercise and weight control. Surgery in these cases is still considered beneficial.

In the immature dog affected only by an OCD lesion, surgery is recommended. The prognosis is slightly less favorable than the dog with an FCP, with recovery highly dependent on the size of the lesion and the degree of incongruity.

The immature dog with severe incongruity and FCP and/or OCD has a very poor prognosis in spite of surgical intervention. However, removal of joint fragments or the OCD flap provides an increase in comfort for the dog. The untreated joint incongruity causes a rapid progression of the osteoarthrosis leading to a crippled patient at an early age (3 to 4 years).

Immature dogs with a UAP have a very guarded prognosis. Although removal of the ununited process may temporarily decrease the discomfort, the persistent instability adds to the progression of the osteoarthrosis. One technique of controlling pain is through stabilization of the free fragment to the olecranon using a lag screw fixation (Herron 1970, Sinibaldi 1975). This, however, does not result in correcting the underlying incongruity in the articular surface. Lag screw fixation performed in a manner that results in an increase in the circumference of the ulnar trochlear notch may be accomplished by providing a space between the UAP and the ulna. Use of a spacer such as cancellous bone graft may be helpful.

Most dogs with a UAP result in a slight distal movement of the proximal ulna that prevents healing. Therefore, another recommended treatment is an osteotomy through the proximal ulna into the trochlear notch that allows for proximal movement of this fragment. The osteotomy results in a decrease of space between the UAP and the proximal ulna and decreased fragment movement that allows for a healing of the UAP. The osteotomy site heals following bridging of the persistent gap. The osteotomy not only reduces motion at the site of the nonunion and permits a bony union of the free fragment but it permits restoration of joint stability as a result of a most important increase in the diameter of the trochlear notch.

Dogs with a combined UAP and FCP have the worst prognosis. Following any form of surgery, a crippling lameness is usually present by the age of 4 to 5 years that may be unresponsive to exercise limitation, weight control, or drug therapy.

## Mature dogs

Mature dogs with minimal to moderate incongruity and osteoarthrosis associated with an MCPD and/or OCD lesion may be considered for surgery, however, with only a guarded prognosis. A portion of the pain in the older dog is due to a persistent sterile synovitis caused by degenerating articular cartilage. Although all surgical invasions into the elbow joint should be accompanied by joint lavage, this procedure is especially of value in the older dog.

In rare instances, an older dog with a chronic FCP may become acutely lame due to dislodgment of the fragment. In this dog, the osteoarthrosis is usually mild and the prognosis for improvement following surgery is quite good.

In dogs with severe osteoarthrosis regardless of the type of dysplasia, the elbow joints are stable, but painful, and should not be operated because of potential interference with this stability. Analgesic medication, arthrodesis, or prosthetic joint replacement should be considered for these patients.

## Heritabilitiy

The incidence of elbow dysplasia has consistently been noted to be higher in certain breeds. In a radiographic study of elbows of 825 middle-sized and large dogs, the incidence of elbow dysplasia was found to be strongly breed specific and was higher in intermediate and heavy-set breeds when compared with sight hounds and setter breeds (Wind 1986, Wind and Packard 1986). In a study comparing the occurrence of elbow dysplasia in 77 Bernese Mountain Dogs and in 30 dogs of other Swiss mountain breeds (Entlebucher, Appenzeller, and Grossen Schweizer), 27.9% of the Bernese Mountain Dogs were affected with elbow dysplasia, compared with only 10% of the other breeds (Bienz 1985).

Other studies have proven an inherited disposition for elbow dysplasia. In Rottweilers, grouped according to the status of the elbows of their parents, an inherited disposition for lesions of the coronoid process was suggested (Grøndalen 1982b). This study of 207 Rottweilers showed that about 40% of the offspring were affected when two affected dogs were mated, whereas 12.5% of the offspring were affected when one of the parents was affected. Another study of 616 Rottweilers confirmed that the Rottweiler as a breed had a genetic predisposition for elbow dysplasia and that certain stud dogs had a higher percentage of affected offspring. The likelihood of elbow dysplasia in the offspring of matings in which one or both parents were affected was 1.8 times higher than in the offspring of matings of non-affected parents. This study also showed that males in this breed were 1.5 times more likely to be affected than females (Grøndalen and Lingaas 1988). Recent reviews left little doubt relative to elbow dysplasia being an inherited disease in pedigree dogs (Wind 1993, Bedford 1994).

The largest study that evaluated heritability of arthrosis of the elbow joint in the Bernese Mountain Dog and Rottweiler breeds clearly showed significant sex effects in both breeds. In Bernese Mountain Dogs, the estimated heritability based on regression of sons on sires was 0.34 and the estimated heritability based on regression of daughters on dams was 0.28. Heritability in Rottweilers based on regression of sons on sires was 0.34 and heritability based on regression of daughters on dams was 0.40 (Swenson, et al 1997; Audell 1990). An inherited basis for elbow disease in general has also been reported in the Labrador Retriever with the dam contributing significantly more variation than the sire (Lavelle and Studdert 1990; Studdert, et al 1991). The differences in the prevalence can be explained by a direct effect of genes on the sex chromosomes or by an effect of secondary sex characteristics such as differences in growth rate, sex hormones, or behavioral patterns. For a polygenic trait, such as osteoarthrosis in the elbow joint, the effect of secondary sex characteristics is a more plausible explanation (Swenson, et al 1997).

A recent study evaluated the results of mating bilaterally affected Labrador Retrievers with both OCD and FCP. The elbows of the offspring were examined at arthrotomy or necropsy for presence or absence of disease and the results strongly support earlier findings that both are multifactorial or polygenic traits (Padgett, et al 1995). This study also showed that OCD and FCP appear to be inherited independently.

The Swedish program for the control of Elbow Dysplasia utilizes a radiographic examination of the elbow joints and has accumulated the largest material available for study of this disease. The program has recorded the frequency of osteoarthrosis in susceptible breeds instead of attempting to record the specific type of dysplasia. The heritability estimates for osteoarthrosis in the elbow joint are between 0.24 and 0.43 for the Bernese Mountain Dog and 0.44 and 0.55 for the Rottweiler if sex, age at diagnosis, and sire or dam are included in the statistical analysis. In addition, the results of different mating combinations further support elbow dysplasia as an inherited disease. In Bernese Mountain Dogs, normal to normal matings resulted in 34% of the progeny having osteoarthrosis while affected to affected matings resulted in 58% of the progeny being affected. In Rottweilers, normal to normal matings resulted in 28% of the progeny having osteoarthrosis while affected to affected matings resulted in 50% of the progeny being affected (Swenson 1972). These figures were changed slightly in a subsequent report (Swenson, et al 1997). These studies show a large percentage of affected offspring from normal to normal breeding, indicating that the disease is present genetically while the phenotype is normal radiographically.

In the German Shepherd Dog, which is a highly predisposed breed for elbow dysplasia, ununited anconeal process was reported early to be an inherited disease (Carlson and Severin 1961; Wamberg 1966; Corley, et al 1968; Hayes, et al 1979).

In summary, breed predisposition to the development of elbow dysplasia indicates that these conditions are genetically influenced (Corley, et al 1968; Hayes, et al 1979; Grøndalen 1979 b; Hazewinkel, et al 1988; Wind and Packard 1986; Guthrie and Pidduck 1990; Grøndalen and Lingaas 1991; Studdert, et al 1991; Swenson, et al 1997). Having established that osteoarthrosis indicative of elbow dysplasia is a multifactorial polygenic threshold trait, then a lowering in prevalence can be expected through selection of breeding stock (Swenson, et al 1972). In addition, knowledge of the status of full- and half-siblings and parents further improves a breeding program along with progeny testing of sires. Progeny testing of dams is of little value because they have already made their contribution to the breed prior to being evaluated (Swenson, et al 1997). A recent study of 41 Rottweilers followed the dogs from 3 months until 12 months of age and determined the relationship between physical signs and radiographic signs of dysplasia. Because a high percentage of dogs were affected (57%), it was suggested that a justification might be made in using dogs classified as having grade I dysplasia to avoid depletion of the breeding pool (Read, et al 1996).

# Ununited Anconeal Process (UAP)

## Introduction

In German Shepherd Dogs and greyhounds, a separate center of ossification within the anconeal process of the

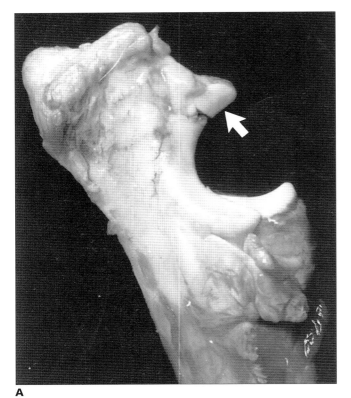 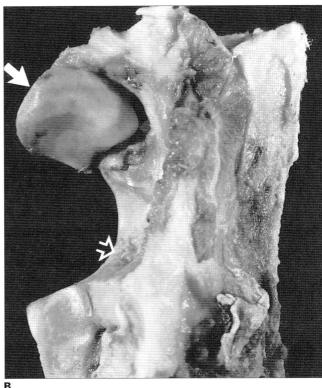

**Figure 3-27**
Photographs of specimens taken from the proximal ulna of two German Shepherd Dogs with failure of union of the anconeal processes. On a medial view of one dog, the ununited anconeal fragment (arrow) has an almost normal position with a remnant of the cartilaginous bridge (A). The articular surface of the medial flange of the trochlear notch appears normal. On a lateral view in the other dog, the large, malformed, ununited fragment (solid arrow) is displaced with loss of the fibrocartilaginous bridge resulting in an empty space (B). The injury to the articular surface of the lateral flange of the ulnar trochlear notch (hollow arrow) indicates loss of normal contact between the humeral trochlea.

ulna may be present at an age that is later than in other breeds. Closure of this center of ossification should occur at 124.5 days (± 17.1 days) in the GSD and approximately 3 weeks earlier in the greyhound (van Sickle 1965). In the GSD, with a relatively high incidence of elbow dysplasia, the combination of a separate center of ossification of the anconeal process and the too small circumference of the trochlear notch creates micro-movement at the cartilaginous bridge between the center of ossification and the ulna. This causes a failure of endochondral ossification of this bridge and results in this particular form of elbow dysplasia (UAP). Chronic movement of the fragment results in modeling of the fragment while incongruity causes injury to the articular surface of the trochlear notch (Bradney 1967) (Figures 3-27, 3-28, 3-29).

The histopathology of bony specimens taken from elbows with UAP shows the cartilaginous bridge or physis between the separate center of ossification of the ulna. The zones within this unusual physis are irregular in width due to the presence of numerous unsuccessful attempts at physeal closure resulting in only a few sites of bony union between the anconeal process and the metaphyseal spongiosa of the proximal ulna. Usually there is evidence of hemorrhage, necrosis, and fibroplasia, which often coalesce to form a "fracture line" through the remnant of the physis.

In other members of the German Shepherd Dog breed, the union of the anconeal process with the ulna occurs prior to the development of the joint incongruity. In these dogs without the micro-movement that causes the nonunion of the anconeal process, an MCPD can develop. In dogs from breeds other than German Shepherd Dog, UAP may also occur probably due to a similar pattern of events as described above.

If the cartilage bridge remains stable, the clinical signs may only be minimal, if present at all. However, if the bridge fractures later in life, pain, instability, and osteoarthrosis result quickly. This fracture may occur early in an active dog, or may remain stable for some time and fracture later in life (3 to 4 years).

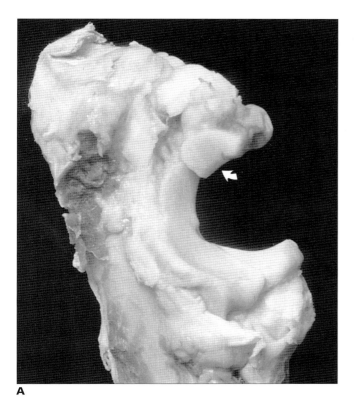 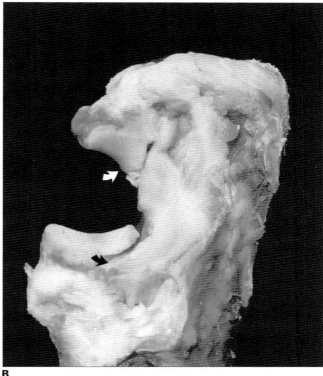

**Figure 3-28**
Photographs of the medial aspect of the elbows of a 6-month-old male German Shepherd Dog. The specimen of the left elbow shows the UAP (arrow) without distal displacement of the ulnar trochlear notch (A). The MCP lies slightly above the level of the radius. Loss of articular cartilage along the central portion of the ulnar trochlear notch is just visible with the major destruction being lateral and not seen on this view. The specimen of the right elbow shows the UAP (arrow) with distal displacement of the ulnar trochlear notch and medial coronoid process (B). The MCP lies below the level of the radius (arrow). Loss of articular cartilage along the central aspect of the ulnar trochlear notch is visible.

In the greyhound, UAP is unknown. This is assumed to be because fusion of the anconeal process occurs earlier and/or because the trochlear notch has a normal circumference and nothing interferes with the normal ossification of the physeal center.

## History

Ununited anconeal process of the proximal ulna is a disease primarily of German Shepherd Dogs that was first described by Cawley and Archibald (1959), Carlson and Severin (1961), and Loeffler (1963, 1964). Cawley and Archibald (1959) "embarked upon a discussion of the elbow lameness of German Shepherd Dogs, which had been earlier described (Stiern 1956) as due to ectopic sesamoid bones". They mentioned that Hare, in 1958 through personal communication, had reported "lines of cleavage" through the anconeal process in dogs that were bred from stock of a kennel in which affected dogs had been noted and that Rhodes (1959) through personal communication, had known of a dog affected bilaterally in the same manner. On lateral radiographs of the elbow joint, triangularly shaped fragments were present adjacent to the ulna with the "lines of cleavage" of varying width. The possibility of a traumatic fracture was discounted and it was thought instead that this represented a failure of fusion of a normally occurring ossification center. It is interesting in this early report that the authors correctly recognized: (1) a frequent bilateral involvement of the disease, (2) a possibility that the process could unite in a normal manner at a later age, and (3) a familial aspect to the disease. They suggested the term "ununited anconeal process of hereditary origin."

Vaughan (1962) later reported the condition as a congenital detachment from the anconeal process in the German Shepherd Dog while Loeffler (1963) additionally reported the condition in 12 members of that breed, 11 of which were males. At an annual meeting of the AAHA, Singleton (1971) reported on the UAP: the nonunion of the anconeus beyond the age of 5 months in German Shepherd Dogs was abnormal and responsible for most obscure and protracted forelimb lameness in

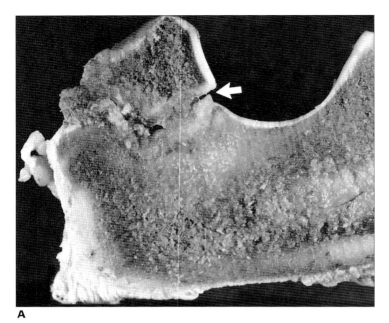 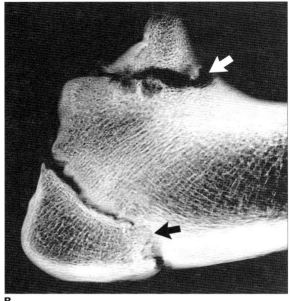

**Figure 3-29**
Photograph (A) and radiograph (B) of a section taken from the proximal ulna from elbows with a UAP (white arrows). The failure of union across the cartilage bridge is more clearly seen on the radiograph because the persistent cartilage bridge is radiolucent. Note the process of closure of the normal apophyseal center of the olecranon (black arrow).

those dogs between the ages of 4 and 12 months. The detachment was also reported in a Basset-Saluki-cross but was incorrectly thought to be congenital (Hare 1962). The condition was reported in another Basset hound as a fracture secondary to a premature closure of the distal metaphyseal plate of the ulna (Herron 1971, Grüll and Henschel 1973, von Hitz 1976). Kasström, et al (1973) thought that the condition when found in chondrodystrophoid breeds was a result of an abnormal pressure on the anconeal process that was directed towards the distal part of the olecranon fossa of the humerus by the shortened ulna. The authors agree with the last assessment and consider this type of UAP to be different from that associated with joint incongruity associated with elbow dysplasia.

Van Sickle (1965) studied the postnatal development of the elbow in the German Shepherd Dogs and in the greyhound and found that both breeds have a distinct center of ossification for the anconeal process. The anconeal process begins to ossify at 12 to 14 weeks and appears to be formed of a number of small discrete ossification centers, which eventually merge into one center. The center has its own blood supply that enters the process on the dorsal aspect. However, in the affected German Shepherd Dog, the process of ossification is slow and a cartilage plate remains separating the process from the body of the ulna.

In the normal German Shepherd Dog, after 6 to 8 weeks from first appearance, the cartilage plate disappears, the two blood supplies unit, and a single bony model is the result. Thus, fusion of this ossification center occurs by 4 1/2 months of age. In the Greyhound, the ossification occurs much faster and bony union is seen regularly within 2 to 3 weeks following appearance of the separate ossification center. It was speculated that the much larger size of the cartilaginous anconeal process of the German Shepherd Dog could account for the slower endochondral ossification as compared with a smaller process in the greyhound.

In another study using controlled matings, the time of first appearance of the anconeal process in the German Shepherd Dog ranged from 81 to 105 days and fusion occurred in the normal dog from 101 to 130 days of age (Hanlon and Spurrell 1967, Hanlon 1969). These ages of closure are somewhat younger than reported before. It is important to understand that in most breeds of dogs, the anconeal process is thought to develop in the proximal ulna without a separate ossification center.

A modern concept of the disease faults the underdevelopment of the ulnar trochlear notch in conjunction with the separate center of ossification within the anconeal process as the cause of UAP (Figure 3-30). This nonunion is most likely due to micro-movement of the

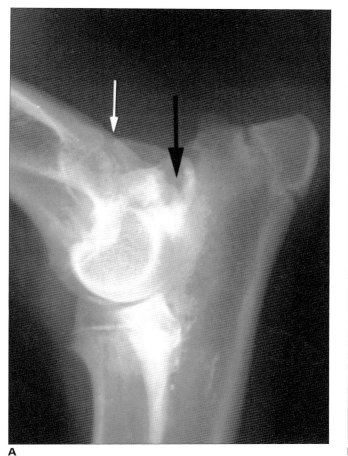 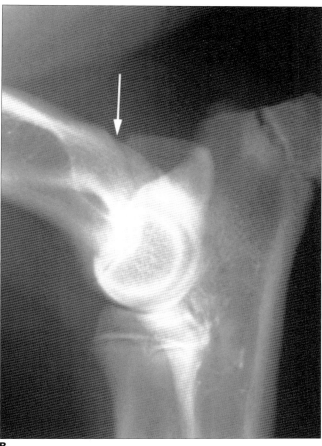

**Figure 3-30**
Lateral radiographs of both elbows of a 6-month-old male German Shepherd Dog. (A) Elbow dysplasia is characterized by an ununited anconeal process. Note the wide fibrocartilaginous band separating the UAP (black arrow) and the marked opening of the trochlear notch. Elbow dysplasia is often characterized by a high-lying coronoid process. (B) The opposite elbow is radiographically normal. The normal growth plate of the medial epicondyle is seen bilaterally (white arrows).

cartilage bridge between the separate center of ossification and the olecranon caused by too tight a fit between the anconeal process and the humerus, the result of the too small curvature of the trochlear notch (Weis 1983, Wind 1986, 1990).

## Clinical signs

Clinical signs are dependent on the stability of the anconeal process (Figure 3-27) and the usual age of referral has been reported to be as early as 5 to 6 months (Hazewinkel, et al 1988; Guthrie 1989b). If the cartilage bridge is stable and non-fissured, clinical signs may be absent or only minimal. When the cartilage union begins to fissure and the joint becomes unstable, clinical signs develop. In the active dog the cartilage bridge fractures rather early (6 to 8 months), but in the less active dog, this fracture may not occur until a much later date (2 to 3 years). This difference in age of onset of pain has been observed earlier and it has been noted that in most patients, the onset of lameness is around 1 year of age, however, in certain dogs, the onset of signs seems to be much later (Loeffler 1963, Mitten and Hoefle 1978).

Lameness resulting from UAP is more distinctive than lameness noted in other forms of elbow dysplasia, however, it is certainly not pathognomonic. In the gait, the limbs are abducted with the feet turned outwardly, resembling that seen in a "tall basset hound". The pain from UAP often causes the dog to incompletely extend the forelimbs. Since this lack of drive is also a symptom associated with hip dysplasia, it is possible for the gait abnormality secondary to UAP to be confused with that seen with a hip dysplasia. If only one elbow is affected, the lameness may be obvious. If both elbows are

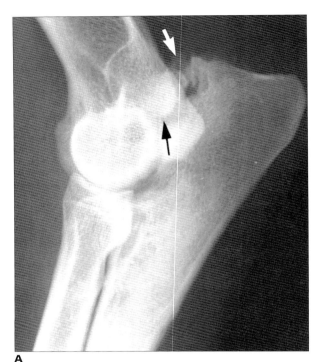 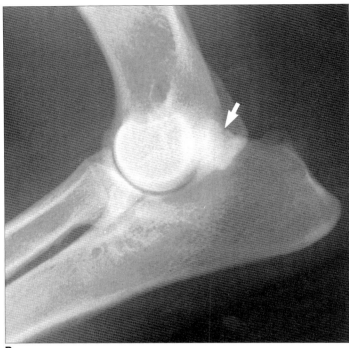

**Figure 3-31**
Lateral radiographs of the elbows from a 10-month-old male German Shepherd Dog in which one elbow shows a radiolucent line that indicates a minimally displaced UAP (arrow) with sclerosis around the cartilaginous bridge (A). Panosteitis in the proximal ulna complicates the clinical signs. The other elbow is normal with an intact anconeal process (arrow) (B).

involved, the resulting altered gait may not be obvious to the casual observer.

## Physical examination

On palpation of the elbow joints, flexion and extension may be limited and crepitus may be noted especially when palpating beneath the triceps tendon. The amount of pain noted on palpation might be difficult to ascertain because of the great variety in the personality of the dogs examined. Joint effusion may be present beneath the anconeus muscle. The detection of joint capsule thickening, increased prominence of the medial epicondyle, and muscle atrophy is dependent on the length of time the lameness has been present.

## Radiographic diagnosis

Ununited anconeal process is the most easily recognized form of elbow dysplasia with the nonunion of the anconeal process readily diagnosed in affected elbow joints on the lateral view. Diagnosis is more difficult if the fragment remains in position (Figure 3-31) and is easier if the fragment is displaced (Figure 3-32). The detached fragment can be identified on either a flexed or extended lateral view. Comparison of these views often shows a range of movement if the fragment is free. Usually the fragment remains with the ulna; however, it has been reported to move with the humerus (Sikkema and Roush 1994).

In the majority of younger patients, the degree of osteoarthrosis is slight and, when present, is characterized by sclerosis and new bone formation surrounding the "fracture site" within the anconeal process. Osteophyte formation may also be present at areas of synovial membrane attachment and is more pronounced medially. The extended lateral view of the elbow positions the anconeal process over the distal humerus in a manner that the open apophyseal growth plate of the medial epicondyle can be superimposed over the radiolucent line separating the anconeal process. This lucent line can mimic the lucent zone present with UAP. On the flexed lateral view, the "fracture line" is separated from the epicondylar apophyseal plate. Careful examination of the radiograph often shows this normal growth plate to extend caudally beyond the anconeal process and helps to avoid an erroneous radiographic interpretation (Figure 3-29).

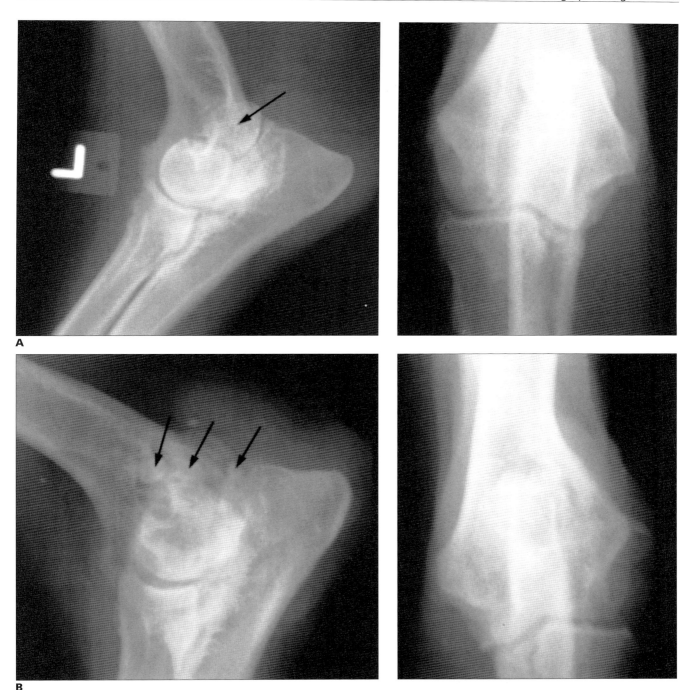

**Figure 3-32**
Lateral and craniocaudal radiographs of the elbows of an 8-year-old male German Shepherd Dog with a history of untreated lameness since puppyhood. The left elbow has a malformed ununited anconeal process (arrow) (A). The osteoarthrosis is moderate with sclerosis of the ulnar trochlear notch and osteophyte formation on the cranial aspect of the humerus and radius and surrounding the UAP. The right elbow is shown below and the ununited anconeal process has taken a different form and appears to have fragmented and shifted into the olecranon fossa (arrows) (B). The osteoarthrosis is more prominent in this limb. It is difficult to imagine the status of the medial coronoid process in these joints.

If secondary bony growth is prominent as a result of joint instability and is seen unilaterally, the UAP may not be hidden. If the secondary changes are extensive, such as might be seen in an 8-year-old dog with a bilateral UAP, the process could be so deformed and hidden by osteophyte formation that it is no longer recognized as UAP. In this case, the diagnosis may be limited to that of an elbow joint osteoarthrosis, etiology uncertain (Figure 3-31). Contrary to this situation, if the UAP causes an osteoarthrosis at an early age, diagnosis of the dysplasia is relatively easy (Figures 3-30, 3-31).

## Differential radiographic diagnosis

UAP not associated with elbow dysplasia can also occur when there is a combination of a separate center of ossification in the anconeal process of the ulna with delayed growth or premature closure in the distal ulnar growth plate. This results in shortening of the ulna but continued growth of the radius and pushes the olecranon fossa of the humerus against the anconeal process making a fracture of the cartilage bridge possible. This event may occur: (1) as a part of the syndrome of chondrodysplasia as seen in the Basset hound, (2) secondary to physeal trauma, (3) in association with a persistent cartilage core in the distal ulna, or (4) because of synostosis between the radius and ulna. Radiographs of the antebrachium are necessary to determine the specific cause for this type of UAP that is not associated with an elbow dysplasia.

Panosteitis is a common cause of forelimb lameness especially in the young German Shepherd Dog, thus, while having a markedly different radiographic appearance, it is an important differential diagnosis clinically. Panosteitis may also be found in conjunction with UAP (Figure 3-31) or other type of elbow dysplasia compounding the clinical signs.

## Treatment

### Conservative treatment

Since surgical treatment may be of marginal value, one may decide to recommend only conservative treatment of UAP with or without the use of analgesics. The affect of conservative treatment is to simply delay the otherwise rapid progress of the elbow osteoarthrosis by controlling body weight and by the selection of an appropriate exercise regimen. The results of medical treatment are variable and may or may not slow clinical lameness and discomfort. This treatment is often not satisfactory in the long term.

### Surgical treatment

Surgical removal of the ununited anconeal process has long been recommended as therapy for the associated lameness (Cawley and Archibald 1959, Loeffler 1963, Grøndalen 1979 c). Most dogs admitted for surgery are between 5 and 12 months of age (Grondalen and Rørvik 1980). Although some have reported relatively good results following surgical removal of UAP (Dietz, et al 1972; Sinibaldi and Arnoczky 1975; Roy, et al 1994), the authors' experience has been that surgical removal of the ununited process does not preclude a progressive painful osteoarthrosis. Although the initial reaction following the surgery may be a lessening of the lameness, this improvement is short-lived. Others have supported this opinion and have suggested that the osteoarthrosis tended to progress with or without surgical treatment (Hanlon 1969) thus questioning the value of the surgery. The degree of arthrosis is reported to increase proportionately to the increase in the time interval between the surgery and re-examination (Grøndalen and Rovik 1980).

Despite any question of the efficacy of surgical treatment for removal of UAP, it often remains the only method of treatment available. Two surgical approaches for removal of the fragment are described in achieving exposure of the elbow joint. The most commonly described technique is through a modified lateral approach with incision of the anconeus muscle and joint capsule along the caudal aspect of the lateral condylar crest. Another approach is used in cases where a MCPD is thought to be present. In this case, the joint can be approached from the medial side via a medial epicondylar osteotomy that provides visualization of the MCP. Incision of the joint capsule along the medial condylar crest permits removal of the UAP. Because of the possibility of medial coronoid disease, the approach that provides better visualization of the joint is strongly recommended. Failure to obtain the best view of the elbow joint has probably had a strong influence on the inaccuracy of reports of surgical findings.

The most common treatment for UAP has been surgical removal of the ununited fragment because of the ease of the procedure. However, lag screw fixation has also been described in an effort to unite the anconeal fragment with the body of the ulna (Herron 1970,1975, Sinibaldi 1975) as has stabilization using cerclage wire (Lewis and Leighton 1995). The results of the lag screw fixation have not been satisfactory because of the persistent progressive arthrosis.

Either removal or stabilization of the UAP has not provided satisfactory treatment because the joint incongruity remains unchanged. Failing to appreciate that the underlying problem is the underdeveloped trochlea, this result is understandable. In the authors experience, the only time the lesion has been effectively treated using the lag technique is when this has been combined with the use of a cancellous graft that has been utilized as a spacer in an effort to treat the malformed trochlea as well as the ununited fragment.

Ulnar osteotomy performed at an extra-articular site 20 mm to 30 mm distal to the plane of the radial joint surface has been described in treatment of an UAP. This treatment was proposed following the observation that the UAP was always displaced cranially from the normal site and the radial head on the affected side was proximal to that measured on the unaffected limb. The cut was made perpendicular to the axis of the ulna. The surgery altered the relative position of the radial and ulnar joint surfaces of the elbow and resulted in a better fit of the trochlear notch around the humeral condyle. The ununited process healed in most dogs with a narrower space between the process and the parent bone noted in the remaining dogs. The osteotomy site healed without problem influenced by the healing occurring in healthy bone in a young dog. Cranial tilting of the proximal ulnar fragment occurred due to triceps pull and the angle of the cut was changed to an angle of 45°. However, this seemed to hasten bony healing at the osteotomy site. Almost all of the 20 dogs described showed marked clinical improvement following this type of treatment in spite of progressive radiographic changes of osteoarthrosis (Sjöström, et al 1995).

## Prognosis

Ununited anconeal process, rather similar to hip dysplasia, can produce some variation in severity of clinical lameness between dogs with lesions that have a similar appearance radiographically. Some affected dogs may show no clinical signs even after developing osteoarthrosis, while others with only minimal osteoarthrosis are markedly lame. Following surgery in which the fragment is removed, the osteoarthrosis continues to progress because the surgical removal of the fragment does nothing to relieve the underlying incongruity or instability within the joint. Simple lag screw fixation is also of questionable value because of the failure to correct the malformed trochlea. Thus, the prognosis for many of these patients must be guarded, with or without surgery.

However, since it is not possible to predict how the dog will react clinically to this problem, the presence of a UAP should not automatically lead to a decision for euthanasia. Some of these affected dogs can have an acceptable quality of life and be a happy companion for its owner (Lavelle and Studdert 1990).

## Heritability

The heritability of this condition, especially in the German Shepherd Dog, was reported early and conclusively (Carlson and Severin, 1961, Corley, et al 1968, Hayes, et al 1979). The lesion in other breeds has not been so well studied; however, it is thought that it is probably inherited in these dogs as well.

# Medial coronoid process disease (MCPD)

## Introduction

Since 1974 (Olsson), an increasing number of dogs of various large and giant breeds are being presented with unilateral and/or bilateral elbow lameness caused by fissuring with partial to complete separation (fragmentation) of the medial coronoid process of the ulna. The MCP lies at the mediodistal edge of the trochlear notch of the ulna. In some breeds, the frequency of this type of elbow dysplasia approaches 40%. While some reports have recognized the high incidence of this disease, others have commented that the condition "is not a commonly diagnosed and recognized cause of osteoarthrosis of the canine elbow joint." This contradiction in frequency is the result of difficulty in radiographic diagnosis and lack of familiarity with the condition (Berzon and Quick 1980).

## History

An ununited coronoid process (UCP) was first described (Olsson 1974) as a new type of elbow dysplasia in the dog. At that time, use of the term elbow dysplasia was limited to an ununited anconeal process (UAP) and the resulting osteoarthrosis. Olsson suggested a causal relationship between the presence of a UCP that resulted in an unstable elbow joint and the subsequent development of secondary joint disease (OA). The term ununited was thought to be inappropriate since there was no evidence that the medial coronoid process of the ulna formed from a separate center of ossification (Guthrie, et al 1992). Therefore, the term was replaced with that of a fragmented coronoid process (FCP) (Olsson 1976). This condi-

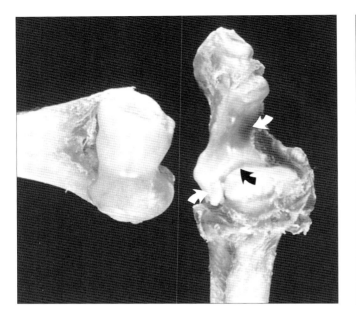

**Figure 3-33**
Photograph of the elbow of a dog with elbow dysplasia characterized by a high-lying medial coronoid process and a marked "step" between the distal portion of the trochlear notch of the ulna and the radial head (black arrow). The fracture fragment of the lateral aspect of the medial coronoid process remains "in situ," but has increased in size (note how far the cranial tip of the enlarged fragment lies relative to the radial head) (white arrow). Articular cartilage is lost on the lateral flange of the trochlear notch of the ulna due to loss of contact with the humeral articular cartilage (white arrow). Abrasion of the articular cartilage of the humeral condyle opposite the coronoid fragment is difficult to identify in the photograph.

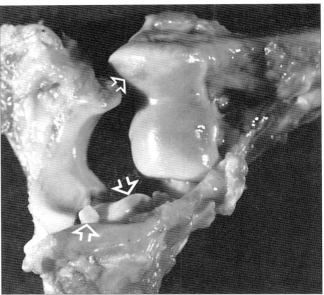

**Figure 3-34**
Photograph of the elbow of a dog with elbow dysplasia made at such an angle that the relationship between the distal portion of the trochlear notch of the ulna and the radial head (arrow) cannot be appreciated. The lateral aspect of the medial coronoid process has fractured and is displaced (arrow). Articular cartilage wear on the medial aspect of the humeral trochlea is evident (arrow).

tion was increasingly recognized in many young, rapidly growing dogs (Grondalen 1976).

The authors subscribe to the belief that elbow dysplasia is caused by temporary or persistent lagging in growth of the ulnar trochlear notch resulting in underdevelopment of the trochlear notch that may also be temporary or persistent. This underdevelopment causes the anconeal process and the medial coronoid process to become too closely associated with the humeral trochlea while the center of the trochlear notch of the ulna loses contact with the opposing humeral articular cartilage. Radiographically, this is seen as a cranially subluxating humeral condyle. The lagging growth of the trochlear notch of the ulna begins at the time when the process is still cartilaginous and is pliant and prior to the time it gradually ossifies. Damage to the medial coronoid process is explained by the fact that it rises slowly above the level of the downward sloping of the medial aspect of the radial head. In this position, it is subjected to unusual weight bearing forces. The damage to the MCP varies widely. It may remain cartilaginous, have a delayed ossification, or may ossify at a more normal time. The lesion may appear as a fissure within the cartilage, with complete separation of the cartilage fragment(s) (Figure 3-33) or it may appear as a fissure within the bone, with an incomplete fracture or complete separation of a bony fragment(s) (Figures 3-34, 3-35).

The pieces may remain in situ (Figures 3-33, 3-36, 3-37) or may be displaced (Figures 3-34, 3-35). Olsson (1975 b) reported that a fragmented medial coronoid process might be separated from the fracture bed and remain viable because it is loosely attached to the joint capsule from which it continues to maintain its blood supply. Thus, if displaced, the fragments may remain unchanged or, because of a persistent blood supply, the fragments of cartilage may become larger and may ossify or fragments of bone may enlarge (Figures 3-33, 3-36, 3-37). Because of the many faces of this disease, the term MCPD is suggested rather than a more specific term. Because, the underdevelopment of the trochlear notch places the MCP above the head of the radius, the high-lying MCP can damage the opposing articular cartilage of the humeral

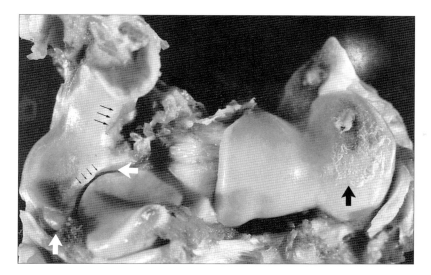 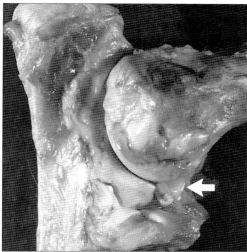

**Figure 3-35**
Photographs of the elbow of a dog with elbow dysplasia characterized by a high-lying medial coronoid process and a marked "step" between the distal portion of the trochlear notch of the ulna and the radial head (white arrow). Note the thickened dead cartilage at the lateral edge of the ulnar trochlear notch (small arrows). The cranial tip of the medial coronoid process is fractured and the fragment has rounded with a slight increased in size (white arrows). Loss of articular cartilage and destruction of the subchondral bones present on the lateral flange of the ulnar trochlear notch (medium arrows). Note the "kissing lesion" on the opposing articular surface of the trochlea of the humerus (black arrow). Differentiation between a "kissing lesson" and an OCD is difficult in this elbow.

condyle resulting in an abrasion called a "kissing lesion" (Figures 3-34, 3-36). This contributes to the resulting osteoarthrosis.

MCPD is reported in many breeds, however, certain ones are reported to be over represented consistently and include the German Shepherd Dog, Labrador Retriever, Rottweiler, Bernese Mountain Dog, and Golden Retriever (Olsson 1983; Carpenter, et al 1993). Other breeds are known to have this condition as well and include the Newfoundland, Saint Bernard, Giant Schnauzer, Shar Pei, and Sheltie. While this lesion has been described usually in dogs produced by breed fanciers, it has also been reported in a survey study of dogs in Iran that included crossbred dogs (Tirgari 1974, 1980). Lesions occur more in the male with a ratio of 2:1 (Grøndalen 1979 b; Olsson 1983; Carpenter, et al 1993) and occur bilaterally in most patients (Grøndalen 1979 b, Olsson 1983).

The fracture line and/or the fragment are not always easily identified grossly and close inspection of the joint is required. Because of this difficulty surgeons often overlook the fragment(s) and the condition is seriously underreported. More than one type of lesion may be present within the elbow joint. A series of eight cases was described with both osteochondrosis and UCP (Wissler and Sumner-Smith 1977).

## Clinical signs

Dogs tend to show the first signs of elbow lameness due to medial coronoid disease at the age of 5 to 6 months. This follows a very rapid growth spurt that occurs between the age of 4 to 5 months. Most patients are seen prior to 1 year of age and, according to the owners, have been lame for only 3 or 4 weeks prior to first admission (Grøndalen 1979 b, Bienz 1985). However, the age of referral for treatment may range as late as 2 years of age (Hazewinkel, et al 1988). In a young dog with this disease, the lameness may be unilateral or bilateral. The pain is probably associated with a cartilaginous or bony fracture with a secondary synovitis. Because of pain, exercise endurance may be limited especially with bilateral involvement. The pain may also affect the personality of the dog and cause it to appear quiet.

Older dogs seem to be stiff in the joints of the forelimbs, especially after rest. After a short period of exercise, they usually move more easily, but after prolonged exercise, the lameness becomes more severe. This type of lameness is due to the arthrosis and not due to pain from MCPD. When the dog has bilateral lesions, obvious lameness may not be present. Instead, the lameness may be characterized by an abnormal gait with supination of the foot during the forward stride. The owner often has problems deciding which limb is affected (Wind 1982).

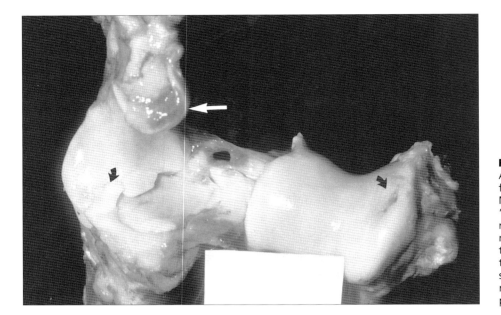

**Figure 3-36**
A photograph of the elbow joint from an 11-month-old male Bermese Mountain Dog with MCPD. The large "step" between the ulnar trochlear notch and radius is seen with fragmentation of the edge of the trochlear notch and lateral edge of the MCP (arrow). A "kising" lesion is seen on the medial aspect of the humeral condyle (arrow). The anconeal process is identified (straight arrow).

## Physical examination

On physical examination of the younger dog, pain may be demonstrated on both flexion and extension of the elbow joint. In more severe cases, joint effusion may be palpable beneath the anconeus and extensor muscles, and may become more pronounced after physical activity. In chronic cases, thickening of the joint capsule is noted along with increased prominence of the medial humeral epicondyle due to osteophyte development. Muscle atrophy if evident due to the dog's inactivity.

In very chronic cases, flexion and extension of the elbow joint may be limited due to further thickening of the joint capsule and new bone production rather than because of pain. When palpating the elbow in the region of the MCP, one has to be certain that the pain elicited originates from the lesion and not from the application of pressure on the ulnar nerve.

## Radiographic diagnosis

In the normal dog, the humeroulnar joint space forms a symmetrical, semi-circular, radiolucent shadow. The articular surface of the radial head is located adjacent to the coronoid process so that the trochlear notch forms a continuous arc with the radial head (Figure 3-38). No evidence of periosteal new bone formation or periarticular lipping is present. The radiographic diagnosis of MCPD is based on detection of joint incongruity and/or secondary osteoarthosis (Figure 3-39). On a lateral radiograph of an affected elbow in the immature dog before the onset of arthrosis made with the limb partially extended, the following abnormalities may be noticed:

(1) an increase in the humeroulnar joint space in the central area of the ulnar trochlear notch,
(2) an increase in the humeroradial joint space,
(3) a break in the normal continuous arc between the ulnar trochlear notch and the radial head with the distal edge of the ulnar trochlear notch lying a step above the level of the radial head, or
(4) a cranial displacement of the humeral condyle relative to the radial head.

Of these, the break in continuity of the arc that represents the continuation of the articular surface of the ulnar trochlear notch and the radial head and the cranial displacement of the humeral condyle are most indicative of disease (Wind 1982, Wind and Packard 1986). Bony changes may also be identified at this age and include:

(1) a delay in ossification of the medial coronoid process that results in its incomplete or irregular outline and
(2) a mild increase in density of the subchondral bone at the distal end of the ulnar trochlear notch (Table 3-8).

It is uncommon that the exact nature of the MCPD is identifiable on the radiograph.

Joint incongruity can be detected by noting that the medial coronoid process and sometimes the distal edge of the ulnar trochlear notch lie slightly above the level of the adjoining radius, creating a step between the radial head and the ulna and causing incongruity within the joint. The height of the step may vary from barely noticeable to a magnitude of 5 to 6mm in severe cases. Joint surface incongruity may become less in the more mature animal due to compensatory adjustments during growth

**Figure 3-37**
Photograph, radiograph, and histopathology section made from the right elbow of a 16-month-old male Bernese Mountain Dog with MCPD. Photograph of the elbow shows the disease characterized by a high-lying medial coronoid process, a marked "step" between the distal portion of the trochlear notch of the ulna and the radial head (black arrow), and a fracture of the entire cranial portion of the medial coronoid process (white arrow) (A). The fragment has remained "in situ" but has increased markedly in size. Note the dead articular cartilage of the distal edge of the trochlear notch above the radial head. Radiograph of a slab section from the distal portion of the ulnar trochlear notch and the radial head showing the "step" between the bony structures more clearly (B). Calcification is seen within the degenerating articular cartilage (arrow) that formed in an attempt to smooth out the "step." The osteophyte on the cranial margin of the radial head is prominent. Histopathology section of the interface between the high lying distal trochlear notch and the radial head (C). The fibrocartilage is seen extending over the "step." The darker staining areas (arrows) indicate calcification of the cartilage.

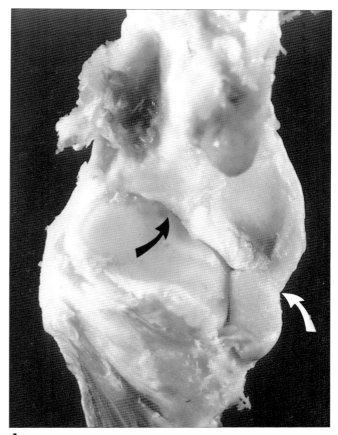
A

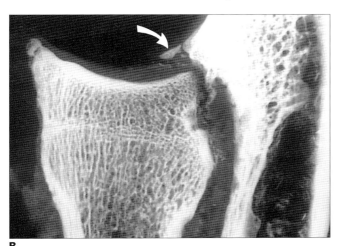
B

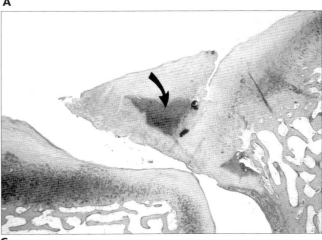
C

that tend to minimize unequal growth rates between the articular growth plate of the distal humerus and the articular growth plate of the ulnar trochlear notch. Despite this compensation, injury to the articular surface has occurred and a continued progression of an arthrosis is expected.

On the craniocaudal view of the normal young dog, the width of the joint space between the humeral condyle and the radial head and the humeral condyle and the ulna (MCP) is equal. In the affected young dog, the width of the joint spaces varies markedly because of positioning and x-ray beam angle and this is not a reliable radiographic finding unless the change is marked. The high lying MCP may be seen projected proximal to the radial head on this view.

The sesamoid bone in the annular ligament lies craniolateral to the radial head and has been confused by some to be a coronoid fragment as seen on the lateral view. On

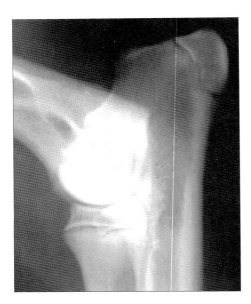
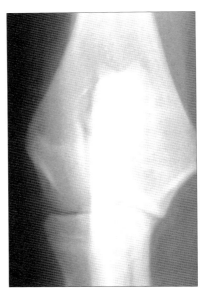

**Figure 3-38**
Lateral and craniocaudal radiographs of a normal elbow joint of a 7-month-old male Collie. The congruity of the joint is characterized by a deeply seated humeral condyle with equal width of the surrounding joint spaces. The shape of the trochlear notch of the ulna is full and it accepts the humeral condyle. No evidence of new bone production is noted.

the craniocaudal view, the bone can be seen lateral to the radial head. This bone is positioned some distance from the medial coronoid process and its margination and density is similar to other sesamoid bones. Detection of this bone in the absence of any other sign indicating elbow dysplasia should make its true identification easier.

#### Table 3-8: Radiographic changes in the young dog with medial coronoid process disease

I. Incongruity
　　A. Increase in width of the humeroulnar joint space
　　B. Increase in width of the humeroradial joint space
　　C. "Stair-step" between the ulnar trochlear notch and the radial head
　　D. Indistinct outline of medial coronoid process
　　E. Cranial displacement of humeral condyle

II. New bone formation
　　A. Distal portion of the trochlear notch
　　B. Proximal surface of the anconeal process

On the lateral radiograph of the chronic dog with MCPD, one of the first signs indicating osteoarthrosis within the affected elbow joint is an increase in bone density at the distal portion of the trochlear notch. This is due to subchondral sclerosis and/or osteophytosis of the medial flange of the ulnar trochlear notch. This change is perhaps the most easily identified change on the radiograph (Wind 1982, Olsson 1983). The osteophytoses on the medial flange of the ulnar trochlear notch are actually enthesophytes and represent a type of periosteal new bone, which forms at the site of attachment of the joint capsule (Figure 3-40). Enthesophytes also form on the medial aspect and proximal border of the anconeal process and on the caudal aspect of the lateral condylar ridge (Grøndalen 1982b). Periarticular lipping occurs on the cranial aspect of the radial head and is the result of an effort to extend the weight-bearing surface of the radial head to control joint instability and is in response to the cranial displacement of the humeral condyle on the radial head. Periarticular lipping is also seen on the cranial lip of the distal humerus also due to joint instability. Uncommonly, formation of small cystic lesions within the subchondral bone is seen.

The craniocaudal view of the elbow with chronic disease permits identification of enthesophytes and periarticular osteophytes along the medial aspect of the coronoid process, on the lateral aspect of the radial head, and on the medial epicondyle of the distal humerus. The width of the humeroradial and humeroulnar joint spaces is also evaluated on this view and may be uneven in width in chronic disease. If the "kissing" lesion opposite the medial coronoid fragment extends through the articular cartilage into the subchondral bone, it may be visible as a small bony defect on the medial aspect of the humeral trochlea. However, changes indicative of elbow dysplasia are more easily detected on the lateral radiograph, the view most recommended for evaluation.

It is helpful to summarize, in particular, the radiographic appearance of the medial coronoid process in this form of dysplasia on the lateral extended view. In the young dog, increased stress on the medial coronoid process delays ossification and may result in a process which is poorly identified radiographically because it remains cartilaginous. Because of this, the exact condition of the pro-

**Figure 3-39**
Lateral radiographs of both elbows of an 11-month-old male Bernese Mountain Dog with MCPD. Incongruity is evident by increase in width of the humeroulnar (double-headed arrows) and humeroradial joint space. New bone formation around the trochlear notch is present bilaterally but is more prominent on the right (A). Enthesophyte formation is evident on the proximal surface of the anconeal process on the right (arrows). The "stair-step" between the ulnar trochlear notch and the radial head is seen more clearly on the left elbow (B). The medial coronoid process on the left is blunted and a radiopaque fragment represents the cranial tip (arrow). Cranial displacement of the humeral condyle is more evident on the left (double-headed arrows).

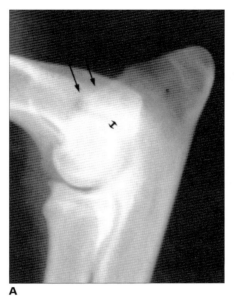
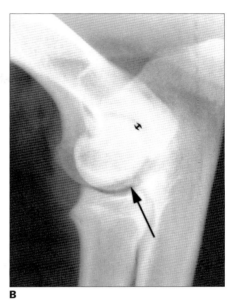

A  B

cess is often not determined. The lateral aspect of the MCP is most frequently fragmented but this bony portion of the process is hidden by the main body of the process and the radial head. If separation of the coronoid process occurs within a transverse plane, the "fracture line" is visible on the radiograph and the fragment is seen to lie cranial to the parent bone on the lateral view. However, a fissure of the coronoid process is the more common variation of MCPD with the fragment remaining in position and this is impossible to see radiographically. In fact, in many diseased elbows, the radiographic appearance of the coronoid process remains normal and a false negative diagnosis is made unless incongruity and arthrosis are considered.

Thus, the radiographic diagnosis of coronoid disease is more readily made from the detection of changes indicative of secondary osteoarthrosis rather than from identification of the injury to the medial coronoid process (Grøndalen 1979 b, 1982 a; Olsson 1975 a, b 1977, 1983; Grøndalen 1979 a; Berzon and Quick 1980; Denny and Gibbs 1980; Robins 1980; Henry Jr 1984; Wind and Packard 1986). In a joint with developing osteoarthrosis, it is not always possible to differentiate on routine radiographs between OCD and MCPD (Denny and Gibbs 1980) or to determine if the two forms of the dysplasia occur concurrently. Often the diagnosis is best made through consideration of clinical and radiographic findings plus consideration of the breed and age of the dog (Grøndalen 1979 b). These facts seem to have been recognized and accepted by many investigators.

The craniocaudal oblique projection with the limb rotated laterally demonstrates the relationship between the medial coronoid process and the articular surface of the medial humeral condyle and permits evaluation of the MCP. The craniocaudal oblique projection with the limb rotated medially demonstrates the relationship between the radial head and the articular surface of the lateral humeral condyle. That view also displays the ectopic sesamoid bone adjacent to the radial head that lies within the annular ligament of the lateral collateral ligament. However, fragmentation of the lateral edge of the MCP will not be seen. These oblique views, while strongly recommended by some to permit diagnosis of elbow dysplasia, have been found by the authors to not materially add to information already obtained from the extended lateral and CrCa views. However, these views may provide an opportunity to visualize radiographic change on another study making a clinician more secure in a diagnosis.

## Diagnosis using other radiographic imaging techniques

Xeroradiography, linear tomography, and computed tomography (CT) have all been used in an effort to obtain better visualization of the fragmented medial coronoid process. Computed tomography has the highest accuracy in diagnosis. Routine radiography plus linear tomography closely approached the accuracy found with computed tomography (Carpenter, et al 1993). However, that study was directed toward the detection of an irregularity of the medial coronoid process and the principle criterion used in evaluation of these imaging techniques was identification of a fragment. If the fragment remains partially cartilaginous, its visualization on any type of radiographic imaging technique is compromised. Linear tomography alone has been used in examination of coro-

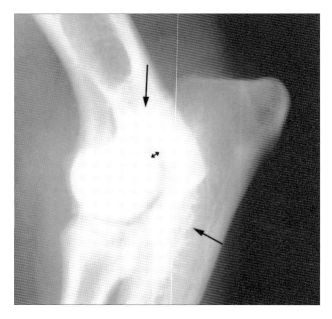 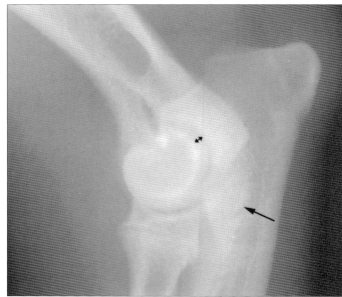

**Figure 3-40**
Lateral radiographs of the elbows of an 8-month-old male Bernese Mountain Dog with MCPD. Incongruity of both joints, increased width of the joint spaces (double-headed arrows), and cranial displacement of the humeral condyle are prominent. The osteophytosis on the medial flange of the ulnar trochlear notch is an early diagnostic change and one that is relatively easy to see (arrows). Note the failure of ossification of the medial coronoid processes bilaterally. New bone has formed on the proximal margin of the anconeal process in one elbow (arrow).

noid disease (Voorhout and Hazewinkel 1987, Fox and Roberts 1987) and has been reported to be more accurate in the detection of a fragmented coronoid process than routine radiography.

The authors believe that the diagnosis of MCPD can be made from the: (1) detection of joint incongruity, (2) form of the ossified medial coronoid process, and (3) pattern of new bone production as an indication of osteoarthrosis and that routine diagnostic radiography thus remains the most useful diagnostic tool. This is especially true when these findings are combined with the appropriate history of forelimb lameness and clinical findings of an elbow pain in a young dog of a highly susceptible breed.

Positive-contrast arthrography of the cubital joint was evaluated as a possible alternative to more sophisticated imaging techniques that require extensive technical expertise or expensive equipment (Lowry, et al 1993). Contrast arthrography is more commonly known for its routine use in the detection of cartilage flaps in OCD of the shoulder.

An upcoming method of diagnosis is arthroscopy in which the character of the articular surfaces can be examined (Bardet 1997). Using this method, fissures, fragments, and "kissing" lesions can be visualized and if present, the fragments can be removed during the procedure using arthroscopic instruments (van Bree, et al 1992; McCarthy 1994)

## Differential radiographic diagnosis

In a middle or larger breed dog with bilateral osteoarthrosis in both elbows, elbow dysplasia should be the first etiology considered. The osteoarthrosis noted following the developmental disease of elbow dysplasia is similar to that caused by a traumatic or chronic inflammatory event. Thus, it may be difficult in all cases, especially with unilateral disease, to determine the specific cause of the arthrosis in the older dog radiographically (Figure 3-41).

In the event of a healed articular fracture, the old fracture line and resulting fragment malunion are often identified making it possible to determine the exact etiology of the osteoarthrosis. Destructive changes within the subchondral bone commonly associated with an infectious arthritis are not present in osteoarthrosis secondary to elbow dysplasia and they serve as a method of differentiation of this uncommon cause of elbow arthrosis.

Other developmental anomalies of the elbow joint that might be bilateral and cause joint pain in a young patient are usually characterized by unique anatomical changes that separate the lesions from elbow dysplasia. However, as the dog ages, the resulting secondary osteoarthrosis may resemble that seen following elbow dysplasia.

## Treatment

If the incongruity is minor, often OCD, MCPD, or UAP may occur and the osteoarthrosis is minor and of no clinical significance. With greater incongruity, an associated medial coronoid process lesion is commonly seen and both the incongruity and the coronoid lesion contribute to the severity of the osteoarthrosis.

Regardless of the age at which the dog is presented for treatment, common therapy for any orthopedic disease includes weight control, intelligent nutrition, and a wise selection of the exercise program. All of these influence the progression of the osteoarthrosis.

However, analgesics are often the only method of diminishing the dog's discomfort and therefore need to be given. Because the pain reducing affect, the dog may over exert physically and thus may adversely influence the positive effect that exercise and weight control have. This may have a negative enhancing influence on the progress of the osteoarthrosis. Intermittent or long-term medical treatment with analgesics may be necessary if the osteoarthrosis is the main cause of the discomfort.

### Conservative treatment

Mildly affected dogs that are treated conservatively using weight control and limited exercise along with analgesics when the dog is obviously in pain manage to cope with the problem quite adequately. However, the osteoarthrosis is most likely progressive because of the combined effect of the joint incongruity and the presence of an FCP and the need for analgesics can increase. Dogs with severe FCP that are not operated show a rapid progression of osteoarthrosis, which leads to a crippling disease often at an age of 3 years.

### Surgical treatment

Surgical treatment consists of the removal of bony or cartilaginous fragment(s). This diminishes the pain caused by movement of the fragments or the synovitis caused by the ingress of the synovial fluid. The surgery encourages the sealing off of the lesions in the host bone through creation of a fibrocartilaginous covering. However, the underlying incongruity remains unaltered and a decrease

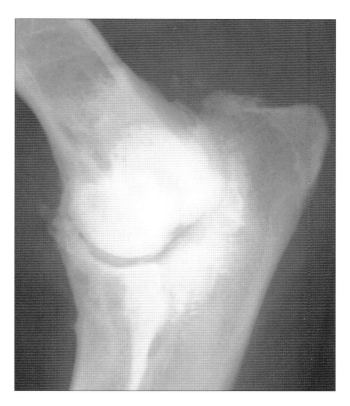

**Figure 3-41**
Lateral radiograph of the elbow of a 5-year-old male Saint Bernard with extensive osteoarthrosis. The extent of new bone formation makes it difficult to determine the specific cause of the joint disease.

in discomfort, not normalcy, is the goal of the surgery. It is imperative that the surgical approach allows a thorough inspection of the MCP because many of the lesions are inconspicuous. Often overlooked is the presence of a very minimal crease in the overlying articular cartilage that often denotes a partial fracture of the underlying bone.

It is advisable prior to surgical treatment to conduct a careful examination of the dog and search for other developmental bone disease, such as hip dysplasia, to more accurately counsel the owner about treatment.

## Prognosis

If the fragmented coronoid process is small and the degree of incongruity is minor, conservative treatment can give satisfactory results although lameness may remain a recurrent problem. However, surgery in this type of patient with removal of the fragment may permit healing of the fracture line and complete disappearance of clinical signs. Even with surgery, progression of the osteoarthrosis is expected but of a character the dog can cope with at an older age.

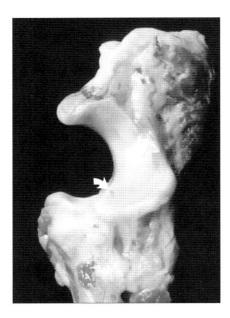
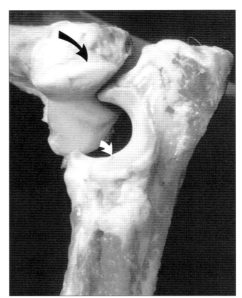
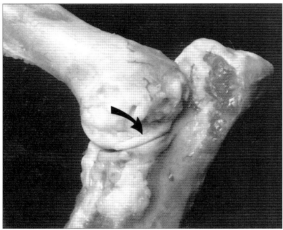

**Figure 3-42**
Photographs of an elbow joint of a 6-month-old male Labrador Retriever with osteochondritis dissecans of the distal medial humeral condyle (curved arrows). The dead cartilage within the fragment is identified grossly by its whiter color. The fragment remains "in situ." The medial coronoid process is greatly increased in size, is flattened and has an upward slope toward the medial edge instead of the normal downward slope away from the "keel" of the trochlear notch. The shape of this MCP suggests a greater weight bearing function of the ulna in contrast to the normally accepted shape that enables the radial head to be the main weight bearing bone. This anomaly should be considered a form of MCPD. Note the "crease" within the cartilage in the MCP adjacent to the radius (arrows). It is tempting to speculate that this "crease" represents the first stage of a cartilage fissure.

In the dog with a larger fragment and more severe incongruity, the opposite articular surface of the humeral condyle is damaged causing a more painful lameness. This dog is still a good candidate for surgery in an effort to decrease the pain but the osteoarthrosis can be expected to be more rapidly progressive. Even with surgery, the prognosis is guarded and the dog may be crippled by 4 to 5 years of age.

## Heritability

MCPD seems to occur to a high extent in some families and this was first found by examination of litters in which the disease was noted more often than in a randomly selected material (Olsson 1976; Hayes, et al 1979). A major survey of Rottweilers in Norway based on the presence of osteophytes determined that 50.5% had abnormal elbows at 12 to 18 months of age on radiographic examination. The survey showed that hereditary factors are important in influencing the presence of elbow dysplasia because puppies from two affected parents had a significantly greater chance of having dysplasia than those from two normal parents (Grøndalen and Lingaas 1991). The study to determine a possible familial tendency was actually difficult to perform in certain breeds because of the problem in finding breeding animals that are free of disease.

A study using breeding data from the Guide Dogs for the Blind association in the UK examined heritability of osteochondrosis and coronoid disease in the elbows of Labrador and Golden Retrievers and found factors of 0.77 and 0.45 respectively (Guthrie and Pidduck 1990). Another study of Labrador Retrievers in Australia reported coronoid disease to be inherited, but at a lower level of heritability (0.27). This study also suggested that the genetic contribution of the dam might be significantly greater than the genetic contribution of the sire suggesting a maternal affect that was most likely to be of a non-genetic origin (Studdert, et al 1991). In addition, clinically normal dogs were found to sire numerous affected females, tending to rule out a sex-linked recessive trait (Boudrieau, et al 1983) since an affected male is required to produce a female having a sex-linked recessive trait.

A recent study evaluated the results of matings between dogs bilaterally affected with both OCD and FCP. The elbows of the offspring were examined by arthrotomy or surgically for the presence or absence of disease. The results strongly support earlier findings (Guthrie and Pidduck 1990) that both traits are multifactorial or polygenic (Padgett, et al 1995). This study also showed that FCP and OCD are inherited independently. No difference in the frequency of these disorders was noted among the sexes.

## Osteochondrosis of the medial aspect of the humeral condyle

### Introduction

Osteochondrosis of the medial aspect of the humeral condyle is similar to that in other parts of the body with a thickened articular cartilage in a developing epiphysis in which there is a delay in endochondral ossification (Alexander, et al 1981; Guthrie and Vaughan 1992; Guthrie, et al 1992). It involves the medial portion of the humeral condyle in the dog and is frequently identified in conjunction with medial coronoid disease. As described earlier, osteochondrosis may progress to an osteochondritis dissecans (OCD) and this is the case within the elbow joint. By the time the lesion is identified in the humeral condyle, it is an OCD with a single or fragmented cartilage flap. The lesion is identified radiographically as a bony defect on the medial aspect of the medial condyle. This lesion lies opposite the medial coronoid process. The fragment may remain "in situ" (Figure 3-42). If the flap is not removed surgically it gradually becomes free and comes to lie within the cranial radial fossa where it sometimes becomes attached to the joint capsule and ossifies. They also may detach and are present in the distended medial joint space (Figure 3-43).

This OCD lesion should not be confused with a "kissing lesion" as described earlier, which is an abrasion of the articular cartilage that sometimes may extend into the underlying bone. Both lesions may be located opposite

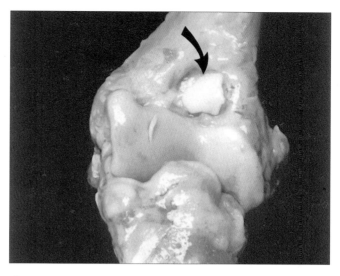

**Figure 3-43**
Photograph of the cranial aspect of the elbow joint of a 6-month-old male Labrador Retriever with an osteochondritis dissecans of the distal medial humeral condyle that appears to have partially healed following displacement of the fragment into the radial fossa (arrow).

the medial coronoid process, however, the OCD lesion lies opposite the main body of the process while the "kissing lesion" lies opposite the coronoid fragment which is further lateral. The OCD lesion probably develops at a younger age and is most likely the result of the tight contact forces between the cartilage of the high-lying coronoid process and the opposite articular cartilage on the humerus. The "kissing lesion" probably develops after ossification of the high-lying coronoid process and is the result of its abrasive effect. The slightly earlier appearance of the clinical signs in the OCD support this view. OCD is most likely the result of two separate problems, a breed pre-disposition for osteochondrosis combined with a breed pre-disposition for underdevelopment of the ulnar trochlear notch. Although, in the author's experience, the humeral condyle OCD has usually been associated with joint incongruity and an MCPD, a primary OCD may also be possible.

The lesions are more commonly found in the male dog (Olsson 1974; Hazewinkel, et al 1988; Guthrie 1989 a). In the authors' experience, certain families in Labrador Retriever, Rottweiler, and Newfoundland breeds are more commonly affected by this form of elbow dysplasia.

### History

The distal humerus is one of four major sites of osteochondrosis in the dog and was reported as a separate lesion in the elbow and was also frequently identified

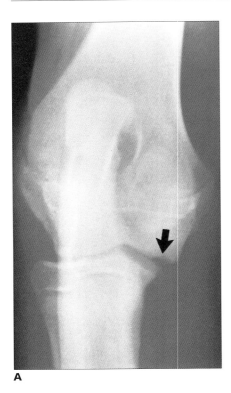 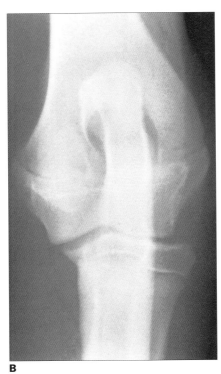

**Figure 3-44**
Craniocaudal radiographs of both elbows of a 6-month-old dog show an OCD lesion in the medial aspect of the humeral condyle on the right (arrow) (A) and a normal contour on the left (B). Failure to detect the defect in the articular contour using this CrCa view does not exclude the presence of a lesion further caudally.

in conjunction with coronoid process disease (Olsson 1974). A single case was described by Wood, et al (1975). Osteochondrosis of the humeral condyle is not as common as MCPD (Olsson 1976).

In osteochondrosis in the humeral condyle, it is rather easy to demonstrate histologically that the basic pathogenesis is a failure of the growth function of the immature joint cartilage. The cartilage fails to undergone provisional calcification, and it is not replaced by bone. This failure of endochondral ossification leads to retention and thickening of the cartilage followed by necrosis of its deeper parts and by dissecting fissures within the deeper layers (Figure 3-42).

The process of endochondral ossification may be disturbed at certain sites in fast growing animals because of mechanical factors. The joint surface of the medial aspect of the humeral condyle seems to be particularly vulnerable in certain breeds and leads to formation of a cartilaginous flap or, eventually, a loose body of thickened cartilage that does not ossify because of the lack of a vascular supply. The cartilage flap gives rise to mechanical irritation of the opposing joint cartilage causing fibrillation, cleft formation, and erosion at that location. The changes are age related. The resulting inflammatory reaction leads to painful synovitis and lameness. The irregularity in the joint cartilage leads to an osteoarthrosis, the severity of which depends on many factors (Olsson 1983).

This description of the pathogenesis does not include the fact that the underdeveloped trochlear notch of the ulna is associated with the medial coronoid process that lies above the level of the radial head. This fact is considered by the authors to be the single most likely underlying cause for the development of the OCD lesion in the humeral condyle in breeds predisposed to OCD. This does not mean that this single explanation for OCD applies to other sites of OCD lesions in the body.

## Clinical signs

The first clinical signs of pain and lameness may appear at 3 to 4 months of age (Olsson 1974; Hazewinkel, et al 1988) although the average age at the time of referral for treatment is between 5 and 8 months (Hazewinkel, et al 1988). The lesions are predominantly bilateral with right and left limbs affected to a similar degree (Guthrie 1989 a). In general, the clinical signs are similar to those described in a dog with an MCPD, however, the lameness is often severe.

## Physical examination

On physical examination at approximately 6 months of age, pain is demonstrated on both flexion and extension of the elbow joint. If the lesion is large, crepitus may be detected within the joint and joint effusion is noted at an

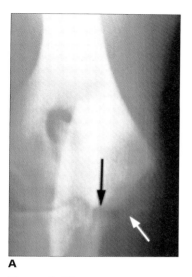 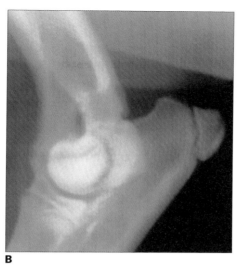 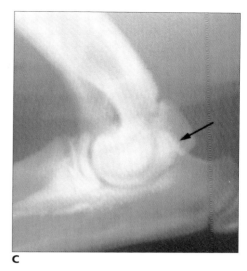

**Figure 3-45**
Radiographs of the left elbow of a 6-month-old male Labrador Retriever with lameness for 3 days. On the craniocaudal view, a defect in the medial aspect of the humeral condyle indicates an osteochondrosis (black arrow) (A). A linear soft tissue opacity is present adjacent to the lesion (white arrow). The widened joint space demonstrates the underlying incongruity. On the extended lateral view (B) and the flexed lateral view (C), the lesion is not identified; however, enthesophyte formation is present on the proximal aspect of the anconeal process (black arrow). At surgery, the 0.5 x 4 x 2 cm displaced cartilage flap was removed from the medial joint space and the defect in the humeral condyle was curetted. The MCP was examined and appeared stable.

early age. The findings on physical examination are similar in elbows with MCPD and OCD.

With time, the osteoarthrosis is characterized by development of a marked thickening of the joint capsule. These changes result in a limitation of motion within the joint causing a mechanical lameness rather than one associated with pain.

## Radiographic diagnosis

The OCD lesion is seen radiographically as a somewhat flat triangular radiolucent area on the surface of the medial aspect of the humeral condyle. The defect in the bony contour may be seen on the craniocaudal view, craniocaudal medial oblique view (lateromedial craniocaudal oblique view), or either the flexed or extended lateral views. If the lesion is somewhat cranial in location, it can be identified on the more conventional craniocaudal view made with the x-ray beam only slightly angled. However, many lesions are more caudal in location and the conventionally angled craniocaudal views do not project them in a tangential manner. These lesions are seen more completely when the x-ray beam is angled to a greater degree distoproximally.

On a lateral view, the lesion may create a flattening of the cranioventral portion of the medial aspect of the humeral trochlea. Careful examination on a lateral view for the three curvilinear lines that represent the articular surfaces of the distal humerus may permit detection of the defect created by the OCD lesion in the line representing the medial condyle (Figures 3-44, 3-45).

The radiographic changes associated with the secondary osteoarthrosis are indicative only of instability within the elbow joint and are not uniquely diagnostic for an OCD lesion. These secondary changes are progressive and their magnitude is dependent on the size of the lesion, degree of joint incongruity, and the age, weight, and athletic use of the dog. If an osteochondral flap becomes detached, calcifies, and remains as a large osteochondral body or ossicle this may be identified radiographically. Loosened pieces of cartilage may migrate cranially into the radial fossa where they remain hidden from the examiner (Figure 3-41) or into the medial aspect of the joint capsule (Figure 3-43). The most consistent early radiological feature reported is osteophyte development on the proximal aspect of the anconeal process (Figure 3-43) (Robins 1980; Bennett, et al 1981) but this is not a unique change seen in this form of elbow dysplasia. In most patients with an OCD lesion, a wider radioulnar joint space in the affected elbow joint demonstrates the underlying incongruity.

## Differential radiographic diagnosis

The main differential diagnosis is a "kissing lesion" caused by a rather large fragmented coronoid process that has caused cartilage and subchondral bone destruction. This is slightly lateral to the location of a typical OCD lesion. This lesion occurs because of the underdevelopment of the trochlear notch that places the MCP above the head of the radius. In this position, the high-lying MCP can damage the opposing articular cartilage of the humeral condyle resulting in an abrasion called a "kissing lesion." This contributes to the resulting osteoarthrosis. Often both MCP and OCD can occur in the same joint and if the resulting lesion is large, it may be impossible to separate an OCD from a "kissing lesion" (Figure 3-34).

## Treatment

The dog with an OCD lesion is usually presented for treatment at an earlier age than is a dog with other forms of elbow dysplasia. If the lesion can be identified radiographically, surgery is recommended at that time. If the owner chooses to delay the decision to perform surgery, conservative treatment, with or without the use of drugs, is the only alternative.

Surgical removal of a small flap should be considered, however, the surgery only removes the flap that is secondary to the underlying cause and does not address the joint incongruity. During surgical exploration, the joint space should be closely examined for a fragmented coronoid process with removal of a fragmented or fissured coronoid process being recommended.

## Prognosis

Without surgery, the prognosis is rather poor depending on the size of the lesion. However, the tightness of the joint often prevents the cartilage fragment from separating into the joint pockets where it would create more synovial irritation. This is contrary to what is experienced with an OCD lesion in the humeral head in which the cartilage fragment typically falls into the caudal pouch of the joint capsule. However, if the fragment remains in position, it can delay healing of the underlying defect.

If the joint shows osteoarthrosis typical for FCP and OCD, severe clinical signs of lameness that is unilateral or bilateral, and conservative treatment has not been helpful, surgery should be performed. Because FCP and OCD are both accessible through the same surgical approach, surgery has the chance to affect treatment of both lesions. With surgical removal of the flap, the prognosis is partially dependent on the size of the lesion. Because the surgery only removes the flap and does not address the joint incongruity, the prognosis remains guarded. During surgical exploration, the joint should be closely examined for a fragmented coronoid process, which can be removed. However, identification of an intact, but high-lying coronoid processes offers no opportunities for the corrective surgery.

## Heritability

A recent study evaluated the results of mating between dogs bilaterally affected with both OCD and FCP. The elbows of the offspring were examined at arthrotomy or necropsy for presence or absence of disease. The results strongly support earlier findings (Guthrie and Pidduck 1990,1991) that both traits are multifactorial or polygenic (Padgett, et al 1995). This study also showed that OCD and FCP are inherited independently. No difference in the frequency of these disorders was noted among the sexes.

# References

ALEXANDER JW. Malformation of canine forelimb due to synostosis between the radius and ulna. JAVMA 173:1328-1330,1978.

ALEXANDER JW, RICHARDSON DC, SELCER BA. Osteochondritis dissecans of the elbow, stifle, and hock - A review. JAAHA 17:51-56,1981.

Anomymous. Elbow group recommends protocol. JAVMA 205:1376-1377,1994. Anonymous. Canine elbow arthrosis registries encouraged. JAVMA 197:1269,1990.

AUDELL L. Heredity of elbow dysplasia: Can elbow dysplasia be controlled by judicious breeding. AAHA Scientific Proceedings 730-733,1990.

AUDELL L. System of classification of elbow arthrosis. Meeting of the International Elbow Working Group, Berlin1993.

AUDELL L. Personal communication,1995.

BARDET JF. Arthroscopy of the elbow in dogs - Part 1. The normal arthroscopic anatomy using the craniolateral portal. VCOT 10:1-5,1997.

BEDFORD PGC. Control of hereditary elbow disease in pedigree dogs. J small Anim Pract 35:119-122,1994.

BENNETT D, DUFF SRI, KENE RO, LEE R. Osteochondritis dissecans and fragmentation of the coronoid process in the elbow joint of the dog. Vet Rec 109:329-336,1981.

BERZON JL, QUICK CB. Fragmented coronoid process: Anatomical, clinical, and radiographic considerations with case analyses. JAAHA 16:241-251,1980.

BIENZ HA. Klinische und Radiologische Untersuchungen über den fragmentierten Processus coronoideus medialis im Ellbogengelenk des Berner Sennenhundes und der anderen Sennenhunde-Rassen. Inaugural-Dissertation Zürich,1985.

BINGEL SA, RISER WH. Congenital elbow luxation in the dog. J sm Anim Pract 18:445-456,1977.

BOUDRIEAU RJ, HOHN RB, BARDET JF. Osteochondritis dissecans of the elbow in the dog. JAAHA 19:627-635,1983.

BRADNEY IW. Non-union of the anconeal process in the dog. Aust Vet J 43:215-216,1967.

CAMPBELL JR. Nonfracture injuries to the canine elbow. JAVMA 155:735-744,1969.

CAMPBELL JR. Congenital luxation of the elbow of the dog. Vet Annual 19:229-236,1979.

CAWLEY AJ, ARCHIBALD J. Ununited anconal processes of the dog. JAVMA 134:454-458,1959.

CARLSON WD, SEVERIN GA. Elbow dysplasia in the dog: A preliminary report. JAVMA 138:295-301,1961.

CARPENTER LG, SCHWARZ PD, LOWRY JE, PARK RD, STEYN PF. Comparison of radiologic imaging techniques for diagnosis of fragmented medial coronoid process of the cubital joint in dogs. JAVMA 203:78-83,1993.

CARRIG CB. Growth abnormalities of the canine radius and ulna. Symposium on orthopaedic diseases. J sm Anim Pract 13:91-114,1983.

CARRIG CB, MORGAN JP, POOL RR. Effects of asychronous growth of the radius and ulna on the canine elbow joint following experimental retardation of longitudinal growth of the ulna. JAAHA 11:560-567,1975.

CARRIG CB, MACMILLAN A, BRUNDAGE S, POOL RR, MORGAN JP. Retinal dysplasia associated with skeletal abnormalities in Labrador Retrievers. JAVMA 170:49-57,1977.

CAWLEY AJ, Archibald J. Ununited anconeal processes of the dog. JAVMA 134:454-458,1959,

CORLEY EA, CARLSON WD. Radiographic, genetic and pathologic aspects of elbow dysplasia. Abstract JAVMA 147:1651,1965.

CORLEY EA, SUTHERLAND TM, CARLSON WD. Genetic aspects of canine elbow dysplasia. JAVMA 153:543-547,1968.

DE HAAN JJ, GORING RL, BEALE BS. What is your diagnosis? (fragmented medial coronoid process) JAVMA 201:927-928,1992.

DENNY HR, GIBBS C. The surgical treatment of osteochondritis dissecans and ununited coronoid process in the canine elbow joint. J sm Anim Pract 21:323-331,1980.

DIETZ O, NAGEL E, LI E. Zur Klinik der Ellenbogengelenkdysplasie (isolierter Processus anconeus) des Hundes. Monatsh Vet Med 27:734-735,1972.

FLO GL, BLOOMBERG MA, TVEDTEN HW. Review of five clinical cases of osteoarthrosis of the canine elbow due to the avulsion of the medial epicondyle and posterior medial supracondylar ridge of the humerus. Proceedings. Vet Orthop Soc p.1,1978.

FOX SM. Premature closure of distal radial and ulnar physes in the dog. Part1. Pathogenesis and diagnosis. Compend Contin Educ Pract Vet 6:128-138,1984.

FOX SM, ROBERTS RE. Linear tomography in diagnosing fragmented coronoid processes in canine elbows. Compend Contin Educ Pract Vet 9:60-65,1987.

FOX SM, BLOOMBERG MA, BRIGHT RM. Developmental anomalies of the canine elbow. JAAHA 19:605-615,1983.

GORING RL, BLOOMBERG ME. Selected developmental abnormalities of the canine elbow: radiographic evaluation and surgical management. Compend Contin Educ Pract Vet 5:178-188,1983.

GRØNDALEN J. Malformation of the elbow joint in an Afghan hound litter. J sm Anim Pract 14:83-89.1973.

GRØNDALEN J. Lidelser i skulder og albueledd hos unge hurtigvoksende hunder. Norsk Vet Tidning 88:309-316,1976.

GRØNDALEN J. Arthrosis with special reference to the elbow joint of young rapidly growing dogs. 1. A review of the literataure. Nord Vet Med 31:62-68,1979a.

GRØNDALEN J. Arthrosis with special reference to the elbow joint of young rapidly growing dogs. 11. Occurrence, clinical and radiographical findings. Nord Vet Med 31:69-75,1979b.

GRØNDALEN J. Arthrosis in the elbow joint of young rapidly growing dogs. 111. Ununited medial coronoid process of the ulna and osteochondritis dissecans of the humeral condyle. Surgical procedure for correction and postoperative investigation. Nord Vet Med 31:520-527,1979c.

GRØNDALEN J. A generalized chondropathy of joint cartilage leading to deformity of the elbow joints in a litter of Newfoundland dogs. J Sm Anim Pract 22:523-538,1981.

GRØNDALEN J. Arthrosis in the elbow joint of young rapidly growing dogs VI. Interrelation between clinical, radiographical and pathoanatomical findings. Nord Vet Med 34:65-75,1982a.

GRØNDALEN J. Arthrosis in the elbow joint of young rapidly growing dogs. VII Occurrence in the Rottweiler dogs. Nord Vet Med 34:76-82,1982b.

GRØNDALEN J, BRAUT T. Lameness in two young dogs caused by a calcified body in the joint capsule of the elbow. J sm Anim Pract 17:681-684,1976.

GRONDALEN J. Arthrosis in the elbow joint of young rapidly growing dogs. A pathoanatomical investigation. Nord Vet Med 33:1-16,1981.

GRONDALEN J, LINGAAS J. Arthrosis in the elbow joint among Rottweiler dogs Results from investigations into hereditary disposition. Tijdschrift voor Diergeneeskunde 133:Supplement 1,1988.

GRONDALEN J, LINGAAS J. Arthrosis in the elbow joint of young rapidly growing dogs: a genetic investigation. J sm Anim Pract 32:460-464,1991.

GRONDALEN J, RORVIK AM. Arthrosis in the elbow joint of young rapidly growing dogs. IV Ununited anconeal process. A follow up investigation of operated dogs. Nord Vet Med 32:212-218,1980.

GRÜLL F, HENSCHEL E. Distractio cubiti beim Bassethound. Kleintierprax 18:217-223.1973.

GUTHRIE S. Use of a radiographic scoring technique for the assessment of dogs with elbow osteochondrosis. J Sm Anim Pract 30:639-644,1989a.

GUTHRIE S. Some radiographic and clinical aspects of ununited anconeal process. Vet Rec 124: 661-662.1989b.

GUTHRIE S, BUCKLAND-WRIGHT JC, VAUGHAN LC. Microfocal radiography as an aid to the diagnosis of canine elbow osteochondrosis. J Sm Anim Pract 32:503-508,1991.

GUTHRIE A, PIDDUCK HG. Heritability of elbow osteochondrosis within a closed population of dogs. J Sm Anim Pract 31:93-96,1990.

GUTHRIE S, PIDDUCK HG. Arthrosis in the elbow joint of young rapidly growing dogs: A genetic investigation. J Sm Anim Pract 32:460-464,1991.

GUTHRIE S, PLUMMER JM, VAUGHAN LC. Post natal development of the canine elbow joint: a light and electron microscopical study. Res in Vet Sci 52:67-71,1992.

GUTHRIE S, VAUGHAN LC. Aetiopathogenesis of canine osteochondrosis: A study of loose fragments removed at arthrotomy. Res Vet Sci 52:284-291,1992.

HANLON GF. Additional radiographic observations on elbow dysplasia in the dog. JAVMA 155:2045-2046,1969.

HANLON GF, SPURREL FA. Elbow dysplasia with reference to the maturation of the processus anconeous in the German Shepherd Dog. Minn Vet 7:11-15, 1967.

HARE WCD. The ages at which the centers of ossification apper roentgenographically in the limb bones of the dog. Am J Vet Res 22:825-835,1961.

HARE WCD. Personal communication 1958.

HARE WCD. Congenital detachment of the processus anconeus in the dog. Vet Rec 74:545-546,1962.

HAYES HM, SELBY LA, WILSON GP, HOHN RB. Epidemiologic observations of canine elbow disease (Emphasis on dysplasia). JAAHA 14:449-453,1979.

HAZEWINKEL HAW, KANTOR A, MEIJ B, VOORHOUT G. Fragmented coronoid process and osteochondritis dissecans of the medial humeral condyle. Tijdschrift voor Diergeneeskunde 113: suppl. 41-46,1988.

HENRY WB Jr. Radiographic diagnosis and surgical management of fragmented medial coronoid process in dogs. JAVMA 184: 799-805,1984.

HENSCHEL E. Zur Anatomie und Klinik der wachsenden Unterarmknochen mit Vergleichen zwischen der Distractio cubiti des Hundes und der Madelungschen Deformität des Menschen. Arch Experim Vet Med 26: 741-745,1972.

HERRON MR. Ununited anconeal process in the dog. A new approach to surgical repair. Mod Vet Pract 51:(6)30-34,1970.

HERRON MR. Ununited anconeal process in the dog. Vet Clinics of NA. 1:417-428,1971.

HERRON MR. Ununited anconeal process in the dog. In: Bojrab MJ (ed). Current Techniques in Small AnimalSurgery, Lea & Febiger, Philadelphia, 1975. pp526-529.

HOULTON JEF. Osteochondrosis of the shoulder and elbow joints in dogs. J sm Anim Pract 25:399-413,1984.

KASSTRÖM H, LJUNGGREN G, OLSSON S-E. Growth disturbances of the ulna in dogs. Abstract J Am Vet Rad Soc 14: 6,1973.

KELLER GG, KREEGER JM, MANN FA, LATTIMAR JC. Correlation of radiographic, necropsy and histologic findings in 8 dogs with elbow dysplasia. Vet Rad and Ultrasound 38:272-276,1997.

KENE ROC, LEE R, BENNETT D. The radiological features of congenital elbow luxation/subluxation in the dog. J sm Anim Pract 23:621-630,1982.

LAVELLE RB, STUDDERT VP. Elbow dysplasia (osteochondrosis) A report. 2nd Internat Elbow Working Group Meeting, San Francisco. March 1990.

LEWIS DD, PARKER RB, HAGER DA. Fragmented medial coronoid process of the canine elbow. Compend Contin Educ Pract Vet 11:703-715,1989.

LEWIS DD, MCCARTHY RJ, PECHMAN RD. Diagnosis of common developmental orthopedic conditions in canine pediatric patients. Compend Contin Educ Pract 14:287-301,1992.

LEWIS R, LEIGHTON RL. Surgical stabilization of the ununited anconeal process in the dog using cerclage wire. Cal Vet 49; May/June:10-11,1995.

LJUNGGREN G, CAWLEY AJ, ARCHIBALD J. The elbow dysplasias in the dog. JAVMA 148:887-891,1966.

LJUNGGREN G. Osteoarthrosis of the shoulder and elbow joints in the dog. A radiographic and pathologic study. Abstract J Am Vet Rad Soc 14: 5,1973.

LOEFFLER K. Der isolierte Processus anconaeus beim Deutschen Schäferhund. Dtsch tierärztl Wschr 70:317-321,1963.

LOEFFLER K. Gelenkanomalien als Problem in der Hundezucht. Dtsch tierärztl Wschr 71:291-297,1964.

LONG RD, ROGERS AJ. Letters to the editor. J sm Anim Pract 18:157,1977.

LOWRY JE, CARPENTER JG, PARK RD, STEYN PF, SCHWARTZ PD. Radiographic anatomy and technique for arthrography of the cubital joint in clinically normal dogs. JAVMA 203:72-77,1993.

MARCILLIN-LITTLE DJ, DEYOUNG DJ, FERRIS KK, BERRY CM. Incomplete ossification of the humeral condyle in Spaniels. Vet Surg 23:475-487,1994.

MASON TA, LAVELLE RB, SKIPPER SC, WRIGLEY WR. Osteochondrosis of the elbow joint in young dogs. J sm Anim Pract 21:641-656,1980.

MCCARTHY TC. Arthroscopy of the canine elbow. Proceedings of the 21st Annual Conference of the Veterinary Orthopedic Society. Snowbird/Alta, Utah.1994.

MILTON JL, HORNE RD, BARTELS JE, HENDERSON RA. Congenital elbow luxation in the dog. JAVMA 175: 572-582,1979.

MITTEN RW, HOEFLE WD. Ununited anconeal process: Unusual presentation in two dogs. JAAHA 14:595-596,1978.

MORGAN JP, WIND A, DAVIDSON AP. Bone dysplasias in the Labrador Retriever: A radiographic study. JAAHA; in press 1999.

O'BRIEN TR, MORGAN JP, SUTER PF. Epiphyseal plate injury in the dog: A radiographic study of growth disturance in the forelimb. J sm Anim Pract 12:19-36,1971.

OLSON NC, CARRIG CB, BRINKER WO. Asynchronous growth of the canine radius and ulna: Effects of retardation of longitudinal growth of the radius. Am J Vet Res 40:351-355,1979.

OLSSON S-E. En ny typ av armbågsledsdysplasi hos hund? En preliminär rapport. Svensk Vet tidn 26: 152-157,1974.

OLSSON S-E. Osteochondritis dissecans in the dog. Proc AAHA 42 Ann Meeting p362.1975a.

OLSSON S-E. Lameness in the dog. A review of lesions causing osteoarthrosis of the shoulder, elbow, hip stifle and hock joints. Proc AAHA 42 Ann Meeting p363-370,1975b.

OLSSON S-E. Osteochondrosis- A growing problem to dog breeders. Gaines Progress 1-11,Summer,1976.

OLSSON S-E. Osteochondrosis of the elbow joint in the dog: Its manifestations, indiations for surgery. Archives of ACVS 6:46-47,1977.

OLSSON S-E. The early diagnosis of fragmented coronoid process and osteochondritis dissecans of the canine elbow joint. JAAHA 19:616-626,1983.

OLSSON S-E. General and etiologic factors in canine osteochondrosis. Vet Quart 9:268-278,1987.

OLSSON S-E, REILAND S. The nature of osteochondrosis in animals. Acta Radiol (Suppl) 358:299-305,1978.

PADGETT GA, MOSTOSKY UV, PROBST CW, THOMAS MW, KRECKE CF. The inheritance of osteochondritis dissecans and fragmented coronoid process of the elbow joint in Labrador Retrievers. JAAHA 31:327-330,1995.

PASS MA, FERGUSON JG. Elbow dislocation in the dog. J sm Anim Prac 12:327-332,1971.

PAATSAMA S, ROKKANEN P, JUSSILA J. Etiologic factors in osteochondritis dissecans, Acta Orth Scand 46:906-918,1975.

POBISCH R, GERES V, ARBESSER E. Ellbogengelenkdysplasie beim Hund. Wiener tierärztl Mschr 59:297-307,1972.

PROLE JHB. Letter to the editor. J sm Anim Pract 14:309-310,1973.

READ RA. Osteochondrosis and elbow arthrosis in young dogs: Incidence, diagnosis and management. Waltham Intern Focus 3:2-10,1993.

READ RA, ARMSTRONG SJ O'KEEFE JD EGER CE. Fragmentation of the medial coronoid process of the ulna in dogs: A study of 109 cases. J sm Anim Pract 31:330-334,1990.

READ RA, ARMSTRONG SJ, BLACK AP, MACPHERSON GC, YOVICH YC, DAVEY T. Relationship between physical signs of elbow dysplasia and radiographic score in growing Rottweilers. JAVMA 209:1427-1430,1996.

REILAND S. Morphology of osteochondrosis and sequelae in pigs. Acta Rad (Suppl) 358: 45-90,1978.

RHODES WH. Personnel Communication,1959.

RISER WH, SHIRER JF. Normal and abnormal growth of the distal foreleg in large and giant breeds. JAVRS 6:50-64,1965.

ROBINS GM. Osteochondritis dissecans in the dog. Aust Vet J 54:272-279,1978.

ROBINS GM. Some aspects of the radiographical examination of the canine elbow joint. J sm Anim Pract 21:417-428,1980.

ROY RG, WALLACE LJ, JOHNSTON GR. A retrospective long-term evaluation of ununited anconeal process excision on the canine elbow. VCOT 7:94-97,1994.

SEER G, HUROV L. Elbow dysplasia in dogs with hip dysplasia. JAVMA 154:631-637,1969.

SIKKEMA DA, ROUSH JK,. Unusual presentation of an ununited anconeal process in a six-year-old Great Dane. VCOT 7:177-179,1994.

SINGLETON WB. Excerpts from AAHA scientific presentations. JAVMA 159:19,1971.

SINIBALDI KR. Ununited anconeal process. In: Bojrab M (ed). Current Techniques in Small Animal Surgery, Lea & Febiger, Philadelphia, 1975. pp719-722.

SINIBALDI KR, ARNOCZKY SP. Surgical removal of the ununited anconeal process n the dog. JAAHA 11:192-198,1975.

SJÖSTRÖM L, KASSTRÖM H, KÄLLBERG M. Ununited anconeal process in the dog. Pathogenesis and treatment by osteotomy of the ulna. VCOT 9:170-176,1995.

STEVENS DR, SANDE RD. An elbow dysplasia syndrome in the dog. JAVMA 165:1065-1069,1974.

STIERN RA. Ectopic sesamoid bones at the elbow (Patella cubiti) of the dog. JAVMA 128:498-501,1956.

STUDDERT VP, LAVELLE RB, BEILHARZ RG, MASON TA. Clinical features and heritability of osteochondrosis of the elbow in Labrador retrievers. J sm Anim Pract 32:557-563,1991.

SUNDGREN PE. Hundavel met ansvar. Hundsport, no. 8-9,6-7, 1980.

SWENSON L. Personal communication,1972.

SWENSON L, AUDELL L, HEDHAMMAR Å. Prevalence and inheritance of and selection for elbow arthrosis in Bernese Mountain Dogs and Rottweilers in Sweden and benefit: cost analysis of a screening and control program. JAVMA 210:215-221,1997.

THOMSON MJ, ROBINS GM. Osteochondrosis of the elbow; a review of the pathogenesis and a new approach to treatment. Australian Vet J 72:375-3787,1995.

TICER JW, KERR LY, HAMILTON HB. Elbow dysplasia in the Shar Pei dog. Cal Vet May-June 1991, pp25-26.

TIRGARI M. Clinical, radiographical and pathological aspects of arthritis of the elbow joint in dogs. J sm Anim Pract 15:671-679,1974.

TIRGARI M. Clinical, radiographical and pathological aspects of ununited medial coronoid process of the elbow joint in dogs. J sm Anim Pract 21:595-608,1980.

VÄÄNÄNEN M, SKUTNABB K. Elbow lameness in the young dog caused by a sesamoid fragment. J sm Anim Pract 19:363-371,1978.

VAN BREE H, Van Ryssen B, Desmidt M. Osteochondrosis lesions of the canine shoulder: Correlation of positive contrast arthrography and arthroscopy. Vet Rad and Ultrasound. 33:342-347,1992.

VAN SICKLE DC. A comparative study of the postnatal elbow development of the greyhound and the German Shepherd Dog. Abstract JAVMA 147:1650,1965.

VAN SICKLE DC. The relationship of ossification to canine elbow dysplasia. JAAHA 2:24-31,1966.

VAUGHAN LC. Congenital detachment of the processus anconeus in the dog. Vet Rec 74:309-311,1962.

VOORHOUT G, HAZEWINKEL HAW. Radiographic evaluation of the canine elbow joint with special reference to the medial humeral condyle and the medial coronoid process. Vet Radiol 28:158-165,1987.

VON HITZ D. Obligatorische Röntgenuntersuchung der Ellbogengelenke auf Dysplasia beim Bassethound. Schweiz Arch Tierheilk 118:167-172,1976.

WAMBERG K. Atlas Radiologica, The Medical Book Company, 1966 pp.370-376.

WEBBON JM and CLAYTON-JONES DG. Radiological refresher –6: The elbow. J sm Anim Pract 17:395-401,1976.

WEIS M. Knochenwachstumsuntersuchungen mittels fluoreszenzmikroskopischer, mikroradiographischer und phasenkontrastmikroskopischer Techniken am Ellbogengelenk sowie distal an Radius und Ulna beim jungen Hund. Thesis. Zurich 1983.

WIND AP. Incidence and radiographic appearance of fragmented coronoid process (in the Bernese Mountain Dog). Cal Vet 6:19-25, 1982.

WIND AP. Elbow incongruity and developmental elbow diseases in the dog. Part I. JAAHA 22:711-724,1986.

WIND AP. Etiology and pathogenesis of elbow dysplasia; a hypothesis. AAHA 57th Ann Meet Proceed, pp 725-727,1990.

WIND AP. Elbow dysplasia. In: Slatter D (ed). Textbook of Small Animal Surgery, 2nd ed, W.B. Saunders, Philadelphia,1993 pp1996-1977.

WIND AP, PACKARD ME. Elbow incongruity and developmental elbow diseases in the dog. Part II. JAAHA 22:724-730,1986.

WISSLER J, SUMNER-SMITH G. Osteochondrosis in the elbow joint in the dog. JAAHA 13:349-354,1977.

WOLFE DA. Surgical correction of osteochondritis dissecans of medial humeral condyle and ununited coronoid process in the dog. VM SAC 71:1554-1557,1976.

WOOD AKW, BATH ML, MASON TA. Osteochondritis dissecans of the distal humerus in a dog. Vet Rec 96:489-490,1975.

WOOD AKW, MCCARTHY PH, HOWLETT CR. Anatomic and radiographic appearance of a sesamoid bone in the tendon of origin of the supinator muscle of dogs. Am J Vet Res 46:2043-2047,1985.

ZONTINE WJ, WEITKAMP RA, LIPPINCOTT CL. Redefined type of elbow dysplasia involving calcified flexor tendons attached to the medial humeral epicondyle in three dogs. JAVMA 194:1082-1085,1989.

# Chapter 4

# Retained cartilage core

## Introduction

Between the diaphysis and the epiphysis of long bones are cartilaginous plates that are referred to as metaphyseal growth plates that furnish most of their length. On the side of the growth plate nearest the epiphysis, cartilage cells multiply and grow in columns toward the metaphysis. As the cartilage cells extend into the metaphyseal side of the growth plate, they become vesiculated, die, and their intercellular matrix is calcified. At the same time, some of the calcified matrix cartilage is removed by a specialized cell population that is derived from a population of circulating mononuclear cells. These cells, osteoclasts, open channels into which vessels penetrate.

A second population of bone forming cells originates from osteoprogenitor cells that lie adjacent to bone surfaces. They are capable of cell division and produce osteoblasts that synthesize bone matrix. They deposit osteoid on the walls of the channels in the cartilage, followed by deposition of mineral salts within the osteoid matrix, resulting in formation of immature bone tissue. Once formed, the early bone becomes more mature in character by forming trabecular and cortical bone that supports the increasing weight of the growing dog. This mechanism of bone growth is referred to as endochondral ossification (bone formation from an earlier cartilage model).

However, if the blood supply is deficient, the cartilage matrix does not become mineralized and it is not replaced by bone. In the distal ulna, the metaphysis is flared and is of a large diameter. This may influence the blood supply to the cartilage that is normally found on the metaphyseal side of a physis and may cause a large core of cartilage to accumulate within the metaphysis. The failure to convert to bone results in an altered growth rate of the distal ulna. The slower growth results in a shortened ulna that causes bowing of the adjacent radius or, in some dogs, causes a failure of normal development of the elbow joint characterized by distal subluxation of the proximal ulna. Retained cartilage core within the distal ulna occurs frequently in giant breeds, generally causing first clinical signs between the ages of 4 and 7 months of age and is usually bilateral.

## History

A retained endochondral cartilage core was described as a distinct pathological condition of the metaphyseal region of the ulna that affected longitudinal bone growth (Riser and Shirer 1965). The etiology was suggested to be an insufficient blood supply that results in interference with endochondral ossification within the distal ulnar metaphysis. Because of the deficient blood supply, the cartilage matrix produced by the distal ulnar physis is not replaced by bone. Three factors may influence this problem in blood supply in the distal ulna. One is the large diameter of this physeal region in comparison with other long bones that compromises invasion of the metaphyseal-physeal blood supply to the center of the growth plate. At the time of rapid growth in the dog, this width is approximately twice that seen in the adult dog. Second, the fact that the nutrient vessel enters the ulna proximally may lessen the contribution of blood through this vessel to the distal ulnar growth plate. The third factor is the growth requirement of the distal ulna. Because 85% of the growth of that bone is derived from the distal growth plate, a large blood supply is required. Each of these factors may influence the blood supply that is available or required by the distal growth plate. The resulting deficiency in blood supply may result in a slower ulnar growth.

In dogs with a retained cartilage core, the diameter of the cone may vary from a small core (Figure 4-1) to one involving over 50% of the cross-sectional area of the distal metaphysis. This suggests the severity of the mismatch of the blood supply from the metaphyseal-physeal ring of vessels between the periphery of the metaphysis and the core. The size of the cartilage core is inversely related to the area of viable growth plate in which there is a more normal conversion of cartilage to bone. The area of the cartilage core determines the decrease in rate of longitudinal growth of the ulna. In some dogs, the core is of equal diameter as it extends proximally toward the shaft while in others, the core tends to be have a smaller diameter near the physis and a broader diameter within the diaphysis. This shape may tend to reflect a change in the character of the metaphyseal blood supply during the

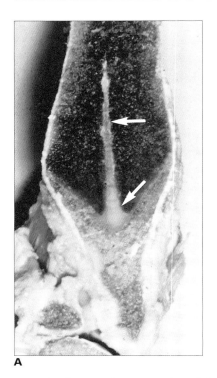 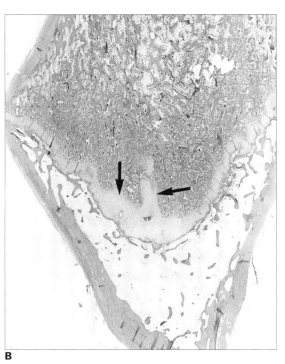

**Figure 4-1**
Photograph of (A) a sagittal section of the distal ulna with a persistent cartilage core (white arrows) and (B) a histological section of the distal ulna with a much smaller persistent cartilage core (black arrows). Neither of these is sufficient to affect the length of the ulna and cause clinical disease. Note how the shape of the distal ulnar growth plate resembles an inverted cone.

growth phase and suggests that if the nature of the blood supply improves, the diameter of the core will narrow.

## Course of the disease

The radial and ulnar physes grow at different rates. The distal ulnar physis grows at a rate equal to that of the proximal and distal radial physes combined. It is considered to contribute 85% of the total length of the ulna, 100% of the length of the ulna distal to the humeroradial joint. Growth in length of the ulna proximal to the humeroradial joint is by the apophysis (traction physis) of the proximal ulna and by the cartilage covering the proximal end of the olecranon. The distal radial physis contributed 65% of the total length of the radius and the proximal radial physis contributes 35% of the total length.

Points of contact between the radius and ulna are the annular ligament and collateral ligaments proximally, the radial ulnar ligament distally, and the interosseous membrane and ligament centrally. The proximal and distal ligaments retain the same anatomical relationship throughout normal growth. The interosseous ligament runs in a transverse direction that gradually changes with ulnar growth to a more downward oblique direction from ulna to radius as the ulna slides proximally along the radius.

Decreased growth of the distal ulnar physis due to retention of a cartilage core may occur because of failure of the metaphyseal-physeal blood supply. This may be influenced by the unique cone shape of the distal ulnar epiphysis that prevents the epiphysis from shearing from the distal metaphysis. Instead, the apex of the ulnar metaphysis tends to be forced down into the epiphysis leading to a crushing type of injury to the blood supply.

Normal development of bones and limbs is not only dependent on normal physes, but also on normal mechanical forces acting on these physes. Unequal stresses of weight-bearing, muscle or tendon pull can result in unequal growth rates within a normal physis. In general, compressive forces such as weight bearing decrease the growth rate while a decrease in compressive forces or creation of tension across a growth plate increases the growth rate. In the case of decreased ulnar growth because of injury to the distal ulnar physis, the shortened ulna lying caudolateral to the radius acts via the radialulnar ligament and the interosseous ligament and creates a compressive force on the caudolateral part of the radial physis, resulting in decreased growth, especially of that part of the physis. The craniomedial part of the radial physis is under the least influence of this compressive force. Therefore, it has the greater growth rate and a craniomedial bowing of the radius is the result. Lateral deviation of the paw (valgus deformity) results initially, but as the bow string effect of the shortened ulna increases, the distal radius pivots laterally around the ulna resulting in external rotation of the carpus and paw toward the position of supination. The articular surface of the distal radius that shifts from a transverse plane to one that begins to slope cranially adding materially to the deformity of the craniomedial radial bowing. In spite of the apparent craniomedial overgrowth, the distal radial physis as a whole has a decreased growth rate and is shorter than seen on the normal limb.

Depending on the strength of the humeroulnar joint and the ulnarocarpal joint, the lagging ulna may subluxate distally (downward) at the elbow joint or the styloid process of the ulna may become proximally displaced at the carpal joint or both may occur. If the anconeal process is still ununited or breaks off, the subluxation at the elbow joint may become severe and may minimize the degree of craniomedial bowing of the radius.

## Clinical signs

Retained distal ulnar cartilage core occurs frequently in a subclinical stage because the viable portion of the growth plate is large enough to sustain normal ulnar growth. However, if the diameter of the core is large enough, growth of the ulna is slowed and first clinical signs are seen between the ages of 4 and 7 months of age. A shortening effect within the ulna may have important clinical consequences for the dog with secondary changes within the radius that are characterized by external rotation of the foot, lateral deviation of the foot (valgus deformity), and craniolateral bowing of the radius (Olson, et al 1979) (Table 4-1). While the presence of the cartilage core is not painful, pain is eventually produced depending on the age of onset of the lesion and the severity of the decrease in growth rate of the ulna.

**Table 4-1: Clinical signs of a distal ulnar retained cartilage core**

I. Cranial and medial bowing of the radius
II. Lateral deviation and external rotation of the paw
III. Shortening of the limb
VI. Lameness
    A. Due to an altered relationship of the radiocarpal joint
    B. More severe with downward subluxation of the ulna
V. Altered gait

Usually, the strong interosseus ligament and the articulation of the radius and ulna with the humerus allow for little longitudinal movement between the radius and ulna proximally. Thus, all of the deformity secondary to retained cartilage core may occur distally with proximal displacement of the styloid process and resultant bowing of the distal radius. Uncommonly, the interosseous ligament seems to fail and the ulna shifts in position distally with marked subluxation of the elbow joint characterized by a marked disruption of the articulation between the radius and ulna and the distal humerus, with deformation of the anconeal process. This releases the pressure on the radius and it grows in a straight, more normal manner. Thus, the limb remains straight however, the dog shows gait abnormality and pain that originates in the elbow joint.

## Physical examination

The lesions may be unilateral or bilateral. In a dog that is affected bilaterally, the size of the retained cartilage core may be similar or markedly different, meaning that the effect on the development of the ulna can vary markedly. The age of onset of the disease influences the findings on the physical examination.

In the middle-sized breeds, the presence of a retained cartilage core is usually an incidental finding without clinical signs. These dogs are normal in appearance, have a normal gait, and do not elicit pain on physical examination. These lesions are detected on radiographic examination made for other reasons.

In the giant breeds in which the lesion develops early, a large core diminishes the growth rate of the ulna so that the physical signs may vary from slight to severe bowing of the radius with minimal to marked lateral and external rotation of the paw. The change from a straight limb to a bowed limb can occur rapidly in a matter of weeks and is of great surprise to the owner. In severe cases with abnormal stresses on the antebrachiocarpal joint, the gait may be painful. If the elbow joint is involved secondarily with slight distal subluxation, pain may be elicited on passive movement of the elbow and the gait may be more painful. Radiography that evaluates for this lesion must include the entire antebrachium (forearm) plus the elbow and antebrachiocarpal joints to determine the full extent of the disease.

## Anatomy and development of the distal ulna

The beginning of ossification of the distal ulnar epiphysis first appears between 7 and 9 weeks of age and continues to enlarge in size changing from a shape that appears as a slightly tapering cylinder within the middle of the epiphysis to one that resembles an inverted cone with a distal apex. Complete ossification of both the base and tip of the ulnar epiphysis does not occur until the age of 16 weeks. Although the ulnar metaphyseal growth plate is

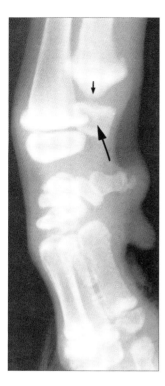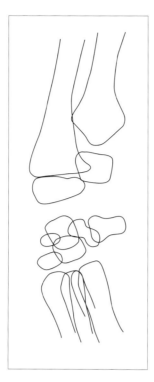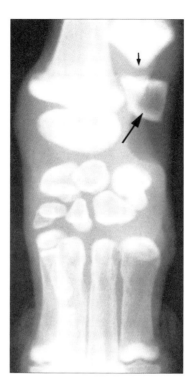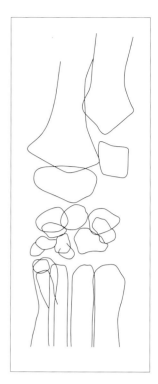

**Figure 4-2**
Radiographs and drawings of the distal ulna of a 10-week-old puppy show the unusual shape of the growth plate of the distal ulna. The metaphysis is conical with the tip of the cone directed distally into the growth plate (small arrows). The distal ulnar epiphysis is a slightly tapering cube at this age (large arrows), but it will develop a more pointed distal tip as ossification progresses. The large discoid shape of the distal radial epiphysis and the adjacent plate-like physis are seen in comparison.

equal in width, the slow ossification of the ulnar epiphysis makes it appear as if the growth plate has an unequal width. It is thought that the cone shape of the distal ulnar epiphysis may cause it to be vulnerable to injury because it can not displace in a transverse plane when traumatized. Based on information gained from traumatic injuries to the distal ulna, injury to this metaphyseal plate is more likely to result in an insult to the blood supply affecting growth.

The distal radial epiphysis appears first between 7 and 9 weeks and enlarges maintaining a discoid shape throughout development. At this time, the distal radial metaphysis and epiphysis are separated by a physeal growth plate that is equal in width. Thus, the radius shows the more commonly seen characteristic pattern with a metaphysis that has a flattened border, a physis that is plate-like, and an epiphysis that is discoid in shape (Figure 4-2). Physeal closure of both distal ulna and distal radius occurs between 8 and 10 months of age and the bones tend to model toward a tubular shape seen in the adult, although the ulnar metaphysis remains widened for sometime after physeal closure (Figure 4-3).

## Radiographic diagnosis

Diagnosis of distal ulnar lesions is made on a radiograph that includes the entire antebrachium (forearm) plus the joints both proximal and distal to the suspect lesions (Morgan 1972). The craniocaudal view is made with the dog in sternal recumbency while the lateral view is made with the dog laying on its side with the limb to be studied dependent (Figure 4-4). The resulting radiographs permit evaluation of joints both proximal and distal and comparison studies of the opposite limb (Figure 4-5).

Both craniocaudal and lateral views clearly show the radiolucent cone of cartilage extending proximally into the ulnar metaphysis from the distal ulnar physis, however, the lateral view is without superimposition of the distal radius (Figures 4-6, 4-7). The cone usually has a dense fine line indicating the interface between the cartilage core and the surrounding cancellous bone. The cone may occupy only a small percentage of the cross-sectional area of the physis or may be large enough to involve the greater portion of the physis. The diameter of the core may be consistent throughout, or it may vary with a broadened "lollipop" appearance with a narrow "stick"

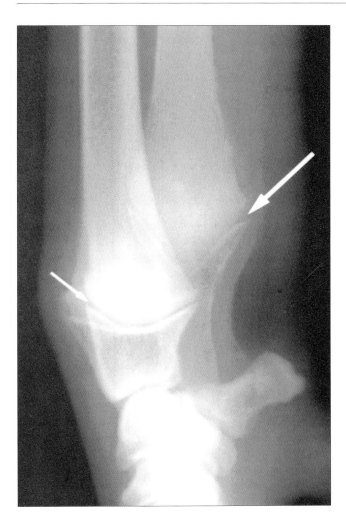 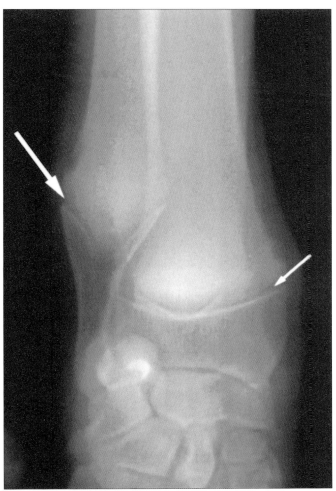

**Figure 4-3**
Radiographs of the distal antebrachium (forearm) of a 7-month-old Bernese Mountain dog with normal skeletal development. The distal ulnar metaphysis remains cone shaped. At its widest part it has a greater diameter than is seen in the diaphysis. The distal ulnar epiphysis is almost completely ossified and the metaphysis fits tightly creating a thin radiolucent physeal zone (long arrows). The distal radial metaphysis is also wider than the diaphysis and the radiolucent physeal plate is identified (short arrows). Note the straight appearance of the diaphyses of both the radius and ulna.

or base. The width of the unaffected portion of the physeal plate is normal but is only identifiable at the periphery and not seen in the center at the depth of the cone. The distal ulnar epiphysis is normal in appearance early in the disease. The comparative thickness of the radial cortices reflects changes in weight bearing and reflects radial bowing (Table 4-2) (Hanlon 1961; O'Brien, et al 1971; Carrig and Morgan 1975).

Secondary changes are dependent on the severity of the ulnar lesion. In the patient with only minimal disease, the only secondary change may be a slight bowing of the radius. Minimal bowing can be detected by noting the slight increase in the thickness of the caudal cortex of radius on comparison with the thickness of the cranial cortex. Further bowing causes the lines of stress to increase and the change in weight-bearing results in a further thinning of the cranial cortex and greater thickening of the caudal cortex. These changes are seen more easily on the lateral view. In the patient with more extensive secondary changes, external rotation of the radius is noted. The radius bows slightly as seen on the craniocaudal view creating a slight varus deformity with external rotation. This is despite the deformity of the limb being one of valgus as the foot is deviated laterally. The cortical shadows within the ulna become thickened uniformly and the bone becomes larger as weight-bearing increases. Generally, the ulna remains straight. The antebrachiocarpal joint subluxates as the styloid process is displaced proximally reflecting the shortened length of the

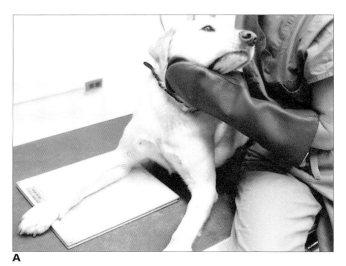

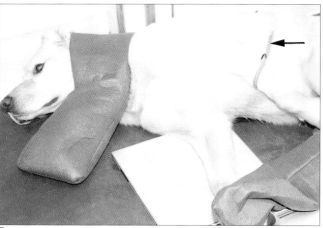

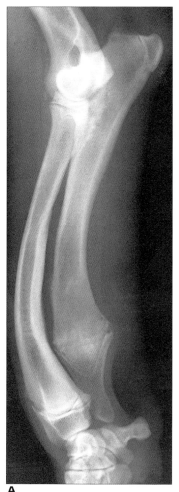

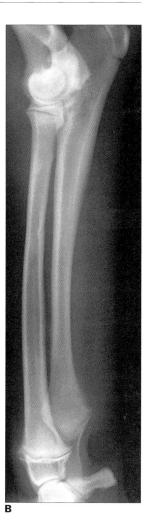

**Figure 4-4**
Photographs show the positioning of the dog used in radiography of the distal ulna. (A) The craniocaudal view of the antebrachium (forearm) is made with the dog in sternal recumbency, the limb extended, and the head and neck flexed so they are removed from the primary beam. (B) The lateral view of the antebrachium (forearm) is made with the dog on its side and the limb extended. Positioning of the patient can be accomplished by use of sandbags. Note the use of a tie-down rope (arrow) to remove the upper limb from the x-ray beam.

**Figure 4-5**
Lateral radiographs of the antebrachium (forearm) include the joints proximal and distal and permit comparison with the opposite limb. (A) A retained cartilage core in the distal ulna on one limb has resulted in shortening of the ulna and has caused marked bowing of the adjacent radius. (B) The distal ulna in the opposite limb is normal. Both elbow joints are normal.

ulna. The radial articular surface seems to "flow" cranially over the radial carpal bone and becomes slanted cranially as the subluxation accommodates the bowing of the comparative longer radius (Figures 4-5, 4-6).

Tertiary changes are seen if the elbow becomes unstable with a distal shifting of the proximal ulna with deformity of the anconeal process. The medial coronoid process lies distal to the radial head but is difficult to observe because of an expected delay in ossification. The trochlear notch is abnormal because of a lack of congruity of articular surfaces (Carrig, et al 1975). The clinical importance to the changes in the antebrachiocarpal joints is not given the attention it deserves. The collapse of the radial carpal bone as the distal radial epiphysis slides cranially leads to an arthrosis of the antebrachiocarpal and intercarpal joints. All of the changes secondary to the external rotation of the paw and bowing of the radius result in a tilting of the joint surfaces and progression of the osteoarthrosis.

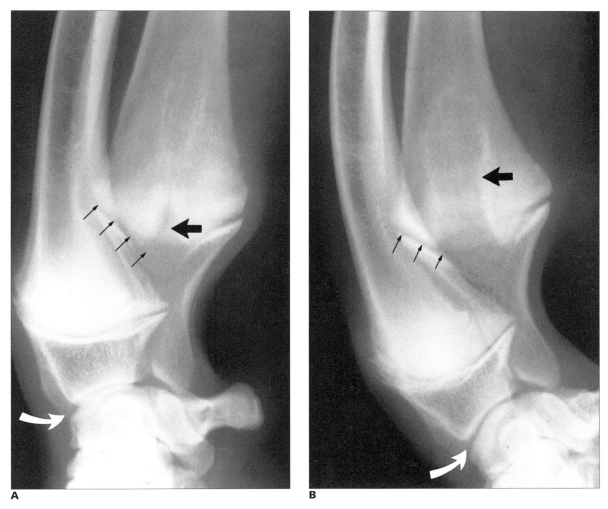

**Figure 4-6**
Lateral radiographs of the distal radius and ulna of both forelimbs of a 6-month-old Great Dane show (A) a small and (B) a much larger retained cartilage core. The radiolucent cartilage (large black arrows) represents a tongue of tissue extending into the metaphyses and is bordered by a shell of mineralized tissue. The influence on the growth rate of the ulna is directly proportional to the size of the lesion. Note the curvature of the radius, the unequal thickness of the radial cortices, and the manner in which the radiocarpal joint space is angled (white arrows) as a result of the distal radial articular surface "rolling" cranially over the radial carpal bone in both limbs. All changes are more severe in (B). The wide distal ulnar metaphyseal plate is partially superimposed by the distal radius (small black arrows).

Without treatment, the changes in the patient following skeletal maturation remain as seen on the radiograph of the immature dog except that the distal ulnar metaphysis narrows with closure of the growth plate. With time, the cartilage core in all stages of the disease is replaced with bony tissue. With the disappearance of the radiolucent core, the specific cause of the bowed radius cannot be determined retrospectively (Figure 4-8).

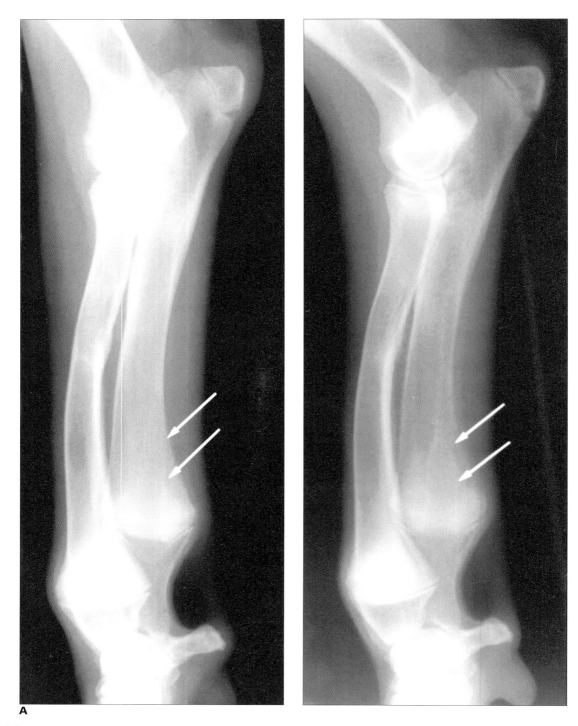

**Figure 4-7**
A-6-month-old male Irish Wolfhound had acute pain of the left forelimb. The forelimbs were sightly bowed with lateral angulation of the forefeet. Radiographs of the shoulders showed bilateral OCD more severe on the left and this was thought to be the cause of the pain. Lateral radiographs of the antebrachia demonstrate retained cartilage cores within the distalulnas (arrows). The comparative over growth of the radii remains minimal at this time; however, the radiocarpal joints spaces are "tilting" with collaps of the radial carpal bones dorsally causing minimal bowing. Note the comparative thickening of the caudal cortices of the radii. The elbow joints remain normal.

Craniocaudal radiographs demonstrated proximal displacement of the styloid processes more servers on the left and "tilting" of the radial physeal plate causing the lateral rotation of the forefeet. The retained cartilages cores within the distal ulnas are not easily identified on the lateral view.

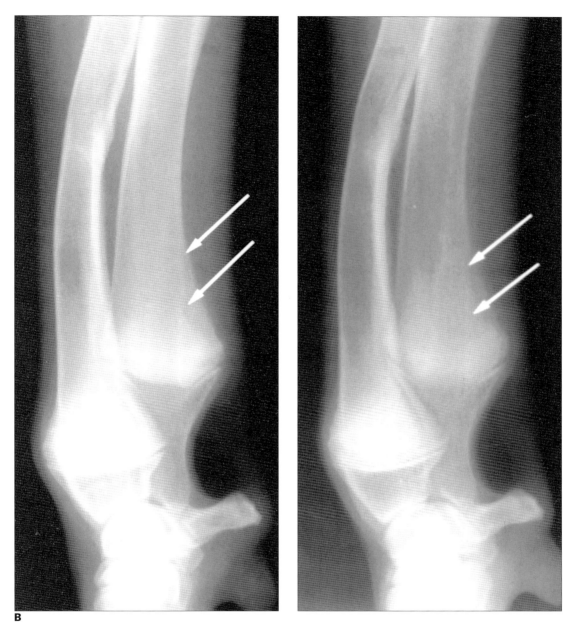

**Figure 4-7**
Enlargement of the distal radius and ulna show the cartilage cores (arrows) with a failure of ossification of the central portion of the distal ulnar metaphyses. This creates an apparent widening of the physes because of the increase in thickness of the growth cartilage. The proximal displacement of the styloid processes and the malalignment of the bones at the radiocarpal joint account for the bowing and lateral angulation of the forefeet.

These lesions are not painful until the arthrosis from the injury to the antebrachiocarpal joint becomes severe.

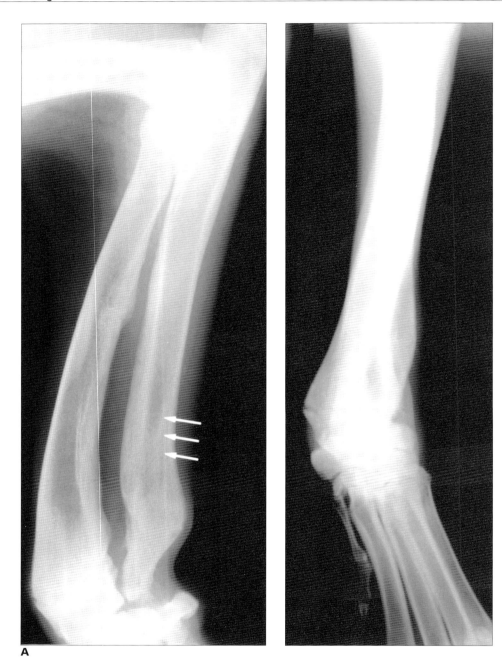

**Figure 4-8**
Radiographs of both antebrachia include joints proximal and distal of a 10-month-old male Great Dane that presented with marked forelimb deviation. The secondary affects of altered ulnar growth are present bilaterally but are more severe on the left (A) than on the right (B). Overgrowth of the radius results in radial bowing causing a change in weight bearing that results in a thinner cranial cortex and a thickening of the caudal cortex. In this patient with more extensive secondary changes, the radial bowing occurs along with external rotation of the radius. The extent of radial bowing as seen on the craniocaudal view varies on the two limbs. This is despite the general valgus deformity of the limb influenced by lateral angulation of the foot. The distal radial articular surface seems to "flow" cranially over the radial carpal bone as this form of subluxation accommodates the bowing of the comparatively longer radius. The distal physeal growth plates are in the stage of closure. The cortical shadows of the ulna are thickened and the bone has become larger as weight bearing by the ulna has increased. The antebrachiocarpal joint has subluxated as the styloid process is displaced proximally reflecting the shortened length of the ulna. The elbow joints remain normal.

Determination of the cause of the forelimb deformity is difficult in this dog. An ulnar diaphyseal bone pattern suggests healing of a retained cartilage core bilaterally (arrows). The secondary changes are compatible with those expected in a case of retained cartilage core. No evidence of trauma induced injury is present, however, a fracture with fragment displacement is not needed to produce a delay of ulnar growth since a crusting injury to the ulnar metaphyseal plate can suffice.

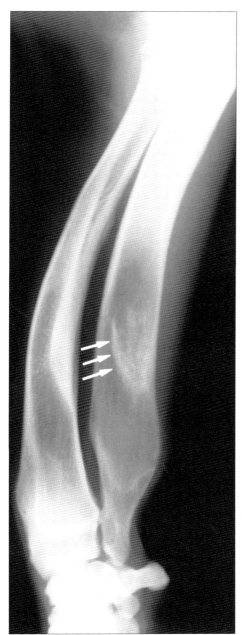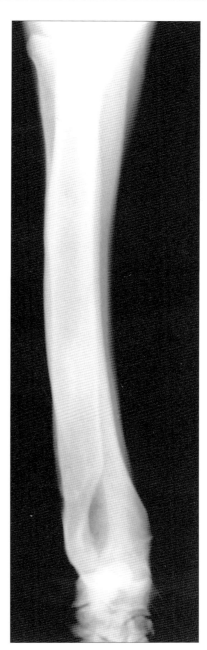

**Table 4-2: Radiographic changes seen with retention of the distal ulnar cartilage core**

I. Primary changes
    A. Retained cartilage core may vary in size
    B. Narrowed joint space between head of radius and lateral part of the humeral condyle (capitulum)
    C. Proximal displacement of the styloid process of the ulna

II. Secondary changes
    A. Retained cartilage core may vary in size
    B. Narrowed joint space between head of radius and lateral part of the humeral condyle (capitulum)
    C. Proximal displacement of the styloid process of the ulna
    D. Cranial and medial bowing of the radius
    E. Thickening of caudal radial cortex
    F. Slanting of radiocarpal joint
    G. Thickening of the ulna due to increased weight-bearing

III. Tertiary changes
    A. Retained cartilage core tends to model and disappear
    B. Elbow joint arthrosis
        1. Downward subluxation of the trochlear notch of the ulna
        2. Anconeal process
            a. Non-union of the separate center of ossification
            b. Fracture
    C. Antebrachial deformity
        1. Cranial and medial bowing of the radius
        2. Thickening of caudal radial cortex
        3. Thickening of the ulna due to increased weight-bearing
    D. Antebrachiocarpal arthrosis
        1. Proximal displacement of the styloid process of the ulna
        2. Slanting of radiocarpal joint

# Differential radiographic diagnosis

In the younger dog, the retained cartilage core is associated with an error in growth and the etiology of the lesion cannot always be determined from the radiograph. With bilateral symmetry, the disease is assumed to be idiopathic which may include minimal repeated trauma. With evidence of a healed fracture, the disease is assumed to be associated with that traumatic event. The central location of the retained core makes it possible to separate these lesions from those due to a developmental enchondroma that are usually unilateral and asymmetrical.

In the older dog, the retained cartilage core within the distal ulnar metaphysis may have been resorbed, however the secondary changes may remain constant (Figure 4-8). Healing may result in an ulna that appears normal in diameter, cortical thickness, and medullary lucency. In the more severe case, the modeling of the cartilage core may leave residual changes within the medullary cavity. With instability of the elbow joint, severe injury to that joint may result in a progressive osteoarthrosis. The arthrosis in the distal portion of the limb is more difficult to characterize. At this time, determination of the etiology of the radial bowing or the secondary joint injury may be difficult to determine.

# Treatment

## Conservative treatment

It has been suggested that delaying the growth rate of the affected dog by altering the feeding regimen may provide the opportunity for conversion of the retained cartilage core to bone tissue and for straightening of the radius to occur. This treatment might be sufficient for a dog in which only minimal deformity has occurred. In most patients, any form of conservative treatment is not deemed to be of value in the correction of the deformity.

## Surgical treatment

If the degree of bowing is still progressive and the cartilage core is moderate in size at the age of 6 months (past the age of rapid growth) in any breed, surgery can be contemplated. The surgery consists of partial ostectomy to remove the effect of the shortened ulna on the radius and allow for more normal development. This may be done with or without derotational radial osteotomy. Even under these favorable circumstances, a normal appearing forelimb should not be the expected result. Osteotomy of the ulna may also relieve the subluxation forces on the elbow joint and joint movement may gradually return to near normal congruity. The malalignment of these articular surfaces may never be completely corrected and will lead to a progressive osteoarthrosis.

In the event of severe deformity, surgical treatment in the form of corrective osteotomy is required if straightening of the limbs is to result. The surgery is complicated by the necessity to correct the rotational deformity as well as the radial bowing. Osteotomy or partial ostectomy of the distal ulna and an aligning osteotomy of the radius are necessary to correct the joint subluxation and to realign the weight-bearing planes of the elbow joint and carpus. Following osteotomy, a lengthening device may be used to gradually increase the length of the radius. Surgery should be performed prior to the age at which the dog is fully-grown. If the surgery is delayed until the deformity becomes severe, the damage to the either elbow or antebrachiocarpal joints may have become permanent.

## Prognosis

The prognosis is dependent on the severity of change present at the time of presentation. It is fair to good when the conformational abnormality is noted later in a medium-sized dog if the degree of bowing is minimal and the elbow joint remains intact. This dog may persist in having a slight radial curvature, but this may only cause a gait abnormality that is not painful.

For all practical purposes, spontaneous repair in the form of ulnar lengthening does not occur and the owner should understand that any deformity is probably a permanent feature. Theoretically, a temporary and minor slowing of ulnar growth rate in a dog with subsequent slight bowing of the radius may correct itself if the ulnar growth rate returns to normal. These cases are probably not brought to the attention of the clinician.

If the primary lesion is severe, little spontaneous repair is evident and the dog completes skeletal maturity with a severely deformed radius and ulna. In either event, the restored blood supply of the distal diaphysis of the ulna ultimately removes the cartilage core and it is replaced by ossified tissue. This means that the retained cartilage core is not identified in the mature dog, however, the resulting curvature of the radius and shortened ulna remains.

The prognosis of correction of a limb deformity is extremely poor when it is first noted in a 3-month-old Great Dane, if the degree of bowing has developed rapidly. Probably no amount of surgical repair can compensate for the loss of length seen in the limb as well as to correct the limb deformity. In spite of surgery, a singly affected limb most likely will not touch the ground after the dog reaches skeletal maturity. If surgery is attempted to correct the limb deformity, the prognosis is very much dependent on the skill of the surgeon. Limb lengthening procedures may be necessary to achieve maximum results requiring a lengthy and costly procedure for the owner to undertake. The severe injury to the antebrachiocarpal or elbow joint may be irreversible and a progressive osteoarthrosis develops. Since this lesion occurs in dogs prone to other developmental lesions in bone, it is important to evaluate other anatomical sites to permit the most accurate prognosis.

## Heritability

Heritability of distal ulnar lesions has not been thoroughly studied and the major evidence for the condition being inherited is found in its occurrence in certain breed and family lines. Because of the assumed important role of blood supply to the growth plate and the possibility of repeated trauma influencing this blood supply, the role of growth rate, weight and size of the immature dog, and trauma from normal athletic activity during skeletal maturation must be strongly considered in the etiology.

## References

CARRIG CB, MORGAN JP, POOL RR. Effects of asynchronous growth of the radius and ulna on the canine elbow joint following experimental retardation of longitudinal growth of the ulna JAAHA 11:560-567,1975.

CARRIG CB, MORGAN JP. Asynchronous growth of the canine radius and ulna - Early radiographic changes following experimental retardation of longitudinal growth of the ulna. J Am Vet Rad Soc 16:121-129,1975.

HANLON GF. Normal and abnormal bone growth in the dog. J Am Vet Rad Soc 3:13-16,1961.

MORGAN JP. Retained hypertrophied enchondral cartilage in the ulnar metaphysis of the dog. p350-351 Radiology in Veterinary Orthopedics, Lea and Febiger, Philadelphia 1972.

O'BRIEN TR, MORGAN JP, SUTER PF. Epiphyseal plate injury in the dog: A radiographic study of growth disturbance in the forelimb. J Sm Anim Pract 12: 19-36,1971.

OLSON NC, CARRIG CB, BRINKER WO. Asynchronous growth of the canine radius and ulna; effects of retardation of longitudinal growth of the radius. Am J Vet Res 40:351-355,1979.

RISER WH, SHIRER JF. Normal and abnormal growth of the distal foreleg in large and giant dogs. J Am Vet Rad Soc 6:50-64,1965.

# Chapter 5

# Hip dysplasia

## Introduction

Dysplasia of the hip joint is another of the inherited developmental diseases of bone. It was the first of the developmental bone and joint diseases to be recognized and thus has been most widely studied in the dog. It was originally thought to affect only larger breeds, but now, it is known to occur in small, medium, large, and giant breeds. Hip dysplasia (HD) is not a congenital disease and cannot be diagnosed by conventional methods at birth (Henricson, et al 1966; Lust, et al 1973). Thus, the abbreviation CHD, refers to "canine hip dysplasia" and not "congenital hip dysplasia." The hips are normal at birth but uneven growth between the skeletal system and muscular system results in a femoral head that is forced out of the acetabular cup dorsally and laterally. The abnormal development of the hip joint is thought to be caused by a delay in development of muscle mass in conjunction with too rapid growth of the skeleton (Riser and Shirer 1967, Riser 1974). Subluxation of the femoral head occurs at an early age when the components of the joint are still cartilaginous and thus soft and malleable. This results in deformation of the acetabulum ("shallow" acetabulum) and modeling of the femoral head leading to the development of a painful osteoarthrosis. The course of the disease in a particular dog is influenced by growth rate (Lust, et al 1973; Hedhammer, et al 1974; Lust and Farrell 1977), body weight (Kealy, et al 1997), and pattern of exercise, as well as other environmental factors. With few exceptions, starting with the breeds with the highest percentage of hip dysplasia and progressing to the breeds with the lowest percentage of hip dysplasia, there is a gradual shift from poorly muscled giant breeds to those breeds that are well muscled (Riser and Larsen 1974).

Hip dysplasia is well recognized as a polygenic trait (Swenson, et al 1997) and this hereditary disease of the coxofemoral joint certainly belongs in this monograph of developmental bone diseases, because of the pattern of clinical signs, and the creation of a secondary osteoarthrosis that often is crippling. "More dogs are put to sleep because of HD and related orthopedic problems than for most other reasons outside of cancer and accidents" (Willis 1990).

## History

The term hip dysplasia means literally the faulty development of the hip and was first described in 1935 (Schnelle). The word dysplasia is formed from the Greek "dys," meaning abnormal, and the Greek "plassein," meaning to form. A more descriptive definition of CHD is "a varying degree of laxity of the hip joint permitting subluxation during early life, giving rise to varying degrees of shallow acetabulum and flattening of the femoral head, (and) finally inevitably leading to osteoarthritis" (Henricson, et al 1966). The impact of this disease on the dog world can be noticed by talking with any of the many owners who have seen the life of a promising field or show dog cut short by the disease. Reviewing data from observations on military working dogs indicates that in the past, hip dysplasia accounted for rejection of approximately 20% of the total number of dogs evaluated for procurement, and approximately 60% of the total number of dogs rejected for medical reasons (Stunkard, et al 1969; Olson 1971; Townsend 1972).

Strong evidence was found that the primary feature of hip dysplasia was a joint laxity present early in life (Månsson and Norberg 1961) that leads to subluxation of the femoral head resulting in the failure of the acetabulum to develop as a deep cup that would adequately hold the femoral head in position. Irregular modeling of the acetabular margin, femoral head, and femoral neck followed. All of these factors lead to the development of incongruous articular surfaces that caused development of a secondary osteoarthrosis. The early phase of the disease is typically an asymptomatic dysplasia characterized by a mild nonsuppurative synovitis characterized by: (1) an increased volume of synovial fluid, (2) thickening of synovium, (3) thickening of the joint capsule, (4) thickening of the round ligament of the femoral head, (5) prominence of the cartilaginous acetabular lip, and (6) focal degenerative articular cartilage lesions (Figure 5-1). Subluxation at this early age can not always be accurately detected radiographically using non-stressed techniques (Lust and Summers 1981, Morgan 1992, 1997).

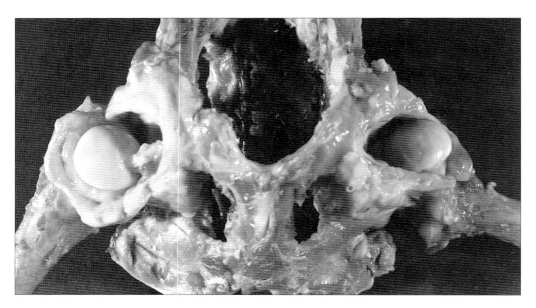
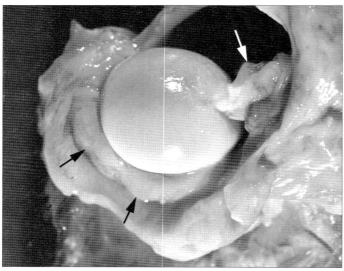

**Figure 5-1**
Photographs of a specimen with early features of hip dysplasia including thickening of the joint capsule, synovial hypertrophy (black arrows) and thickening and tearing of the round ligament of the femoral head (white arrow). These soft tissue changes are not identified on the radiograph made using non-stressed techniques.

Any factor that influences the proper fit of the femoral head into the acetabulum can, singly or in concert with other factors such as rapid body growth, cause development of an osteoarthrosis. One important factor in development of the osteoarthrosis is that the hip joint of the dog is placed under loads much greater than the superimposed body weight (Kealy, et al 1997). During a 3-legged stance without forward action, the hip joint of the dog is subjected to a force of almost 1.5 times the body weight (Arnoczky and Torzilli 1981). Thus, the femoral head is trapped with the body weight forcing downward while the muscle forces are pulling the head of the femur into the acetabulum, both causing a load on the joint surfaces.

Riser (1973 b) suggested that if a puppy were placed in a confining cage during the development of the hip joint, it would be forced to sit "on its haunches." In this position, the femoral head is forced into the acetabulum enhancing the development of a deep acetabular cup with a normally formed femoral head. It is interesting that treatment of suspect congenital hip dysplasia in children incorporates the placement of double or triple diapers that force the limbs into abduction, resulting in the femoral heads being "pushed" into the acetabula. Children treated early eventually develop a normal joint without joint instability or secondary osteoarthrosis. In the non-ambulatory child, there are no weight bearing forces on the hip, whereas the dog is ambulatory from the time of birth with progressively increasing weight-bearing forces. Unfortunately this conservative treatment used in children is not practical in the dog and by the time the disease is recognized, abnormal development of the acetabulum is well advanced.

Hip dysplasia might well be considered to be the result of a duel between weight-bearing forces and the maturation of cartilage to bone. If the cartilage can convert to bone forming a normal shaped hip joint prior to abnormal stresses being placed on the hip joint, dysplasia can be avoided. However, if the cartilage model becomes malformed prior to the final conversion to bone, the joint will be dysplastic. It has been suggested that delayed ossification of the femoral head often leads to the presence of CHD at an older age (Madsen, et al 1991, Todhunter, et al 1997).

Many have demonstrated that the rate of body growth in larger breeds influences the development of the hip joints (Riser, et al 1967; Lust, et al 1973, 1985; Hedhammer, et al 1974; Kasström 1975; Kealy, et al 1992). This is reported in studies of colonies of dogs that are assumed to have a genetic predisposition for HD. A slower rate of growth seems to provide an opportunity for more normal development of the hip joints, while more rapid body growth resulting from a higher energy level within the diet results in a higher frequency of dysplasia. It was also noted that with a rapid weight gain caused by increased caloric intake, the disease occurs earlier and is more severe. It is important to consider that rapid body growth can be influenced genetically as well as by the energy level of the diet in a particular dog.

The effect of diet has been studied in a smaller breed, the Beagle. It was shown that the inclusion or exclusion of carbohydrate in an otherwise nutritionally adequate diet did not statistically influence the frequency of hip dysplasia in female beagles, nor did the 2-fold elevation of dietary protein significantly alter the frequency of hip dysplasia (Tvedten, et al 1977). These factors did not alter the energy level of the diet. This supported the concept that it is the energy level in the diet and not a particular aspect of the formulation that influences the development of HD in genetically predisposed breeds.

In a conference on comparative pathology of arthritis and rheumatism, Riser (1987) described how Lent C. Johnson proposed that HD was a biomechanical disease resulting from a disparity between primary muscle mass and too rapid skeletal growth. He proposed that a lag or failure of the muscle to develop and to reach functional maturity at the same rate as the skeleton allowed a major joint like the hip (which depends on muscle power for stability) to pull apart, triggering a series of events that terminated in hip dysplasia and osteoarthrosis. This idea received further support when a comparison of muscle mass between the greyhound, German Shepherd Dog, and the July hound showed marked differences that cor-

responded with the frequency of dysplasia noted within the three breeds. The higher the muscle mass, the more normal was the development of the hip joints. This was recently reconfirmed in a study that further analyzed earlier data in which pelvic muscle mass was greatest in Greyhounds and least in German Shepherd Dogs (Cardinet III, et al 1997).

The iliopsoas muscle is one of the most powerful muscles in the entire body. The two major components are the iliacus arising from the cranial iliac fossa and medial border of the cranial iliac spine and the psoas major arising from the transverse processes of the lumbar vertebrae and surrounding structures. A single muscle belly attaches to the lesser trochanter of the femur. It is the only muscle attached to the lumbar spine, pelvis, and femur. Because it is hidden within the abdomen and pelvis, it has received scant attention. It would seem strange if a muscle possessing such breadth and power did not have an important function and that it did not contribute substantially to disorders of the hip joint. The role of the iliopsoas has been well described in man (Michele 1962; van Dyke, et al 1987). The psoas minor muscle, which inserts on the iliopectineal eminence in man, is not a part of the iliopsoas muscle in the dog. Insufficient length of the iliopsoas muscle due to failure to keep pace with skeletal growth, causes deleterious pressure on the hip joint including the femoral head, acetabulum, and joint capsule, resulting in subluxation.

The pectineus muscle takes origin from the pelvis and inserts on the medial aspect of the femur distally. If this muscle falls behind the bone in development and becomes effectively shortened, the abnormal muscle pull on the femur participates with the iliopsoas muscle in causing subluxation of the femoral head (Bardens and Hardwick 1968). Abnormal histologic composition of the pectineal muscle in the young dog has been interpreted to indicate that the resulting affected muscle growth would result in hip joint laxity and thus may be an important associative or causal factor in development of hip dysplasia (Ihemelandu, et al 1983).

In summary, if the length of the femur increases rapidly, the growth of the muscles, especially the pectineus and the iliopsoas can fall behind. This creates an abnormal tension on the hip joints resulting in subluxation of the femoral head (Bowen, et al 1972).

The idea that skeletal growth can exceed muscle growth is also suggested by a study of normally fed Beagle dogs. Certain families in this small breed have a high frequency of dysplasia (Morgan 1974). Examination of the growth curve as determined by body weight shows that a growth spurt begins at 10 days and is complete at 200 days with a similar rate of growth noted throughout this time period. The increase in wet skeletal weight follows a similar curve with an increase beginning at 10 days and leveling off at 200 days. More importantly, the weight of the wet skeleton determined as a percentage of body weight shows a maximum at 40 days of age that slowly decreases on a downward curve that continues until the time of death. These figures indicate that the growth curve stops at an earlier age in the Beagle than in the larger breeds and that the skeletal growth is much more rapid than body growth. Thus, an opportunity presents itself in which the skeleton seems to "outgrow" the body during an early period in the life of the dog (Goldman 1970) thus placing unusual forces on the developing hip joint.

The manner of development of hip dysplasia can vary in the various breeds. It has been shown in a study of Rottweilers and German Shepherd Dogs that a difference in disease susceptibility between breeds can in part be explained by differences in conformation and the amount of pelvic muscle mass. It is thought that the conversion of passive to functional laxity within the hip joint triggers the onset of osteoarthrosis and can be influenced by body weight and conformation. The GSD has less muscle mass and a higher frequency of dysplasia (Popovitch, et al 1995). This report only stresses the effect of muscle mass and strength of the dog and does not incorporate the importance of a comparison between skeletal and muscle growth rates.

These ideas appears to be a continuation of early thinking that "the development of hip dysplasia is dependent on the amount of inherited pelvic muscle mass or strength each dog possesses to prevent subluxation of the femoral head" (Riser 1975).

Another interesting feature in the history of this disease is how positive were investigators in the early years that with selective control of breeding, the frequency of dysplasia could be decreased rather quickly (Carlson 1961, Olsson 1963). How incorrectly they guessed is the level of dedication of the average dog owner toward the elimination of this disease.

## Affected breeds

HD is identified in the majority of breeds of dogs (Larsen and Corley 1972, Corley 1983, Corley and Hogan 1985). However, it tends to occur more frequently in larger, faster-growing breeds (Priester and Mulvihill 1972; Lust, et al 1973; Freudiger, et al 1973; Corley 1987; Kealy, et al 1992). It is present but seldom a clinical problem in dogs with a mature weight of under 12 kg especially in those with short limbs. If present in those dogs, it is underdetected because of the absence of clinical signs. For example, dysplasia was studied in groups of colony Beagle dogs without obvious clinical signs with an incidence of up to 37% (Morgan 1974; Preu, et al 1975).

The Saint Bernard has the greatest risk of dysplasia while the collie appears to be the only large dog without significant risk (Priester and Mulvihill 1972). The frequency of dysplasia in the Saint Bernard was reported by the OFA to be 47.4% in the United States (Corley and Hogan 1985, Corley 1987). Twenty-four other breeds had frequency in excess of 20% as reported by the OFA. Greyhounds and other sight-hounds have a low frequency and this is possibly because of long standing selective breeding for speed. While breed frequency appears to be influenced by the expected use of the dog, this does not always hold true. A breed of working dog (Yugoslavian Sheep Dog, Sarplaninac) selectively bred for use as a sheep dog had a 25% frequency of HD. Why such a working breed that is being bred for function should have such a high frequency of HD is confusing (Petrovic, et al 1972). In another study, companion dogs bred from a population of Australian Shepherd working dogs were also reported to have a high frequency of HD (Pharr and Morgan, 1976).

While most think of HD in the closely bred dog, it should be understood that the disease exists in crossbreeds as well. A particularly interesting study was the discovery of 42% dysplasia within seven litters of German Shepherd Dog/Greyhound crossbreeds (Cardinet, et al 1983). While most reports of HD are within the breeds of dog in which man has been involved in breeding selection, nine of 14 closely related dingos (Warrigal, regarded by some as a subspecies of domestic dog introduced to Australia from Asia during the later migration of the aborigines perhaps 5000 to 8000 years ago) were diagnosed radiographically to be dysplastic (Christoph, et al 1969).

## Prevalence of hip dysplasia

General information relative to the distribution of HD throughout the dog world can be gained by referring to a report on the control of the disease in Switzerland over the past 24 years where 42% of all purebred dogs remain affected despite control programs for the last 30 years (Flückiger, et al 1995). It is suggested that breeding dysplastic dogs and the failure to study the status of the progeny in the selection of breeding stock are responsible for this lack of progress. Information can be gained by examination of Swedish data from the years 1976 until 1988. During this time, the frequency of dysplasia can be seen to remain high even though some decrease has been seen to result from the radiographic control of breeding dogs. The frequency of dysplasia decreased: (1) in the German Shepherd Dog from 35% to 21%, (2) in the Rottweiler from 36% to 18%, and (3) in the Labrador Retriever from 25% to 15%. In the Saint Bernard, on the other hand, the frequency of dysplasia remained near 60% throughout this period (Swenson 1987; Swenson, et al 1997).

The prevalence is dependent on the sex and HD is significantly more frequent in female than in male German Shepherd Dogs, Golden Retrievers, and Saint Bernards (Henricson and Olsson 1959; Hedhammar Å, et al 1979; Swenson, et al 1997). The sex related difference in prevalence could be explained by a direct effect of genes on the sex chromosomes. However, a more plausible explanation is an effect of secondary sex characteristics coded by genes on the sex chromosomes such as difference in growth rate, sex hormones, or behavioral patterns (Swenson, et al 1997).

## Clinical signs

The diagnosis of hip dysplasia is primarily based on the owner's history of the behavior of the dog plus the clinical and radiographic findings. Techniques used in diagnosis are somewhat dependent on the age of the patient, however, at all ages, the owner's clinical history is always important in suggesting the diagnosis of hip dysplasia. The findings on physical and radiographic examination are of particular importance (Fry and Clark 1992) (Table 5-1).

### Table 5-1: Diagnosis of hip dysplasia based on:

**I.** Owner's history
    A. Gait abnormality
    B. Behavior pattern
    C. Perceived pain in the hip joints
**II.** Clinical findings of joint laxity
**III.** Radiographic diagnosis

Clinical signs can only be discussed in general since they vary so widely between individual dogs and often can be completely absent throughout life in a large number of dogs. Since many affected dogs show no signs indicative of disease that are recognized by the owner, many affected dogs are not examined clinically (Figure 5-2). Even when clinical signs are present, it is difficult to predict the clinical course of the disease (Tomlinson and McLaughlin 1996 a). Clinical signs also vary widely with the age of the dog (Table 5-2).

### Table 5-2: Clinical stages of hip dysplasia

**I.** Puppy stage
    A. Gait can vary widely
        1. Altered gait that is
            a. Painless
            b. Painful
        2. Clinically normal gait
**II.** Pre-adolescent syndrome
    A. Acutely painful joint
    B. Joint instability
**III.** Young dog
    A. Painful joint
    B. Joint instability
**IV.** Young adult dog
    A. Joint disease
        1. Osteoarthrosis
        2. Joint instability
    B. Much less painful joint
**V..** Older adult dog with osteoarthrosis
    A. Altered gait
    B. Chronic joint pain

Radiographic diagnosis is of less value in the puppy and pre-adolescent because of the incomplete ossification of the bones. Thus, in these ages, physical examination is a most important means for diagnosis. Later, in the young dog (>6 months), radiographs become a much more valuable in diagnosis. Stress radiographs may be helpful in diagnosis in the younger dog (Smith, et al 1998).

### Clinical signs in the puppy (Table 5-3)

Pain on palpation of the hips or pain while walking is noted in only a few puppies during the first few months of life. This absence of pain occurs in puppies that can be affected with severe disease later in life. Instead of demonstrating a painful hip joint, this young puppy during the "painless" phase of the disease can express the presence of the disease by showing an altered gait. Others are simply weak in the hind limbs or want to avoid pain and thus are slow to walk or use the hind limbs. The puppy can appear tired and sit and watch littermates play but not join in the physical activities.

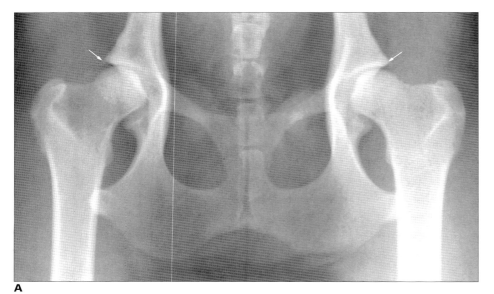
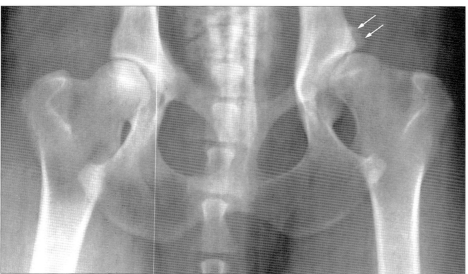

**Figure 5-2**
Radiographs indicate the presence of hip dysplasia in dogs that the owners had assumed to be clinically normal. (A) The owner of this happy and active 18-month-old female Australian Shepherd was surprised to learn that she was affected bilaterally with hip dysplasia characterized by joint laxity and reactive change on the acetabular margins (arrows). (B) This 3-year-old male Rhodesian Ridgeback was presented by the owner with a normal clinical history. The dog was to be radiographed so he "could be judged normal" and used for breeding. The unilateral dysplasia on the left was characterized by subluxation of the femoral head, flattening of the acetabulum, and reactive new bone on the acetabular margin (arrows).

**Table 5-3: Clinical signs seen in puppies with hip dysplasia**

I. Gait
    A. Weak in the hind limbs
    B. Wobbles while walking
    C. "Bunny hops" rather than trots
    D. Stands with hind limbs close together

II. Activity
    A. Sits and watches litter mates play
    B. Runs for a short distance and then sits
    OR

III. Normal gait

IV. Physically active

---

Observation of the standing puppy can be helpful in suggesting the presence of hip dysplasia. By 3 to 4 months of age, the affected puppy, when viewed from the rear, can appear to be broad through the hip area but "caved in" through the thigh and stifle area due to lack of muscle development. When standing, the hind limbs can be close or perhaps even crossed. While these are descriptions of findings of HD in the puppy, their presence is not pathognomonic of hip dysplasia, but may reflect only the action of a young clumsy puppy.

In this "pain free" stage of joint disease, a mild nonsuppurative synovitis, increased volume of synovial fluid, increased size of the round ligament of the femoral head, and focal degenerative articular cartilage lesions are present (Lust, et al 1980; Lust and Summers 1981). Thus, while the dog is without obvious pain, early pathologic changes are present within the joint (Figure 5-1).

Often the owner presents the slightly older puppy because of lameness or pain noticed when the puppy lays down, jumps into the car, or climbs stairs. These signs are often present during the acute stage of the disease when the dog is approximately 6 months of age. Now, the painful dog with HD continues to stand with the hind limbs close together and tucked under the body. Additional clinical signs indicate an altered gait best seen when the dog is run in a large grassy area. At this age, movement is painful and the animal tries to limit motion in the hip joint (Table 5-2). This is accomplished frequently by using an exaggerated movement of the pelvis to become a part of the stride. By swaying the pelvis from side to side as the dog runs, the hind limbs do not need to be extended forward as much as would otherwise be required. At a pace slightly faster than a walk, the animal has a tendency to go over into a hopping gait with both hind limbs being moved forward simultaneously. This is referred to as "bunny hopping" and provides for a longer stride by shifting the pelvis "under the dog" while reaching cranially with the hind feet. This type of movement places increased stress on the lumbosacral disc. Some giant breeds as the Newfoundland and Saint Bernard can extend the length of the stride additionally through hyperextension of the tarsal joints in order to limit the required range of motion in the painful hip joint causing the dog to appear that it has weak hock joints. When this is seen in both hind limbs it is indicative of bilateral hip disease.

In the young dog prior to development of marked osteoarthrosis, joint laxity can be felt by putting one's hands over the dog's hips as it walks. In the affected joint, the femoral head moves into and out of the acetabulum. Actually, it can be possible in the severely affected puppy to visualize the femoral head as it "pops" in and out of the acetabular cup as the puppy walks and runs. Muscle development of the pelvic limbs is lacking in the affected puppy, while thoracic limb musculature can be well developed because of the increased stress from shifting weight to the front. Because of the frequently bilateral nature of the disease, this muscle atrophy is not easily appreciated and a comparison needs be made with the muscular development in the thoracic limb by means of palpation.

## Clinical signs in the preadolescent

As the puppy ages, an acute phase can occur during the period of rapid growth of the dog that might be referred to as a preadolescent syndrome. Many puppies have a rapid burst of growth between 4 to 6 months of age with increased body weight. In addition, physical activity is greatly increased. Pain can be evident upon arising, climbing, or jumping and the dog can object to palpation or even petting of the hindquarters. In fact, the dog can be so affected as to have difficulty in getting up and, when lying down, it "plops" down rather than lying down quietly. If a puppy is from a large breed, it might growl when approached by children intending to ride on the dog's back (Riser 1973 b).

These clinical findings are the result of the changes that occur in the cartilage of the acetabular rim. "The rim is rounded as the result of the delay of chondrogenesis and osteogenesis. Overloading forces on the acetabular rim have delayed the conversion of fibrocartilage to hyaline cartilage and then to bone" (Riser 1973 b). The pain, shown by crying out on movement of the limb during palpation, is probably due to early injury within the rim of the acetabulum. This results from repeated stresses of the loosely fitting femoral head that exceeds the elastic limits of the bone and cartilage (Riser 1973 b, 1975). Painful microfractures can occur at this time within the acetabular rim leading the puppy to suddenly appear to be in pain. Pain shown by lameness can also be due to abnormal stresses placed on the soft tissue components of the hip joint such as the joint capsule and round ligament of the femoral head (Table 5-4).

### Table 5-4: Cause of pain in the dysplastic hip joint

**I.** In the immature dog
    A. Abnormal maturation of the acetabular rim (microfractures)
    B. Stress on soft tissues (joint laxity)

**II.** In the adult dog
    A. Chronic synovitis
    B. Osteoarthrosis

The earliest age at which a puppy can be profitably examined for joint laxity suggestive of hip dysplasia is debatable. Most clinicians are not comfortable in making such an examination prior to 6 months of age. This is because the physical examination is compromised by the behavior of a young puppy in the clinic. Although the examination can be performed following the use of sedation or anesthesia, many owners and clinicians are reluctant to do this. If laxity is detected either in the awake or sedated puppy, its significance is commonly questionable. Is it: (1) a true joint laxity and of what clinical significance, (2) a forced laxity, or (3) an undetected laxity present and not evident because of the gentleness of the examiner. In other words, if joint laxity is detected, is this a sign of dysplasia or just a "normal growing puppy" with "loose" joints? Some clinicians feel the detection of joint laxity can simply be the result of the strength of the examiner when compared to the small size of the puppy and therefore, it is a false positive finding. If palpation is performed without anesthesia, the presence of pain can prevent the detection of joint laxity because of a fear of continuing the physical examination, especially if the palpation is performed by a gentle person. Still, palpation of the puppy with considerable joint laxity due to disease should not be ignored since it can lead to an accurate diagnosis of hip dysplasia at an age of 6 months.

Recently, a distraction index (DI) has been determined in 2 and 4 months old German Shepherd Dogs in an effort to evaluate early radiographic diagnosis. Passive hip joint laxity at 4 months of age was highly correlated with a DI at 24 months of age and early DI was the principal factor associated with development of osteoarthrosis (Smith, et al 1993). The DI was not sufficiently reliable to predict what the DI might be at 4 months of age or 12 months of age (Smith, et al 1993, 1998). These studies are only of one breed and findings may vary from those noted in the German Shepherd Dog.

## Clinical signs in the young dog

In the young dog with hip dysplasia that is 6 to 12 months of age, joint laxity can be recognized radiographically or by palpation. Combining the two techniques in examination of the hip joints is valuable. The radiographic examination can include both neutral and stressed techniques to better determine the extent of movement of the femoral head within the acetabulum. If only the neutrally positioned radiographic examination is used, joint laxity may not be detected using this technique and palpation of the joints is necessary to achieve a thorough examination of the hips. Pain can be evident at this age both during walking and on palpation of the hips, however, the degree of pain can vary from severe to almost nonexistent. Crepitus as an indicator of osteoarthrosis is probably still not present at this age. The gait remains essentially as seen in the younger puppy, with "bunny hopping," pelvic swaying, and decreased excursion of the hip joint.

As the puppy ages, it is possible that other diseases can cause similar clinical signs. These include commonly occurring traumatic injury to the pelvis and hip joints and a generalized bone disease seen commonly in the young adult dog called panosteitis. This inflammatory disease causes a swelling of the periosteal covering over the bone so that when the long bones are grasp in examination of the hip joint, the pain elicited can erroneously be thought to originate from the hip joint. Hip joint infection could cause similar clinical signs but this is an uncommon cause of disease in the puppy. It is possible for these diseases to be present in a dog with normal hip joints where they cause clinical signs similar to those seen in hip dysplasia. Or, they may to be present in conjunction with hip dysplasia, in which case they may cause an increase in clinical signs or a change in the character of the clinical signs. Differential diagnosis for a sudden hind limb lameness or a change in the lameness of a dog with hip dysplasia are listed (Table 5-5).

**Table 5-5: Differential diagnosis for a sudden onset of hind limb lameness in what was thought to be a normal dog or an increase in the degree of lameness in a dog which has had clinical signs of hip dysplasia all its life**

I. In a young dog
    A. Panosteitis (common)
    B. Cranial cruciate ligament rupture (rare)

II. In an adult dog
    A. Cranial cruciate ligament rupture (common)
    B. Idiopathic myelopathy of German Shepherd Dogs (common)
    C. Cauda equina syndrome (common)
    D. Lumbosacral disc disease (common)
    E. Acute infection in one of the hips (rare)
    F. Bone or soft tissue tumor (rare)
    G. Panosteitis (rare)

## Clinical signs in the adult dog

Clinical signs in the adult dog result from a painful osteoathrosis in the hip and are chronic in nature. The signs can appear acutely after either a brisk run or prolonged exercise and are probably due to injury to the soft tissues, with an acute exacerbation of the existing synovitis that was not evident in the resting dog. The dog can evince stiffness of the limbs after periods of rest, however, it will "warm out" of the stiffness, although the stride remains shortened. A continued tendency for "bunny-hopping" persists, as was seen in puppies, since this form of movement of the pelvic limbs decreases the range of movement of the femoral head within the malformed acetabulum through maximum utilization of the lumbosacral joint. Because of the discomfort and pain, the adult dog sits rather than stands when it stops. With time, the thigh muscles can atrophy because pain results in restriction of their use.

While a pattern of clinical signs can be described in a dog with hip dysplasia (Table 5-6), many dogs have a clinical history that varies widely from this pattern.

## Clinical signs of lumbosacral disease

Lumbosacral disease is a particular problem in the adult dog because the clinical signs of a dog affected with chronic hip dysplasia can be similar to those noted in a dog with lumbosacral disease. The disease is caused most commonly by dorsal protrusion of a degenerating LS disc. Diagnosis is complicated by the fact that both dis-

**Table 5-6: Frequent pattern of clinical signs in the course of hip dysplasia**

I. Pain
    A. Often pain free until 5 to 6 months of age
    B. Acute pain develops at 6 months of age
    C. Decreased but comfortable range of motion of the hind limbs
    D. Increased discomfort especially on rising and on exercise at 6 to 7 years
    E. Most hip joint motion painful over 8 years of age

II. Abnormal gait persists throughout adult life
    A. "Bunny hopping"
    B. Pelvic swaying
    C. Decreased caudal extension of hind limbs
        1. Difficult for dog to jump
        2. Difficult for dog to climb stairs
    D. Altered gait

III. Joint instability
    A. Visible or palpable joint instability until 12 to 18 months of age
    B. Joint becomes more stable with onset of osteoarthrosis

V. Osteoarthrosis
    A. Starts slowly during first year
    B. Radiographically evident after 12 months
    C. Causes the acute phase of pain to disappear
    D. Causes joint to become stable

eases are common in the larger breeds as the dog ages and the two conditions can be seen concurrently. Many dogs with dysplasia avoid maximum use of the hind limbs by altering their gait to include "bunny hopping." To accomplish this, the dog relies more on excessive movement of the lumbosacral joint that achieves a cranial placement of the feet while running. By moving the pelvis in this manner, the dog is able to accomplish a near-normal stride of the hind limbs through this exaggerated motion of the lumbosacral joints. This decreases the level of the pain in the hip joints, however, it places unusual stress on the lumbosacral joint and can cause early degeneration of the intervertebral disc at this location. This is one frequent scenario that explains how both LS lesions and hip dysplasia can be found in the same dog.

Regardless of the cause of the LS lesion, a cascading of events can result: (1) degeneration of the lumbosacral disc, (2) formation of heavy bone, referred to as spondylosis deformans, ventral and lateral to the lumbosacral disc, (3) possible dorsal protrusion of the outer anulus fibrosus of the lumbosacral disc, and (4) thickening of the vertebral end plates. These events can lead to creation of instability and/or malalignment between the last lumbar segment and sacrum and can lead to spinal canal stenosis and the clinical signs referred to as the cauda equina syndrome. This syndrome is characterized by: difficulty to rise, tendency to bear weight cranially, disuse atrophy of the muscles in the hind limbs, pain on dorsal pressure over the lumbosacral region, and limitation of forward extension of the hind limbs. Some of these signs are similar to those seen in a dog with only osteoarthrosis in the hip joints due to dysplasia and therefore, the co-existence of lumbosacral disease is often overlooked and it behooves the clinician to examine the lumbosacral area especially in the older dog. In some dogs with lumbosacral disc disease. the cauda equina syndrome is characterized by more severe signs, such as: (1) an inability to elevate the tail, (2) loss of control over urination and defecation, and (3) an inability to flex the hind limbs as expected. These signs can make it easier to distinguish LS disease from hip dysplasia (Bailey and Morgan 1983, Morgan and Bailey 1990). (See Chapter 6).

### Clinical signs in the young dog

A congenital vertebral anomaly at the junction of the lumbar vertebrae and the sacrum can cause an even more rapid progression of the degenerative cycle of the LS disc just described. This vertebral anomaly can assume different appearances, but all are included in the term lumbosacral transitional vertebral segment (Morgan, et al 1968, 1997, 1999). The clinical significance of the lesion lies in the resulting instability and premature degeneration of the lumbosacral intervertebral disc, either of which can lead to spinal canal stenosis. While the anomaly is noted in all large breeds, it occurs frequently in German Shepherd Dogs (Morgan and Rosenblatt 1987). (See Chapter 6).

## Physical examination

The physical examination can be performed with the dog on its side or standing either on the floor or on a table. The size of the dog influences how the examination is to be performed, with the larger dog best examined on the floor. Examination of the dog on its side on a table may be the easiest for the clinician and the dog. The examination can be performed with the dog awake, sedated, or anesthetized. The owner, size, and behavior of the dog, and the time available for examination influence this decision. If you are forced to perform the examination with the dog awake, muscle tension may be strong and prevent detection of pain or abnormal joint movement. If the dog is sedated or anesthetized, greater muscle relaxation is obtained and the examination may be more accurate. Pain is still evident with the dog under sedation, while it is lost under anesthesia. Perhaps the best method of examination would be to accomplish as much as is possible with the dog awake, either standing or lying on its side, and then complete the examination at the time the dog is anesthetized for pelvic radiography.

Palpation during the physical examination permits a determination of the range of motion of the hip joint, detection of pain, and detection of crepitus. The joint can be examined by forcing the limb into: (1) extension and flexion, (2) abduction and adduction, and (3) internal and external rotation. During motion of the limb, crepitus or a feeling of roughened movement of the articular cartilage surfaces may be detected. Both indicate a joint with damage to the articular cartilage. The range of motion should be observed with any limitation indicating joint capsule thickening, however, in the awake dog the limitation may be due to pain. Specific movements of the hind limbs permit an evaluation of joint stability. These are discussed at great length in the paragraphs to follow.

If the dog is awake, the detection of pain during motion is a most important observation. However, in the puppy: (1) traumatic injury to the pelvis and hip joints or (2) panosteitis may also be pain producing. This inflammatory disease is painful and pain can easily be elicited by manipulation of the hind limbs. In the adult dog, painful hind limb movement can be caused by: (1) lumbosacral disease due to disc degeneration causing a cauda equina syndrome and (2) cranial cruciate ligament disease. It is possible that panosteitis can also be seen in older dogs. Consequently, the examination of the hip is performed selectively and the examiner should be aware that depending on the age, other pain-causing lesions may be present. It is necessary to: (1) avoid movement of the stifle (femorotibial) joint that might have painful cruciate ligament disease, (2) avoid grasping the femur that could be painful because of panosteitis, (3) avoid excessive movement of the lumbosacral joint because of a painful LS disc disease, and (4) avoid downward pressure on the back or pelvis of the standing dog, since pain elicited can originate either from the lumbosacral region, the hips, or stifle joints.

## Joint laxity as an indicator of hip dysplasia

Two methods are available for detection of joint laxity: palpation and radiography. It is probable that routine radiography has been too extensively relied upon for detection of joint laxity forgetting that the maximum movement of the femoral head within the acetabulum may not be demonstrated unless some form of distraction is placed on limbs during radiography. Also, joint laxity in some dogs can be hidden on the routine radiographic examination by deliberate attempts to position the hind limbs during radiography into external rotation so that the femoral head is repositioned into the acetabulum.

Detection of the laxity by physical palpation of the hip joint has been described in the past (Norberg 1961, 1962, 1963), however, in contrast to the permanency of the radiograph, owners are hesitant to accept the results of palpation that are: (1) not recorded radiographically, (2) cannot be reproduced at a later time, (3) cannot be reviewed by others, and (4) are not objective. Because of these problems, palpation for the detection of dysplasia has not received the attention it deserves. Also, a fear exists on the part of both the owner and the examiner that it is possible to damage the hip joints in a puppy during palpation, and thus palpation is inadequately performed (ie, performed too gently).

Another problem in palpation has been the thought that the female in heat can have greater joint laxity that is temporary and is not a true reflection of the status of the hip joints. Significant fluxations of estrogen and progesterone occur throughout the phases of the estrous cycle. High estrogen levels (estradiol -17) are present during proestrus while progesterone levels are elevated in diestrous. A comparison of both distraction radiographic techniques (distraction index) and standard Olsson positioning for radiography (Norberg angle) in nine dogs did not document a physiologic joint laxity at the time of estrous (Hassinger, et al 1997). This is contrary to an earlier study that, while unable to demonstrate statistically significant changes in hip laxity associated with estrous, reported a "trend toward coxofemoral subluxation during estrous" (Keller, et al 1993).

The question of whether palpation should be performed in the awake, anesthetized, or sedated patient has not been completely answered. While it is assumed that the examiner has the strength to overcome any resistance to palpation by the muscles in most dogs, in the large adult, anesthesia can be required in an effort to determine the complete range of motion of the femoral head. Stress radiography performed under general anesthesia is probably the most diagnostic technique.

This only discusses some of the problems in palpation and is not meant to suggest that palpation should be ignored, since in the hands of a skilled examiner, true joint laxity is indicative of an abnormal hip.

Early studies by Norberg (1961) did not demonstrate any laxity within the joints at necropsy until about 2 weeks of age. At that age, joint laxity was the first abnormality detected in the dysplastic hip, and it was thought at that time that any technique that positively identified early abnormal laxity would be of great value. Even with the positive detection of joint instability, it is still necessary to establish the degree of laxity beyond which clinical significance is to be attached. Difficulties lie in the area of determining the range of normal laxity and whether this range changes with the age and breed of the puppy or perhaps with the level of muscular development. The older the dog, the easier it is to accept findings of joint laxity as being abnormal and indicative of HD (Smith, et al 1998).

The problem of determining the degree of laxity seems to have been solved, at least in part, by a study in Labrador Retrievers using a compression/distraction technique. This study determined the range of motion of the femoral head from the acetabulum between radiographs made under compression and with distraction (Lust, et al 1993). The index was determined by comparing the two resulting measurements. Normal adults were evaluated to have an index of $0.29 \pm 0.05$ while the dysplastic adults had an index of $0.60 \pm 0.10$. An index of 0.0 indicates that there is no lateral movement of the femoral head detected between the two studies. Any increase in the index indicates an increasing degree of joint laxity. Puppies from normal to normal and dysplastic to dysplastic matings were evaluated at 4 months of age. Those from N x N matings were found to have an index of $0.39 \pm 0.07$ while those from D x D matings were found to have an index of $0.54 \pm 0.04$. It was felt that "distraction indexes between 0.4 and 0.7 were not associated strongly enough with evidence of disease to be clinically reliable in predicting, on an individual basis, the outcome for dysplastic hip conformation when the dogs were older." However, an "index > 0.7 was associated with high probability for developing dysplastic joints and an index < 0.4 predicted normal hips with high probability." In another report, the distraction index was felt to be the most significant determinant of the risk to develop osteoarthrosis of the coxofemoral joint and was thought to be more reliable than the Norberg angle, which has been used in an effort to determine lateral movement of the femoral head as seen on a single, neutrally-positioned radiographic study (Smith, et al 1995).

Generally, it is agreed that laxity in the hip joints in puppies determined through palpation, wedge technique, or by compression/distraction studies is correlated in a positive manner with the radiographic evidence of development of osteoarthrosis in the adults (Lust, et al 1972, 1993; Smith, et al 1995). This strongly supports the concept that joint laxity is an indicator of hip dysplasia.

But, it was also recognized that dogs with minimal laxity can grow to have a normal functioning hip that would be classed normal radiographically, however, the offspring of these dogs might be genotypically dysplastic. Therefore, any technique that tests the stability of the hip joints in addition to examining for secondary bony changes adds information as to the status of the hip joints. The question is what to do with this additional information especially when the laxity is found in a dog with otherwise "normal" radiographic studies. While determination of minimal joint laxity is helpful, knowledge of the status of the hips of the littermates (full or half siblings) and progeny is necessary in the determination of whether small degrees of joint laxity are of genetic importance. This was understood early (Olsson 1974). Obviously, a difference exists in the significance of laxity in a pet when compared with a similar degree of laxity in a potential breeding animal.

**Bardens' technique**

Giardina and MacCarthy (1971) were early in their description of a technique of palpation to determine joint laxity. More complete descriptions of what came to be known as the Bardens' sign followed (Bardens and Hardwick 1968; Bardens 1972 a, b). The 8- to 12-week-old anesthetized puppy was positioned on its side with the pelvis at a right angle to the tabletop. With the acetabula superimposed, the femur to be studied was placed uppermost at a right angle to the spine, and parallel to the tabletop. The thumb was placed on the tuber ischium and the second finger was placed on the wing of the ilium to firmly hold the pelvis in position. The relaxed index finger was placed on the lateral aspect of the greater trochanter so as to detect its upward movement. The middle third of the femur was grasped with the other hand and lifted straight upward with the arm held stiff. In the normal joint, the index finger remained stable, while elevation of the index finger indicated lateral movement of the femoral head and thus, abnormal joint laxity.

A second technique to study the character of the hip joint tested the range of abduction of the hind limb. This method required the dog to be placed on its back with the femurs positioned perpendicular to the vertebral column. The femurs were then permitted to fall laterally (abduction). In the normal puppy, the distal end of the femurs falls to a point between a finger's width of touching the tabletop. Failure to achieve this degree of lateral motion was thought to be due to tightness of the pectineus muscle and recorded as abnormal (Bardens 1972 a, b). In our experience, this description holds true for predisposed breeds, however, it does not apply for the giant breeds, especially the Great Dane. In this breed, abduction of the hind limbs in the normal dog is much more limited. In certain of the smaller breeds, such as the Dachshund, abduction is extreme in dogs with hips that develop normally.

Studies that evaluated the accuracy of palpation of the puppy relied on conformation of the disease by radiographic evaluation of the hip joints at an older age using either joint laxity or early osteoarthrosis as indicative of dysplasia. Since radiographic diagnosis is not without error, these reports must be considered with that knowledge. Giardina and MacCarthy (1971) reported 87% accuracy in detection of abnormal hip joints using palpation of the hips and decreased abduction of the limbs in anesthetized puppies at 7 to 9 weeks when those findings were compared with the radiographic evaluations made at 1 year of age. In another study, only 65% of dogs diagnosed as abnormal by palpation were found to be abnormal radiographically at 1 year of age or older using signs of osteoarthrosis as an indicator of disease (Lust, et al 1973).

Bardens (1972 a) stated the problem of palpation clearly: "The biggest question in my mind today is how much joint laxity does one allow in a puppy as being normal." His experience was that "a truly normal puppy and adult has no joint laxity." In 389 puppies in which 1 or 2 mm of laxity was present at 8 weeks, a normal radiograph was obtained in all puppies at 1 year of age using the standard VD view. However, with use of the wedge view that created distraction of the femoral head, all of these dogs revealed abnormal joint laxity. Therefore, minimal joint laxity noted in a puppy did not result in the development of secondary bony changes that could be detected by that investigator by 1 year of age and a distraction technique was required to make the determination of joint laxity radiographically. However, at 3 years of age, 189 of the 389 dogs had joint laxity and changes of osteoarthrosis on both the standard and wedge view. However, more than one half of the dogs, thought to have minimal joint laxity as a puppy, did not have signs of osteoarthrosis of joint laxity on either a neutral or distraction radiographic study at 3 years.

His study illustrated some of the problems inherent in searching for the correct interpretation of joint laxity as determined by palpation of puppies. The first problem is to appreciate the skill of the examiner necessary to accurately detect the minimal laxity. The second problem is to appreciate the accuracy in positioning and evaluation required in reaching a radiographic diagnosis that is to be used as the confirming study. At the time of these early reports, a complete understanding of the radiographic changes of hip dysplasia and the exact positioning required for these studies was lacking. But, the use of the distraction studies (wedge techniques) was shown to be of great value in confirming the accuracy of the palpation and this was especially helpful to the unskilled examiner.

In the hands of many investigators, palpation has not always been an accurate technique. Of puppies predicted normal by palpation, 15% became dysplastic on later radiographic studies (Bardens 1972 b). Others have found that 51% of dogs predicted to be normal by palpation at 7 to 11 weeks of age, were found to be abnormal when radiographed at 1 year of age or older (Lust, et al 1973). In other studies, Giardina and MacCarthy (1971) reported errors of 7.5% and 20% on puppies palpated between 4 and 10 weeks while Wright and Mason (1977) reported errors of 24.2% and 20% on puppies palpated at 6 to 8 weeks and Lust, et al (1972) simply reported that the data did not correlate significantly with subsequent radiographs. A study by Goddard and Mason (1982) found an accuracy of prediction of HD through palpation of puppies to be only 46%. These studies using Bardens' techniques have shown the possibility of false negative findings. This suggests that the techniques lacked specificity as well as sensitivity.

Others have questioned whether moderate hip joint instability (determined by palpation) is enough of a disorder to cause hip dysplasia especially if the pelvis is wide and relatively horizontal. In one study, a group of 33 puppies of 6 litters were palpated and radiographed with the conclusion that laxity was "not a reliable diagnostic or prognostic sign." "However, tightness of the joints was a good prognostic sign indicating that normal hip joints would develop" (Olsson and Kasström, 1972). Others reported similar problems in the use of joint laxity as a predictive factor for hip dysplasia (Samuelson 1972; Lust, et al 1973).

In spite of variation in correlation between the finding of joint laxity and the later diagnosis of hip dysplasia, palpation should not be ignored and the detection of joint laxity by palpation can be used simply as an encouragement for subsequent re-examination of the dog. Certainly, joint laxity should not be ignored when making a prediction of the future status of the hips. While some have felt that selection of breeding stock based on palpation was not as good in the reduction of the percentage of dogs in the population with HD as was the use of a more conventional radiographic technique (Goddard and Mason 1982), others have more recently proven that use of a distraction index as a measure of joint laxity is a more accurate method of selection of unaffected breeding stock (Smith, et al 1993).

In the discussion of the value of palpation, the goal of the technique should be appreciated. In the puppy with a future as a pet, minimal joint laxity can disappear in the adult resulting in a clinically healthy dog indicating that joint laxity does not always lead to the development of an adult dog with painful hips. The highly selective breeder, however, can appropriately use the detection of joint laxity to eliminate certain dogs from a breeding program, recognizing that minimal joint laxity in the puppy may be an indicator of hip dysplasia and should be selected against. In the puppy to be trained as a working dog, in which the decision relative to the investment of large sums of money for training is important, the finding of joint laxity can be a decisive finding.

## Ortolani technique

Another method of detection of joint laxity is to elicit the Ortolani sign (Ortolani 1937). In palpation of the normal hip joint, the femoral head remains within the acetabulum and there is no outward sign indicating joint laxity (Figure 5-3). The positive Ortolani sign is generated in the dysplastic joint as the femoral head slips forcefully from a dorsally subluxated position as it returns into the acetabulum (Figure 5-4) (Månsson and Norberg 1961; Henricson, et al 1966; Charlman and Butler 1985). A positive Ortoloni sign is an indicator of femoral head luxation and is accepted as being a sign of dysplasia. It is an accurate technique to use in the dog following ossification of the acetabular rim.

This maneuver is easiest performed with the dog in dorsal recumbency, with the femurs perpendicular to the tabletop. This position is near that described for use in the compression/distraction technique used in radiography and places the limbs in a position that permits demonstation of any displacement of the femoral head (Heyman, et al 1993). With one's hands placed around the flexed stifle joint, the femur is adducted and a force applied to the stifle joint is directed toward the tabletop. This causes the femoral head to slip out of the acetabulum in a joint with abnormal laxity. A feeling of "sliding" can be felt on exit by the femoral head in some hips. The femur is then abducted and a "popping" or "clicking" sensation is felt as the head returns into the acetabulum in the affected dog (Figure 5-4).

Some confusion exists as to which movement generates the Ortolani sign. The original description described the sensation or sound felt as the head returns to the

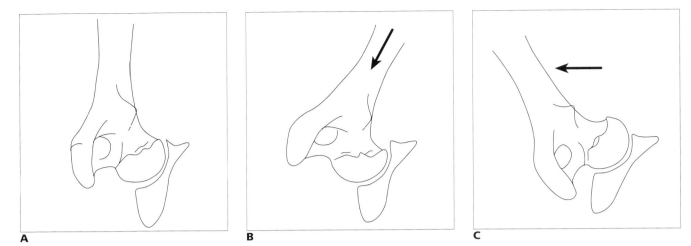

**Figure 5-3**
Drawings of the femoral head as it articulates with the acetabulum in a normal hip joint illustrate a negative Ortolani maneuver. The dog is positioned in dorsal recumbency with the femurs at a 90° angle to the tabletop. (A) The femoral head rests adjacent to the acetabulum in a neutral position. (B) When a force is applied downward on the stifle joint with the limb adducted, the femoral head remains within the acetabulum in a normal joint. (C) When the femur is abducted, the femoral head continues to remain within the acetabulum and no evidence of abnormal movement of the head is noted.

acetabulum. A modification of the Ortolani sign was later described. This was a feeling noted when attempting to luxate the femoral head. "If the femoral head slips out over the posterior lip of the acetabulum and back again immediately," this sensation is indicative of a hip joint that is unstable. This was called Barlow's sign (Barlow 1962).

Position of the femur is critical in performing this technique. A slight cranial positioning of the stifle joint places the femoral head adjacent to the normally underdeveloped caudodorsal portion of the acetabular rim. Since there is only minimal coverage of the head by the acetabulum at this location it may not be possible to produce the clicking sound on re-entry of the subluxated head. With a slight caudal positioning of the stifle joint, a caudal angulation of the femur places the femoral head adjacent to that portion of the acetabular margin that is most developed. Thus, if the head moves over this edge, detection of the clicking sound on re-entry is permitted in the dysplastic hip. While true in theory, in practice use of

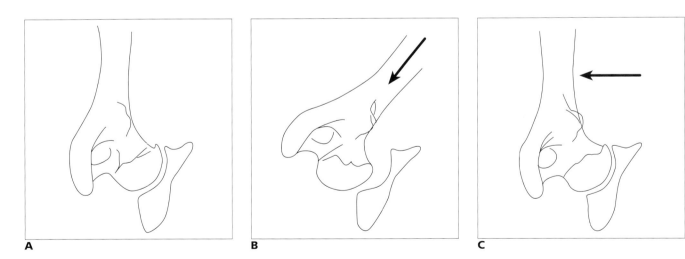

**Figure 5-4**
Drawings of the femoral head as it articulates with the acetabulum in a dysplastic hip illustrate a positive Ortolani maneuver. The dog is positioned in dorsal recumbency with the femurs at a 90° angle to the tabletop. (A) The femoral head rests adjacent to the acetabulum in a neutral position. (B) When the limb is adducted and a force is applied downward on the stifle joint, the femoral head slips out of the acetabulum in a joint with abnormal laxity. A sliding exit can be felt in some hips. (C) The femur is then abducted and a "popping" or "clicking" sensation is noted as the head slides into the acetabulum in the affected dog.

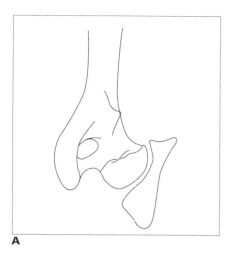 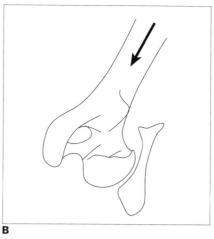 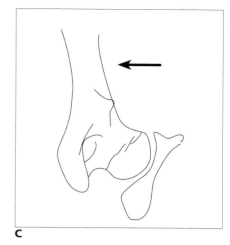

**Figure 5-5**
Drawings of the femoral head and acetabulum in a dog with hip dysplasia in which the acetabular cup is flattened and the sharp margin of the acetabulum has become blunted. In this hip, the Ortolani sign is replaced by a "sliding" sensation. (A) In a neutral position the femoral head is adjacent to the flattened acetabulum. (B) With adduction of the limb, the femoral head slides dorsally and laterally. (C) When the limb is abducted, the rounding of the acetabular margin permits only a "sliding" sensation as the head returns adjacent to the center of the acetabulum

both positions that are only in slight variation from the 90° femoral angle are advised to increase the accuracy of the maneuver.

In some dysplastic dogs, this sign can not be elicited while awake because of pain or size of muscle mass. The examiner can not bring the limb into adduction in order to force the head out of the acetabulum. Consequently, the "re-entry click" cannot be detected because the head remains within the acetabulum. Therefore, anesthesia or sedation should be used in the heavily muscled dog.

This technique of palpation can also be performed with the dog in lateral recumbency. An assistant is required to hold the dog in position during the examination. The dependent limb is pulled caudally and the uppermost limb, which is the one to be studied, is adducted forcing the head lateral to the acetabulum. Pressure is placed on the stifle joint and directed along the femur in an effort to drive the femoral head dorsally. The limb is then abducted permitting the femoral head to fall back into the acetabulum generating the "re-entry click." The dog is more comfortable having the technique performed while in a lateral position, but it requires greater skill to perform the technique accurately.

This sign can also be detected in the young dog by walking behind the dog with hands placed over the greater trochanters bilaterally. Excess movement of the trochanters reflects the abnormal movement of the femoral heads and the "popping" or "clicking" can be detected. If the excess movement is detected while the dog is walking, this is a positive diagnosis of dysplasia.

The dorsal acetabular margin in the severely dysplastic puppy changes from one with a sharp edge to one that is blunted. The rounding of the acetabular margin prevents creation of any exit or entry "click." This is replaced by a "sliding" sensation indicating movement of the femoral head within the flattened acetabulum (Figure 5-5).

With further thickening of the joint capsule, both the Ortolani sign and the "sliding" sensation disappear. A lip no longer exists over which the femoral head can move and the soft tissues thicken to a stage that limits movement of the femoral head (Figure 5-6). Thus, all signs of joint instability disappear and the action of the femoral head is best described as simply that of a restricted movement.

This progression of signs was noted in evaluation of the Ortolani maneuver in a group of 25 German Shepherd Dogs over 1 year of age who were diagnosed as bilaterally dysplastic on detection of secondary bony changes radiographically. In this group, 37 hips had a positive Ortolani sign, while the remaining 13 dysplastic hips had a negative Ortolani sign with only a limitation in movement of the femoral head. The progression of secondary changes prevented detection of the reentry "click" or the "sliding" sensation (Morgan and Stephens 1985).

In some dogs 6 years of age or older with normal or near-normal radiographs, an Ortolani sign can be detect-

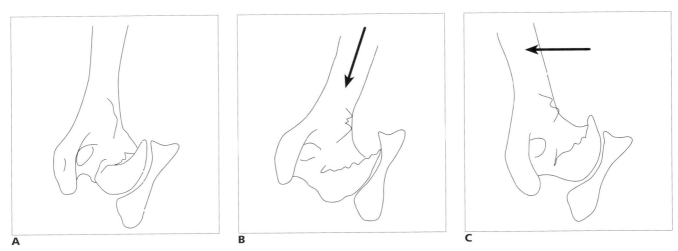

**Figure 5-6**
Drawings of the femoral head and acetabulum in a dog with hip dysplasia in which severe osteoarthrosis causes the absence of both an Ortolani sign and a "sliding" sensation. (A) In a neutral position, the modeled femoral head is adjacent to the flattened acetabulum. (B) With adduction of the limb, the femoral head remains in position. (C) When the limb is abducted, the malformed head continues to remains in position. The only sign detected in this severely affected hip is that of restricted motion because of thickening of the joint capsule. The feeling with movement of the head is similar to that of moving a stick that has been driven into mud.

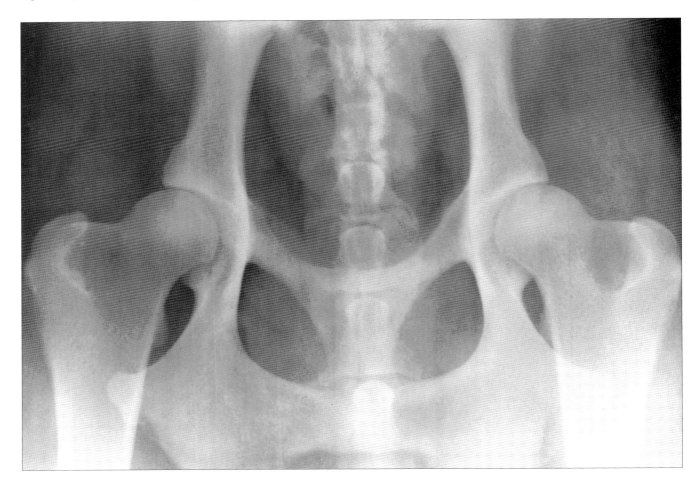

**Figure 5-7**
A pelvic radiograph with tightly fitting femoral heads in a radiographically normal 5-year-old female Great Pyrenees. Note the correct positioning of the pelvis for a conventional radiographic examination.

ed while the dog is under anesthesia. Clinically these dogs are reported to have stable hips while awake and walking. However, the physiologically sound joint can become unstable when the muscles are relaxed under anesthesia (Henry and Park 1972). These dogs should be considered genetically dysplastic.

Routine radiography can not always detect joint laxity and the study should be combined with palpation to more accurately determine the true status of the hip joints. If a positive Ortolani sign is elicited, a diagnosis of hip dysplasia should be made even if the standard radiographs appear within normal limits. If the sign is elicited while the animal is anesthetized, although still controversial in the minds of some, the dog should still be considered genetically dysplastic, even if the standard radiographs appear within normal limits. Palpation becomes of less importance if the radiographic technique includes a form of stress technique, since the use of radiographs made using a wedge or distraction technique can more accurately reveal the degree of joint laxity. Although it is difficult for some to think of these dogs with only joint laxity as dysplastic, they should be considered genetically dysplastic, ie, carrying the genes for dysplasia, even if they remain phenotypically normal.

## Anatomy and development of the hip joint

The normal gross and radiographic anatomy of the hip joint of the dog has been well described (Rhodes and Jenny 1960, Smith 1963, 1964, Lawson 1963) (Figure 5-7). The acetabulum is formed by four bones: the ilium, pubis, ischium, and the acetabular bone. The 3 large pelvic bones, the ilium, pubis, and ischium are partly ossified at birth, while the large triangular area between these bones that will become the acetabular bone begins to ossify at 6 to 8 weeks of age (Figure 5-8). More than one ossification center can be present in the acetabular bone. The acetabular rim remains cartilaginous until 3 to 4 months of age. The dorsocranial rim of the acetabulum can have a separate ossification center that later unites with the ilium (Audell and Gustafsson 1973, Olsson and Audell 1978). Histologically, this rim can have changes similar to those seen in osteochondrosis.

The femoral head is formed by a single ossification center that is preformed of cartilage and is only partially ossified by 2 to 3 weeks of age. Growth plate closure is completed by 9 months of age, except in giant breeds in which it is delayed by 2 to 3 months (Figure 5-9). The radiograph only permits evaluation of the ossified portion of the bone until the time of skeletal maturity. The

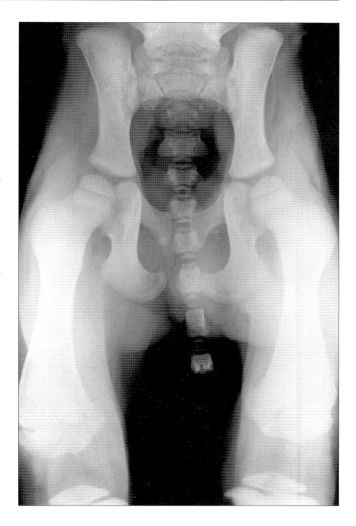

**Figure 5-8**
A radiograph of the pelvis of a normally developing 4- to 5-week-old puppy with ossification of the major pelvic bones and the femoral heads. While the hip joints can be identified, the radiolucent cartilage growth areas cause apparent separation of the pelvic bones and cause the joint spaces to appear widened.

times for appearance and subsequent ossification of all centers are both breed and individual dependent.

The hip joint is unique in that it is the only joint in the dog functioning in both standing and walking positions with a weight-bearing surface on the femoral head having an incomplete horizontal support. This means that the acetabulum does not form a complete cover over the femoral head thus permitting it to more easily escape or luxate dorsally and laterally (Figures 5-7, 5-8).

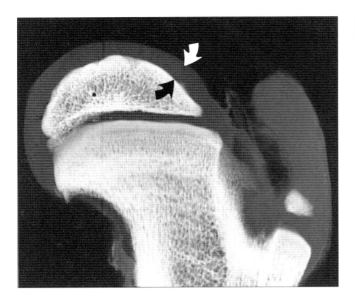
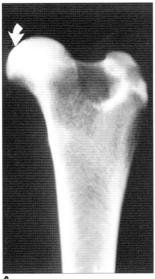
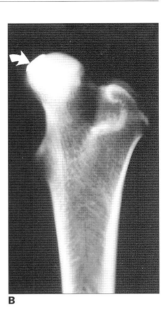

**Figure 5-9**
A radiograph of a slab section of a normally developing femoral head and neck in an 8-week-old puppy. The thickness of the articular cartilage (arrows) causes the joint space on the radiograph to appear much wider than in the adult. The fovea capitis is not identified on this section. Note the small ossification center of the greater trochanter.

**Figure 5-10**
Radiographs of a femoral specimen with the fovea capitis identified with radiopaque markers (arrows). The fovea does not affect the contour of the femoral head if (A) the limbs are positioned in internal rotation. (B) With the limb in external rotation, the fovea is seen to influence the appearance of the contour of the femoral head and cause it to appear flattened.

## Femoral head

The contour of the femoral head is smooth forming approximately two-thirds of a circle and blends smoothly onto the femoral neck. A natural medial defect in the contour of the head is termed the fovea and represents the site of attachment of the round ligament of the femoral head and is visualized on the radiograph dependent on the position of the hind limb. The fovea can be identified on a radiograph in which the limbs are extended caudally with a slight degree of external rotation creating an appearance of a flattened area on the femoral head. On such a radiograph, the fovea has been erroneously described as causing an abnormal flattening of the femoral head and has been thought to be a part of the osteoarthrosis of hip dysplasia. This positioning, while not exactly proper for evaluation of hip dysplasia, nevertheless is frequently accepted for hip evaluation. The fovea is usually not seen if the limbs are more perfectly positioned or if the limbs are partially abducted with external rotation. In either of these positions, the femoral head has the appearance of being round (Figure 5-10).

The femoral head is covered by articular cartilage except at the fovea and on a medially located wedge-shaped area that extends distally from the fovea toward the physeal growth plate and assumes the shape of a "horseshoe."

## Acetabulum

The normal acetabulum is a deep, cup-shaped depression in the pelvis with a prominent dorsocranial rim (margin) and forms from the union of 4 bones: (1) the ilium cranially, (2) the ischium caudally, (3) the small acetabular bone present at the depth of the acetabular cup, and (4) the pubis that plays a minimal role ventrally (Figure 5-11). The open end of the cup is directed laterally and ventrally. A consequence of this is the incomplete dorsal covering of the femoral head. Because of the cartilage content of these bones and the possibility of seeing only the ossified portion of the cup, the acetabular depth is not accurately appreciated on a radiograph until the age of 5 months (Riser 1973 a). Even at that age, because the acetabular rim has not ossified, the acetabulum appears more "open" and not as "cup-shaped" as it appears later in life. Thus, radiographic evaluation of the acetabulum of a puppy is limited.

In the normal adult, the margin of the acetabulum describes a partial circle that is interrupted by the ventrally located acetabular notch that is bridged by the transverse acetabular ligament (Figure 5-11). On the ventrodorsal pelvic radiograph, the cranial margin is seen as a distinct, evenly curving line that extends from the medially and ventrally located acetabular notch toward the craniolateral acetabular margin located dorsally and cranially. The dorsal acetabular margin is seen projected

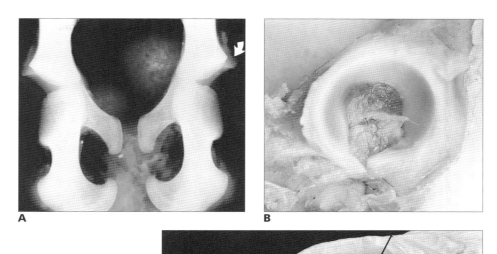

**Figure 5-11**
A radiograph (A) and photographs (B, C) of the acetabulum. (A) A radiograph of the pelvis in a puppy shows the cartilage margin of the acetabulum adjacent to the rim of the bony acetabulum in this specially prepared specimen (arrow). (B) In a photograph of a specimen from a puppy, note the absence of bone at the depth of the acetabular cup and how the cartilaginous margin only forms a lip cranially, dorsally, and caudally. (C) A photograph of a specimen from an adult shows the acetabulum formed of bone (Cr = cranial, Ca = caudal). The dorsocranial area of the rim receives the greatest stress by the femoral head (lines). The "horseshoe" shape of the articular cartilage and subchondral bone can be appreciated (B, C).

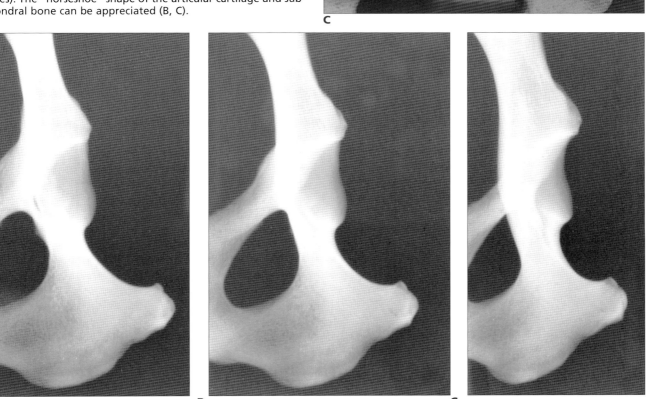

**Figure 5-12**
Radiographs of a pelvic specimen made with the acetabulum angled at (A) 5°, (B) 10°, and (C) 15° to illustrate how the position of the pelvis influences the depth of the acetabulum.

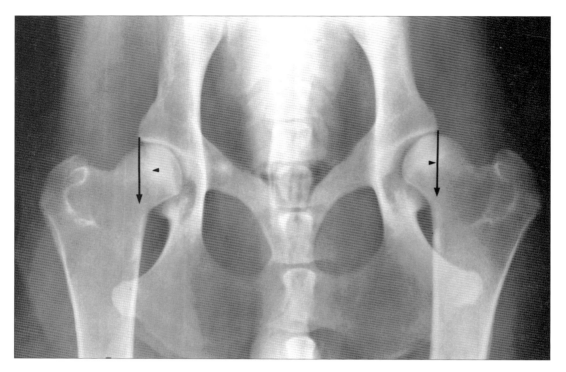

**Figure 5-13**
A ventrodorsal radiograph of the pelvis with arrows directed caudally from the dorsocranial acetabular margin parallel to the spine. The center of the femoral heads is marked with the point of an arrowhead. Note how the center of the head on the right is medial to the line indicating a deeply seated femoral head while the center of the head on the left is almost on the line indicating joint laxity with a femoral head positioned laterally. The location of the femoral head is influenced by joint laxity, positioning of the pelvis, skeletal maturity, and the presence of secondary change on the acetabular rim.

through the femoral head and neck. The caudal acetabular margin is short and underdeveloped.

Determination of the acetabular depth on the radiograph is important in evaluation of the character of the hip joint because it permits a decision as to how deeply the femoral head fits into the acetabulum. The depth of the acetabulum is difficult to determine, even in the adult, because the bottom of the cup, or the acetabular fossa, is not formed of bone (Figure 5-11) and therefore is radiolucent. In addition, detection of the true depth of the acetabulum is dependent on the positioning of the dog during VD radiography. With pelvic obliquity, one acetabular cup appears deeper while the other acetabular cup appears more shallow according to the following rule: The half of the pelvis with the smaller obturator foramen has the more shallow appearing acetabular cup, while the half of the pelvis with the larger obturator foramen has the deeper appearing acetabular cup (Figure 5-12).

## Hip joint

The manner in which the femoral head fits the acetabular cup determines the quality of the hip joint. On the conventional ventrodorsal radiograph made in dorsal recumbency with the limbs extended, the center of the head is located medial to a line extending caudally from the dorsocranial acetabular margin drawn parallel to the spine (Figure 5-13).

Another method of evaluating the correlation between femoral head and acetabulum is to measure the angle created by the intersection of a line extending between the centers of the femoral heads and a line extending cranially from the center of the femoral head through the craniolateral acetabular margin. The angle measured medially is referred to as the Norberg angle and in the normal dog should be equal to or greater than 105° (Norberg 1961). This angle was originally measured on radiographs made with the limbs in a "frog leg" position in which the femoral head was probably forced rather deeply into the acetabulum. Today, its use has been converted to the radiograph made with the limbs extended in which the positioning of the femoral head is more questionable (Figure 5-14). The angle is more accurately measured after skeletal maturation because the angle is artificially decreased in the normal immature puppy because of the lack of ossification of the dorsal rim.

Anatomy and development of the hip joint **129**

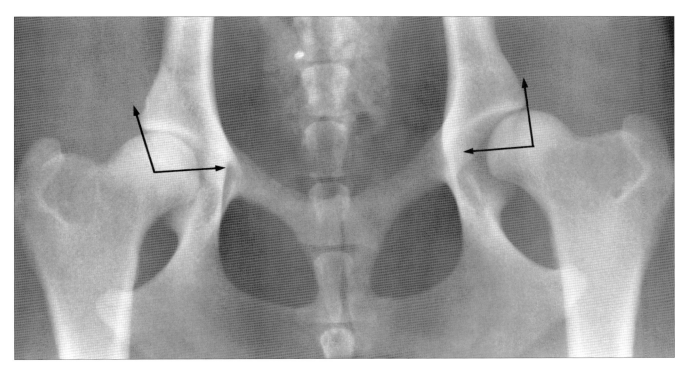

**Figure 5-14**
A ventrodorsal radiograph of the pelvis on which horizontal arrows when connected create a line between the centers of the femoral heads. Near vertical arrows represent the second lines that are drawn from the centers of the femoral head through the dorsocranial acetabular rims. An angle is generated on the medial side and is called the Norberg angle. The normal angle is equal to or greater than 105°. In this dog the measurement is 105° on the right and 87° on the left. Measurement of this angle is greatly influenced by positioning of the pelvis, skeletal maturation of the dog, and by any secondary changes on the acetabular rim.

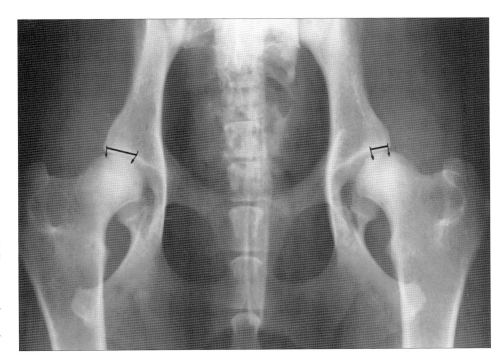

**Figure 5-15**
A ventrodorsal radiograph of the pelvis of a 12-month-old dog in which the articular surfaces on the right are congruent over a greater arc (approximately 60°) than on the left (approximately 30°). The greater the length of this arc (arrows) the deeper the seating of the femoral head and the greater is the joint stability. Joint laxity is also estimated by locating the center of the femoral head relative to the dorsal acetabular margin.

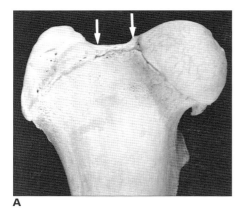 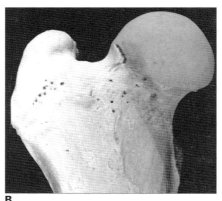

**Figure 5-16**
Photographs of femoral specimens showing (A) the incompletely attached lip of bone along the dorsal aspect of the femoral neck in the immature dog (arrows) and (B) the appearance of the neck in the mature dog following union of the centers of ossification with the femoral neck. Note the fovea capitis in (A).

The measurement is strongly influenced by the position of the femoral head within the acetabulum. This may vary dependent on how the limbs are held. Pelvic obliquity causes the femoral head to be more deeply seated in the acetabulum, generates a smaller Norberg angle, and generates a more normal evaluation. Incomplete acetabular ossification that is age dependent causes a smaller angle to be measured. Changes on the acetabular margin may artificially increase or decrease the measurement of the angle. Thus, erroneous evaluation can result from pelvic position or age of the dog. Determination of an early distraction index (DI) has been shown to correlate better with the subsequent development of osteoarthrosis than the Norberg angle (Smith, et al 1993).

The nature of the joint space can only be estimated on the radiograph because the articular cartilage is radiolucent. An estimation of articular congruity can be made between the arc formed by the acetabular rim and the arc indicating the margin of the adjacent femoral head (Figure 5-15). In the normal hip, the configuration of the cartilage of the acetabulum and that of the femoral head are congruent, one with the other, over an arc of approximately 60°. Consequently, the loading pressures are distributed over as large an area as is possible causing uniformity in the radiographic density of the subchondral bone beneath this arc. As the femoral head luxates laterally, the size of the arc of congruity decreases until it becomes only a contact point and the density within the subchondral bone at this site increases markedly.

## Femoral neck

During skeletal maturation of the femoral neck, a lip of epiphyseal cartilage extends from the ossification center of the head along the dorsal aspect of the femoral neck distally to the ossification center of the greater trochanter. Ossification of the cartilage lip begins from both centers of ossification and advances until they join in the center. The ossification bridge eventually blends with the underlying femoral neck creating a femoral neck with a smooth margin between the head and trochanteric region of the femur (Figures 5-16, 5-17). The joining of these two lips of bone to each other and to the femoral neck occurs as early as 6 months and this causes thickening of the femoral neck on the radiograph of the mature dog. Radiographs made of younger dog prior to physeal

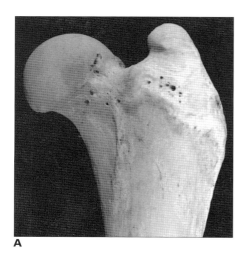 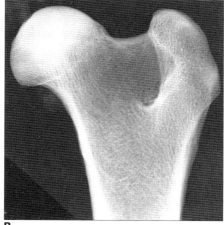

**Figure 5-17**
A photograph (A) and radiograph (B) of the cranial surface of the head, femoral neck, and greater trochanter of a normal mature dog showing the smooth blending of the femoral head with the shaft. Note the vascular channels on the specimen.

closure have a roughened appearance of the dorsum of the femoral neck that can be incorrectly interpreted as secondary bony modeling.

The shape of the femoral neck in the mature dog (Figure 5-17) is characterized by a rather flat dorsal contour and a more arched ventral contour as seen on the VD radiograph with the limbs extended. An increase in stress due to weight-bearing forces creates a plate of strong bony tissue ventrally while strengthening the neck of the femur. This is referred to as the femoral calcar.

### Greater trochanter

The greater trochanter is positioned laterally on the proximal femur and consists of dense trabecular bone (Figures 5-17, 5-18). The gluteal muscles attach to the trochanter with the middle gluteal muscle attaching dorsally, the deep gluteal muscle attaching slightly cranially, and the superficial gluteal muscle attaching more distally. The function of the gluteal muscles and the iliopsoas is primarily extension of the hip joint while the function of the small pelvic association is external rotation of the femur. Neither of these groups contributes to the lateral stability of the hip joint and thus it appears as though the joint capsule and ligament of the head of the femur play the major role in maintaining joint stability in both the normal and dysplastic hip. Differences in morphology of the greater trochanter are breed influenced (Figure 5-18). The deep trochanteric fossae lie between the femoral neck and the greater trochanter caudal to the connecting ridge of bone.

## Radiographic views

Several positions of the patient are used for radiographic evaluation of HD. These positions must be consistent or erroneous conclusions can be reached in interpretation of the radiographs, especially in the younger dog. Patients can be examined awake, sedated, or anesthetized, dependent on the behavior of the dog. There is an unfounded fear that excessive joint laxity can be detected in an anesthetized dog, however, it has been suggested that anesthesia does not create joint laxity but relaxes muscles so that the existing laxity can be more readily detected on the VD radiograph made with the limbs extended (Morgan and Stephens 1985). Another report, in agreement, stated that any increase in the degree of subluxation noted on studies of an anesthetized dog was due to pre-existing laxity of ligamentous structures that had been masked by muscle action on the non-anesthetized study (Keller and Corley, 1990).

A recent study of clinic cases suggested that the use of anesthesia infrequently changed the radiographic diagnosis when compared with radiographs made with the dog awake (Farrow and Back 1989). Finally, the use of chemical restraint was shown to have minimal effect in the radiographic evaluation of clinic cases radiographed without an anesthetic when compared with an immediate follow-up radiograph made using anesthesia (Aronson, et al 1991). The authors examined 10 young adult German Shepherd Dogs awake and anesthetized. The radiographs were evaluated without knowledge of: (1) the identity of the dog, (2) whether it was awake or anesthetized, or (3) which hip was right or left. Following evaluation, the identity of the dogs and each hip was learned. Radiographic evaluations were identical for the two radiographs of each dog and for each hip. All dogs were either normal or with only minimal bony changes and/or slight subluxation.

These studies show that anesthesia provides an opportunity for better positioning and production of a more diagnostic radiograph, lessens patient's discomfort, and

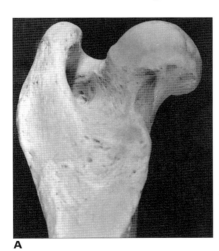 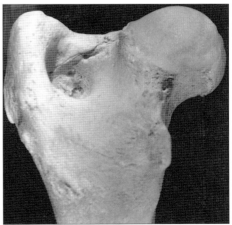

**Figure 5-18**
Photographs of specimens from a (A) mature Afghan Hound and a (B) mature Great Dane show marked differences in morphology of the femoral neck and greater trochanter that are influenced by breed or by difference in growth patterns. Note the prominent trochanteric fossae as seen on the caudal surface.

A   B

## 132 Hip dysplasia

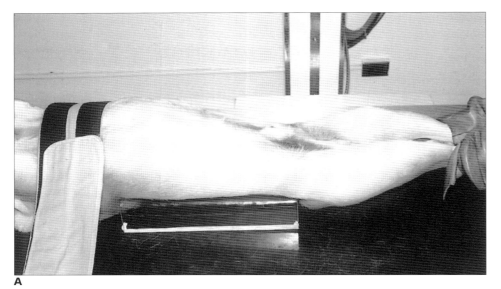

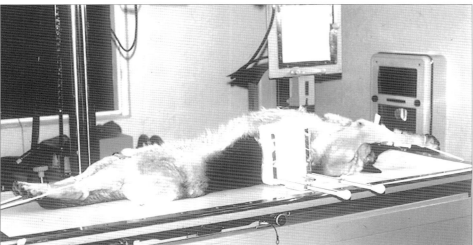

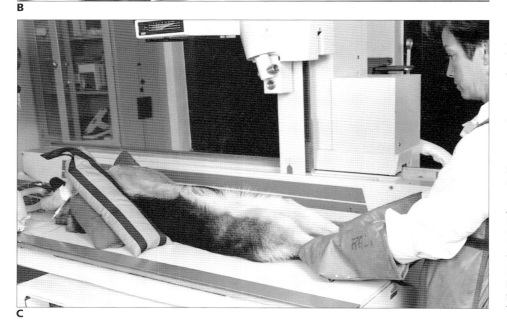

**Figure 5-19**
Photographs of three dogs positioned on their back with the femurs fully extended caudally so they are parallel to each other and as near the table top as possible (probably ~30°). The stifles are rotated internally so the patellae are centrally positioned on the midline of the limb. This is a common positioning used to make a conventional VD radiograph of the pelvis in evaluation of the hip joints for hip dysplasia. The figures illustrate the use of: (A) a restraining band over the abdomen, a trough for positioning, and the feet held with gloved hands; (B) a technique of positioning with the dog having received intravenous anesthetic using restraining devices for the body, tie-down lines for the fore and hind limbs, tape holding the stifle joints together, and a more complete extension of the limbs; and (C) sandbags to achieve positioning of the body with the feet held with gloved hands. Because of the large size of most dogs examined, radiography is easier if the cassette is positioned in an under-table tray along with the grid.

decreases radiation exposure to the assistants participating in the examination. All of these studies were made on VD radiographs with the limbs extended and need to be understood with that in mind. It is the use of stress or distraction techniques that alters the diagnosis so effectively, not the use of anesthesia in radiographic diagnosis.

Accurate radiographic positioning is more important in a dog when the diagnosis is based entirely on the presence of joint laxity. In the dog with secondary bony changes, accurate positioning is not required because the diagnosis is based on obvious bony changes whose detection is not dependent on perfect positioning. However, since the status of the hip joints is not known prior to the examination, the most perfect positioning is the goal of all studies.

It is important that certain rules be followed in association with the radiographic examination. The dog needs to be identified by some recognized system including, a legible tattooing, microchip, or the word of the owner. The minimal identification of the radiographs includes an identification number of the dog (tattoo/microchip/registration), date of the examination, age and sex of the dog, and name of the clinic performing the examination.

Most radiographic studies used to evaluate the status of the hip joints are made with the dog on its back. By convention, the resulting radiographs are viewed with the right hip on the left side of the view box and the left hip on the right side of the view box. Thus, the dog appears to be "standing" and "facing" the viewer.

## Ventrodorsal view

The most commonly used position in the United States is the ventrodorsal (VD) position (Figure 5-19). The dog is placed on its back with the pelvis positioned symmetrically. The femurs are fully extended caudally so they are parallel to each other and as near the tabletop as possible (probably ~30°), and the stifles rotated internally so the patellae are centrally positioned on the midline of the limb (Norberg 1961, Riser 1962, Riser and Rhodes 1966, Corley 1968, Rendano and Ryan 1985). With this positioning, the pelvic canal appears round or symmetrically oval, the iliac wings have equal width, the obturator foramina have equal size, and the sacroiliac joints are similar in appearance (Figure 5-20).

Minimal obliquity of the dog's body causes a difference in appearance in all of these structures. The obturator foramen on the side of the dog nearest to the tabletop appears smaller with an apparent decrease in depth of the

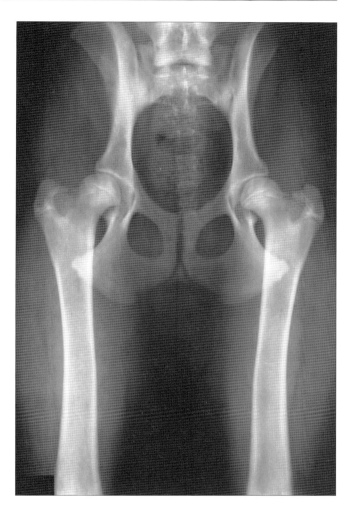

**Figure 5-20**
Routine ventrodorsal pelvic radiograph used for HD examination (Olsson technique) with symmetrical pelvic positioning with the limbs parallel and extended fully. The patellae are correctly centered over the distal femurs. The symmetry between the halves of the pelvis reflects the good patient positioning. Growth plates remain open in this 6-month-old dog.

acetabulum on that side. The obturator foramen on the elevated side appears larger with an apparent increase in depth of the acetabulum on that side. Thus, pelvic obliquity alters the depth of the acetabulum as perceived on the radiograph. With obliquity, the pelvic canal appears asymmetrically oval and one sacroiliac joint appears more open than the other. The width of the iliac wings varies with one more narrow than the other (Figure 5-21). Another form of pelvic malpositioning that influences the apparent depth of the acetabulum results from attempts to position the femurs parallel to the x-ray table surface in heavily muscled dogs. Exerting a great downward pressure on the femurs causes the pelvis to tilt caudally around its transverse axis. As a result, the projected point of intersection between the dorsal and the cranial

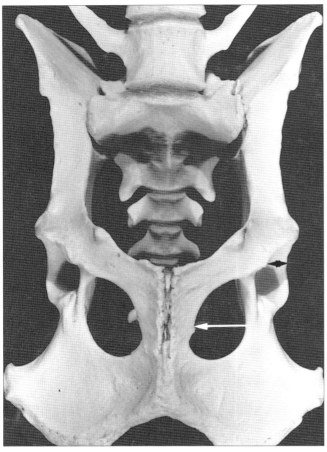 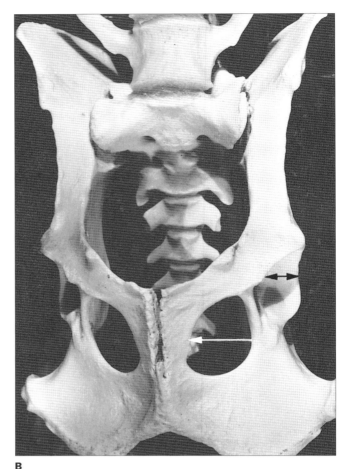

**A**

**B**

**Figure 5-21**
Photographs of a pelvic specimen show (A) correct positioning with the obturator foramina of equal size and shape and (B) oblique positioning with the obturator foramina of different size with an altered depth of the acetabula. The variation in width of the obturator foramina is indicated (white arrows). The variation in depth of the acetabula is indicated by the distance between the dorsal and ventral margins (double-headed arrows).

acetabular rim is thereby moved medially resulting in the projection of a shallower acetabulum.

In the positioning of the dog for radiographic examination, the location of the femurs is as important as that of the pelvis. The correct degree of internal rotation of the limbs, adduction of the femurs, and extension of the limbs is important in obtaining a diagnostic projection of the femoral head and neck. Failure to achieve this correct positioning is characterized by a degree of external rotation and/or abduction of the limbs (Figure 5-22). Positioning the limb in external rotation causes the greater trochanter to be more completely superimposed over the femoral neck and artificially shortens the appearance of the femoral neck. Thus, the femoral neck is projected more "on end" and the angle of attachment of the femoral neck with the shaft (angle of inclination) cannot be accurately ascertained. In addition, the presence of secondary changes on the caudal aspect of the femoral neck cannot be detected preventing knowledge of this important early bony change indicative of joint laxity (Figure 5-23). As a result, early changes of osteoarthrosis such as enthesophyte formation on the femoral neck or thickening of the femoral neck are not seen and a varus or valgus deformity cannot be identified. Abduction of the limbs forces the femoral heads into the acetabula so minimal joint laxity is not identified and the true character of the hip joints is not expressed on the radiograph (Figure 5-24).

Even with the limbs positioned correctly, in the average well-muscled dog, the femurs are not parallel to the tabletop but are at an angle of approximately 30° to 45° to the tabletop. Inclusion of the distal femurs on the radiograph permits evaluation of the location of the patella relative to the trochlear grooves, which serves as an accurate indicator of correct limb positioning for the novice. With increased experience, evaluation of the position of the greater trochanter on the radiograph can serve the same purpose.

Radiographic views **135**

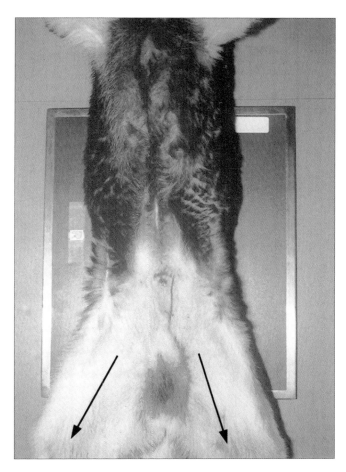

**Figure 5-22**
A photograph showing a dog on its back incorrectly positioned for radiography of the pelvis for hip dysplasia. The abduction of the limbs and external rotation prevents accurate evaluation of minimal hip joint laxity and identification of enthesophytes on the caudal aspect of the femoral neck.

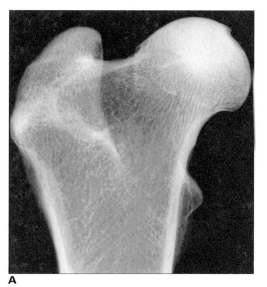

A

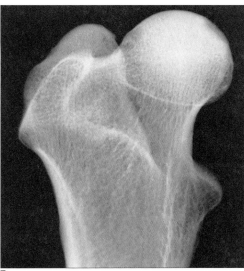

B

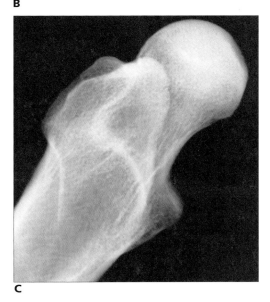

C

**Figure 5-23**
Radiographs of an anatomical specimen of the proximal femur demonstrate the effect of alteration in the positioning of the hind limbs on visualization of the femoral neck. (A) The correct degree of internal rotation of the limbs, adduction of the femurs, and extension of the limbs permits visualization of the femoral neck. (B) A minimal degree of external rotation of the limbs causes the shadow of the greater trochanter to be partially superimposed over the femoral neck preventing evaluation of secondary change in this location. (C) A greater degree of external rotation and abduction of the limb causes the femoral neck to be projected "on end" preventing evaluation of secondary change in this location.

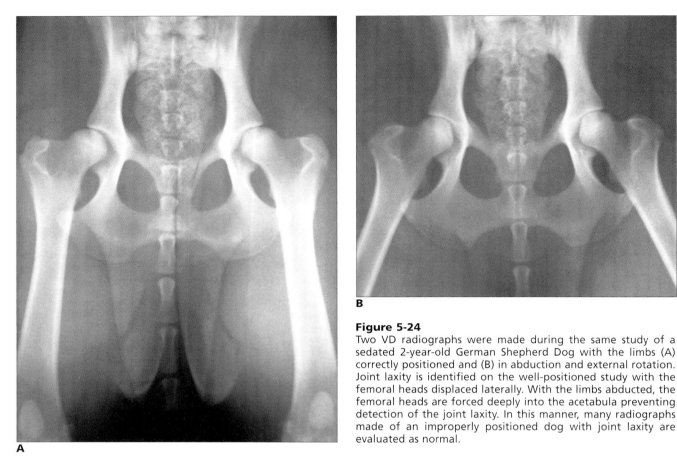

**Figure 5-24**
Two VD radiographs were made during the same study of a sedated 2-year-old German Shepherd Dog with the limbs (A) correctly positioned and (B) in abduction and external rotation. Joint laxity is identified on the well-positioned study with the femoral heads displaced laterally. With the limbs abducted, the femoral heads are forced deeply into the acetabula preventing detection of the joint laxity. In this manner, many radiographs made of an improperly positioned dog with joint laxity are evaluated as normal.

Finally, a study of the effect of positioning on passive hip laxity was made in an effort to try "to characterize the load vs displacement behavior of the canine coxofemoral joint" (Smith, et al 1990; Heyman, et al 1993). The hip possesses three rotational degrees of freedom, those of flexion/extension, adduction/abduction, and internal/external rotation. Passive constraints around the joint are due to the round ligament of the femoral head and the joint capsule and are in a position to permit maximal laxity when the hip is in a neutral orientation. The optimal range of hip position to determine laxity was found to be between 10° of flexion and 30° of extension, between 10° and 30° of abduction, and between 0° and 10° of external rotation. Any degree of extension, adduction, or internal rotation away from this "neutral" coxofemoral orientation serves to tighten the hip presumably by tensing of the fibrous elements around the joint and preventing lateral displacement of the femoral head. This suggests that certain positioning prevents joint laxity and this must be taken into account when evaluating radiographs made in these positions. It should be noted that in this study, the effect of position on the detection of hip laxity was not studied in live dysplastic dogs, however, the effect of limb positioning on the radiographic appearance of the hips of the live young dog with minimal joint laxity should be similar. The study strongly suggests the limb-extended position routinely used for the diagnosis of HP may not be the most correct anatomic position for the detection of joint laxity.

## Ventrodorsal "frog leg" view

The VD "frog leg" view was described early in Sweden (Olsson 1958, 1962 b, Månsson and Norberg 1961) and has been used regularly in many countries in the world (Figure 5-25). Accurate positioning of the pelvis is easily achieved with the dog in dorsal recumbency with the hind limbs flexed to a maximum and abducted so that the stifle joints are held 30 to 40 cm above the tabletop. The tarsi are separated. Equal positioning of the feet avoids rotation of the pelvis and insures that the two halves of the pelvis appear symmetrical (Figure 5-26). This position permits excellent evaluation of the femoral head and neck and detection of early enthesophyte formation on the caudal aspect of the femoral neck, craniodorsal margin of the articular lip of the femoral head, and the dorsal rim of the acetabulum (Morgan and Stephens 1985, Schneider-Haiss and Loeffler 1987). These are anatomical regions that are more difficult to

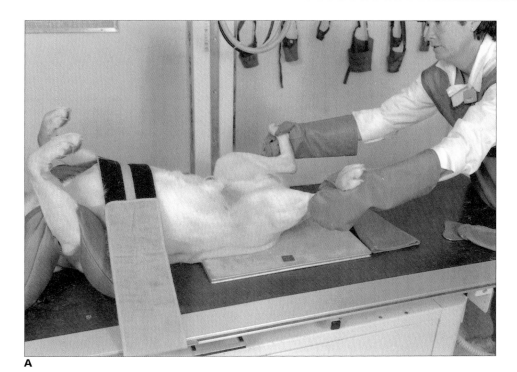

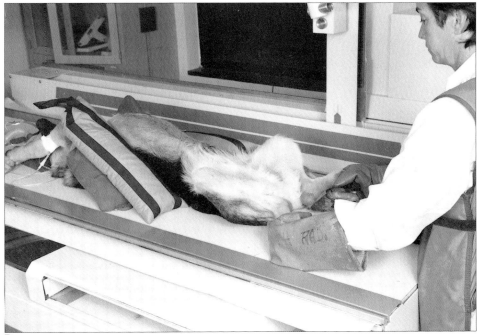

**Figure 5-25**
Photographs of two dogs positioned in dorsal recumbency with the stifles raised 30 to 40 cm above the tabletop with the limbs flexed with the tarsi held somewhat separated. This positioning is used to make a "frog leg" view of the pelvis in evaluation of the hip joints. In one view (A), the restraining band over the abdomen and sandbags over the forelimbs assist in positioning the dog. In the other view (B), sandbags are used to create a trough to support the dog's body. The feet are always held with gloved hands.

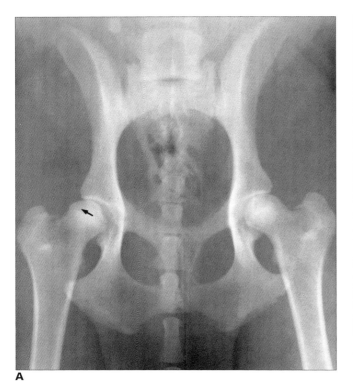 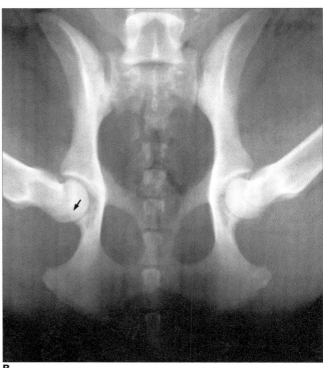

**Figure 5-26**
Radiographs of the pelvis of an 8-month-old Labrador Retriever made in dorsal recumbency permit a comparison between the (A) routine ventrodorsal extended-limb view and the (B) flexed-limb view ("frog leg" view). Note the minimal laxity indicated by subluxation of the head cranially and laterally as seen on the extended-limb view on the right (arrow) is seen differently on the flexed-limb view in which the head is subluxated caudally and laterally (arrow). A marked difference in projection of the femoral head and neck is noted.

evaluate on the conventional VD extended-limb view, especially when the limbs are in external rotation. The "frog leg" view is principally used for the detection of early bony changes and it is often used as an adjunct to the more conventional VD view (Olsson 1962 b).

Since the "frog leg" view tends to force the femoral heads into the acetabula, it can obscure minimal subluxation of the femoral head in the younger dog. However, the positioning of the limbs is probably closer to the neutral positioning described (Heyman, et al 1993) than that found on the limb-extended VD position. Therefore, any suggestion of joint laxity as identified on the "frog leg" view should be considered positive evidence of HD.

### Ventrodorsal wedge view

The VD wedge view is another technique used for evaluation of the hip joints and has been described principally as a method to detect minimal joint laxity (Figure 5-27) (Bardens and Hardwick 1968, Bardens 1972 b, Henry and Park 1972, Flückiger 1997). Any joint laxity produced with the limb in full extension in a joint in which that limb positioning should force the head into the acetabulum, constitutes positive evidence of hip dysplasia. The device to be used as a "wedge" can be any convenient solid object that can be conveniently placed between the distal femurs. A can or jar approximately 10 cm in diameter can be used in a large dog (Henry and Park, 1972). A force is directed medially on the feet so that the wedge becomes a fulcrum creating distracting forces that attempt to displace the femoral heads laterally (Figure 5-28). Distraction can also be created by use of an inflatable bladder (Figure 5-27). The placement of the wedge device between the limbs and the forcing of the feet together causes some difficulty to maintain the symmetrical positioning of the limbs and pelvis. External rotation of the hind limbs is difficult to avoid and a concentrated effort is required to internally rotate the limbs so that the patellae remain centrally positioned.

While the technique has most commonly been used in the mature dog, its use has been described in 1-week-old puppies (Bardens and Hardwick 1968, Bardens 1972 b). The use of a wedge technique or physical examination to detect joint laxity has a greater importance in evaluation

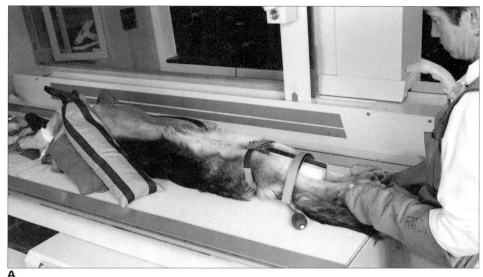
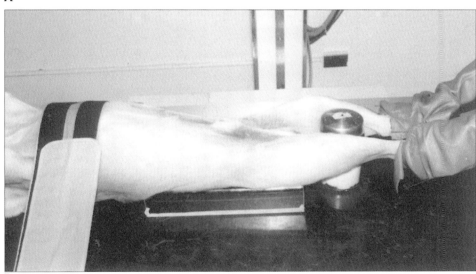

**Figure 5-27**
Photographs of two dogs positioned for a "wedge" technique. The dogs are on their backs with the femurs fully extended caudally and parallel to each other. The stifles are rotated internally so the patellae are centrally positioned on the midline of the limb. (A) An inflatable bladder is secured by Velcro wraps between the upper portion of the hind limbs. When the device is inflated, the femoral heads are distracted from the acetabula. Sandbags are used to position the body. (B) The "wedge" may assume the shape of a sponge canister and is placed between the hind limbs where is serves as a fulcrum. The feet are held with gloved hands with a force directed toward the midline. This distracts the femoral heads from the acetabula. The body is positioned using a trough and a compression band.

of the hips in young dogs, since in older dogs, the detection of secondary bony changes replaces the detection of joint laxity in the diagnosis of dysplasia.

Originally the wedge technique was used in conjunction with the conventional VD view at the time of hip certification. Unfortunately, when the wedge technique was first advocated, the significance of joint laxity as the only evidence of hip dysplasia was not appreciated and the technique fell into disfavor because of the problem created by the detection of joint laxity in what were otherwise radiographically normal hips. This casts doubt on the original diagnosis of normal based on the conventional view, and as often occurs in nature, people would rather not learn of bad news. However, it is encouraging to note a renewed interest in all types of distraction techniques in an effort to detect minimal joint laxity.

## Standing position

Recognition that the dog positioned in dorsal recumbency certainly was not in an anatomical position lead others to question the effect this might have on the radiographic appearance of the hip joints. One of the first proposals was radiography with the patient in a standing position. This was accomplished by use of a curved cassette placed in the inguinal region and the x-ray tube positioned dorsally and caudally. The resulting radiograph was thought to have accomplished two things. The dog was in a natural standing position and the femoral heads, if loose, would tend to be positioned dorsolaterally and joint laxity could be detected (Albrecht and Arnold 1972). At the time of this study, the importance of joint laxity was not recognized. This, plus the tendency to be resistant to change, the additional problems of obtaining

# 140 Hip dysplasia

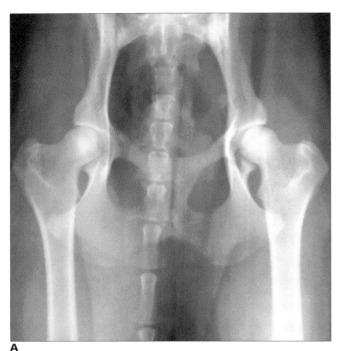
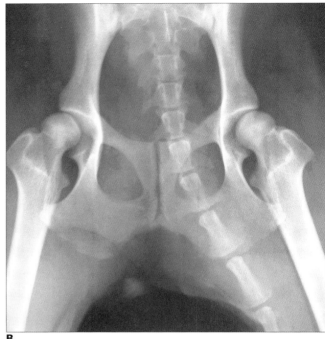

**Figure 5-28**
Two ventrodorsal radiographs are made of the pelvis of a 1-year-old female Retriever. (A) The extended limbs are positioned in a conventional manner and the femoral heads appear to be deeply seated. (B) A wedge is positioned between the limbs and a force is directed on the feet toward the midline causing both femoral heads to be distracted indicating marked joint laxity. Note the external rotation of the limbs indicating the difficulty is maintaining good positioning of the limbs when using the wedge technique. The "wedge" or "fulcrum" used in this patient if larger than necessary.

the positioning required for this type of study, and the increased radiation exposure that resulted in the use of this principally sound technique not being adopted.

## Badertscher view

Another modification of the standard positioning places the dog in dorsal recumbency but positions the limbs in a slightly more normal anatomical position and utilizes a type of wedge. The wedge is a flat wooden lath placed so that the pivot point is close to the pelvic floor. The femurs, while parallel to each other, are flexed to a 60° angle with the tabletop and the tibias are held parallel to each other and parallel to the tabletop. With the wedge placed between the thighs, a force directed medially on the feet causes the femoral heads to displace laterally in an affected dog. Any soft tissue structures that provide extra-articular support are more relaxed with the femurs in this position and subtle joint laxity is more easily detected (Figure 5-29) (Badertscher 1977; Heyman, et al 1993). This positioning seems to be rather easy to perform without the risk of pelvic obliquity. The degree of joint laxity that is seen is greater than is seen on the technique described below.

## Flückiger view

A more recently described technique uses the relaxed positioning of the hind limbs described above (Flückiger 1997). The dog in placed in dorsal recumbence in a Styrofoam trough with the femurs at a 60° angle with the tabletop. The stifles are adducted and the tibiae used as a lever in placement of a force directed craniodorsally (toward the tabletop) at the time of radiographic exposure. With the stifles directed medially, the femoral heads displace in a craniodorsal and lateral direction in the dysplastic dog. The positioning is similar to that used in performing the Ortolani maneuver and results in a similar displacement of the femoral head in the lax joint (Figures 5-29, 5-30). Radiographic technique needs to be increased by 30% because of the increase in thickness of muscle tissue as a result of the special hind limb positioning. The technique is especially attractive since neither a special tool nor special operator training is required. The position of the femoral head can be compared with its position as seen on a radiograph made without any force directed toward the table top or on a radiograph made using a more standard ventrodorsal positioning.

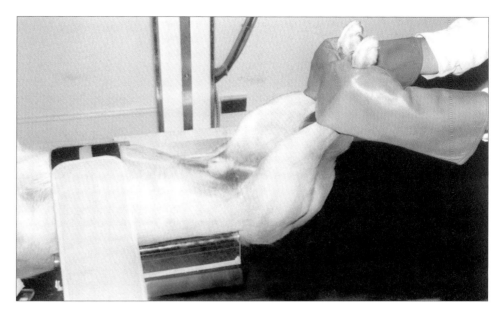

**Figure 5-29**
Photograph of a dog positioned on its back with the femurs partially flexed in a more relaxed manner and the tibiae parallel to the tabletop. A wedge device can be positioned between the thighs and the feet forced together to achieve a type of wedge study or a downward force can be exerted on the limbs to force an Ortolani type maneuver. This uses a more neutral positioning for the dog. Note the compression band and trough that assist in patient positioning. The feet are held with gloved hands.

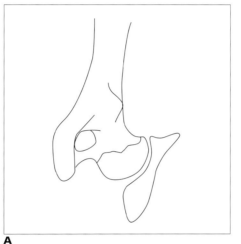 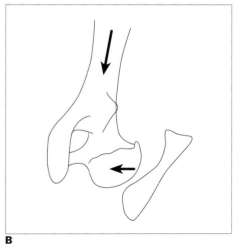

**Figure 5-30**
Drawings of the femoral head and acetabulum that illustrate the effect of downward pressure on the limb in the dysplastic hip. In the (A) neutral position, the femoral head sits in contact with the malformed acetabulum. By (B) placing pressure downward on the femur (large arrow), the femoral head is forced laterally (small arrow) and appears subluxated on the radiograph.

A                              B

Three potential problems are recognized in performing this technique. They are: (1) learning the downward force required by the technician to obtain the subluxation, (2) questioning the affect of potential differences between the strength of technicians, and (3) noting that unequal force placed on the limbs causes tilting of the pelvis and a resulting obliquity on the radiograph. A relatively small force applied by the assistant creates maximal subluxation of the femoral head and evaluation of data showed that no positive correlation existed between the assistant and the resulting laxity meaning that the strength of different technicians did not affect the results. Slight pelvic malpositioning (10° to 15°) had little affect on the final interpretation, however, a greater degree of obliquity produced a non-diagnostic radiograph. By comparing these radiographs with those made in a more conventional manner, the degree of joint laxity, or an index, can be created by measuring the lateral movement of the femoral heads relatively to the acetabula (Figure 5-31).

## Compression-distraction views

A diagnostic method for early (4 months) detection of susceptibility to HD has been developed and tested at the University of Pennsylvania over the past 17 years (Smith 1997). The method requires the puppy to be under deep sedation or general anesthesia and uses two views made with the dog positioned on its back and the hips at a neutral flexion/extension angle. One view is made using a compressive device that "pushes" the femoral heads deeply into the acetabula and a second view is made using a distraction device that "pulls" the femoral heads out of the acetabula. The custom-designed distracter is

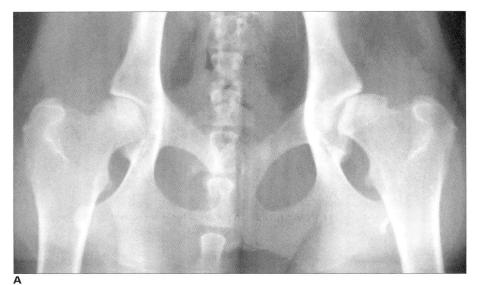

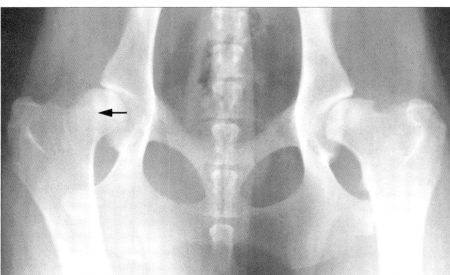

**Figure 5-31**
Ventrodorsal radiographs of the pelvis of 1-year-old female Shepherd-cross made (A) with the partially extended limbs positioned in a neutral position and (B) with downward pressure on the stifle joints causing the lax femoral head on the right to move dorsolaterally. Note how the right femoral head moves from a position of apparent tightness to a position of laxity (arrow). The left femoral head remains with minimal subluxation on both studies, probably because of secondary changes typical of those found with dysplasia. These bony changes, plus thickening of the joint capsule, prevent the femoral head from moving despite forces on the limb. This patient illustrates the two patterns of change used in diagnosis of hip dysplasia. In the right hip, joint laxity is demonstrated only through the use of a distraction technique. In the left hip, joint subluxation and osteoarthrosis are identified without regard to patient positioning.

positioned between the legs at the level of the ventral pelvis and creates maximal lateral displacement of the femoral heads (Smith, et al 1990). The new measurement method utilizes a distraction index (DI) ranging from 0 to 1, with 0 representing a fully congruent hip as seen in the compression view and 1 representing the most extreme joint laxity as might be seen in the distraction of a femoral head. The DI is a ratio scale, meaning that a hip with a DI of 0.6 has twice the laxity of a hip with a DI of 0.3. This technique has been shown in a 3 year longitudinal study of more than 140 dogs followed from 4 months of age to be clearly repeatable with high intraclass correlation coefficients between indices obtained at 4, 6, 12, and 24 months studies (Smith, et al 1993).

A particular problem can be identified in radiographs of the hips made during distraction radiography. That is synovial fluid cavitation, that while uncommon, if present, increases the DI (LaFond, et al 1997). The cavitation, or vacuum sign, results from the lowered intracapsular pressure and represents nitrogen accumulation within the joint. Because of the lower tissue density, the gas causes a radiographic contrast with the articular surface.

Comparison between measurements taken from the two radiographs produces a factor of joint laxity that is judged against what is "normal" for the breed. "Until these important aspects of the CHD research (laxity determination) are completed, the proposed compression/distraction method is not recommended as a clinical tool" (Smith, et al 1990). There is a "need to develop logistic regression curves for all popular breeds of dogs to permit valid application of the distraction index as a selection criterion" (Smith 1994). With further determination of the degree of laxity considered to be normal for each breed, this technique will have great importance in early determination of HD in young dogs being considered for breeding as well as in early progeny testing of phenotypically normal parents.

Another report evaluated the effect of distraction in anesthetized dogs using two different forms of stress techniques compared with conventional studies. The authors agree that "the selection of dogs for breeding must then be based on examination of the dynamics of the joints as well as the static appearance" of the hip joints and "selection for tight coxofemoral joints might be the best way to reduce the frequency of canine hip dysplasia" (Madsen and Svalastoga 1991).

Conventional positioning used for radiographic detection of HD, especially if the limbs are slightly abducted and in external rotation results in a winding of the joint capsule and causes the femoral heads in dogs with lax hip joints to fit more deeply into acetabula. Thus, dysplastic hip joints appear more nearly normal on the radiograph. By the use of an optimal position of the limb during radiography, any of these special techniques permits identification of lateral displacement of the femoral head from the acetabulum greater than is seen when the limbs are fully extended as in the conventional positioning (Heyman, et al 1993). The fulcrum technique in this type dog forces the femoral heads laterally and clearly identifies this previously hidden joint laxity (Figure 5-27). The use of the Flückiger technique identifies the femoral head in a more natural dorsocranial position in the dysplastic dog. The possibility of false negative findings on a conventional VD radiograph have been brought even more clearly into perspective by the use of a technique that takes advantage of both compression and distraction views and evaluates the measurement of joint laxity (Smith, et al 1990). In a young dog with minimal joint laxity, most studies using some type of wedge or distraction device demonstrate a laxity not otherwise detected on standard ventrodorsal radiographs (Belkoff, et al 1989). This creates a most important problem in having to explain to an owner why one positioning technique results in production of a radiograph that is evaluated as normal while another technique produces a radiograph with an evaluation of near-normal or even dysplastic.

With the exception that joint laxity beyond a certain, as yet unknown point is synonymous with genotypic dysplasia, it behooves the clinician to make use of this information when examining the dog for hip dysplasia by using one of the following schemes. These are: (1) comparing the location of the femoral head within the acetabula on routine and fulcrum views, (2) utilizing the compression and distraction views to measure femoral head movement, (3) using the Flückiger technique or (4) comparing findings from a non-distractive radiographic view with those obtained from conscientious palpation for an Ortolani sign. Any of these schemes are recommended for the evaluation of the young dog prior to the onset of secondary joint changes and lead to an earlier and more accurate diagnosis of joint laxity.

## Dorsal acetabular rim view

A special dorsal acetabular rim view (DAR) has been described that proposes to permit more accurate evaluation of the weight-bearing portion of the acetabulum (Slocum and Devine 1989, 1990). With the dog in sternal recumbency the femurs are pulled cranially until they are parallel to the long axis of the body where they are held in position by restraining devices. This causes a marked tilting of the pelvis until it approaches being perpendicular to the tabletop. The vertically directed x-ray beam is thus pointed toward the dorsal margin of the acetabulum and the angle of the acetabular shelf can be determined from the resulting radiograph. In the normal dog, the dorsal rim is sharp and the slope angle had an average of 13.5° (±3.0°) while in a group of dysplastic dog the slope angle had a mean value of 26.3° (±13.4°). With frequent subluxation, the dorsal rim becomes rounded, acetabular filling occurs, and dorsal osteophyte formation is seen. In the event of the dog having secondary changes that have so markedly alter the slope angle, a special radiographic view is not necessary for diagnosis. However, this special view can be helpful to a surgeon in providing additional information needed in determine the appropriateness of doing a triple pelvic osteotomy as well as to determine the degree of acetabular rotation required. The unique positioning of the dog that is required for this view has resulted in it not being used commonly.

## Radiographic diagnosis

Methods of radiographic evaluation for hip dysplasia vary depending on the individual viewer and the certifying registry in which the results of the study are to be recorded. One method is to evaluate the radiograph and mentally record the appearance of a variety of anatomical regions. The sequence of examination of the radiograph varies as can the weight given to change noted in each of the anatomical regions. After completing the review of the radiograph, a subjective evaluation is recorded that can be limited to a statement of normal or dysplastic, or can include other modifiers that indicate the degree of normalcy or abnormality. The subjective evaluation is strongly influenced by past experience of the reviewer and can be influenced by the rules promulgated by the certifying registry. While a subjective evaluation seems to lack objectivity and therefore might be questionable, it should be remembered that most radiographic evaluations, not only of the status of the hip joints but of all disease conditions, are made in this manner.

A second method of film evaluation follows a more directed examination of the radiograph in which a series of parameters are studied in a standardized sequence and each parameter is assigned a number. It has been suggested that standardized forms should be used in recording specific changes or measurements (Lawson 1963, Müller and Saar 1966). The report can include an evaluation of the status of each hip, and scores, if assigned, can be added to obtain a total score for the dog (Lawson 1963, Müller and Saar 1966, Willis 1984, Flückiger 1993). Another protocol might use the status of the most affected hip as indicative of the severity of the dysplasia. In most systems, if one hip is dysplastic and the other normal, the dog is judged to be dysplastic.

Lawson (1963) stressed the need for a method of examination "... in which each part of the hip joint is scrutinized in turn and any changes are noted." Acetabular contour and depth, shape of femoral head and neck, and overall joint structure and conformation were considered individually and the total change recognized as a pattern. The British hip dysplasia control used such a system and assigned a point value between 0 and 6 to nine selected parameters on each hip. The more severe the changes the higher the point value assigned. The total score was tabulated and was used to provide a comparison of hip status with other individual members within the breed and with a breed "average" (Willis, 1984, 1986, 1990, 1997 a). This technique and its results have been recently reviewed (Willis 1997 b) and are discussed more fully elsewhere (see Chapter 10).

A more recent plan has scored the Norberg angle, width of joint space, craniolateral acetabular edge, cranial subchondral acetabular bone, femoral head and neck, and presence of the Morgan-Line and has been proven to be simple, reliable, reproducible, and an efficient protocol (Flückiger 1993). Each structure is assigned a point value from 0 to 5 depending on the degree of severity of change. A total score of 0 to 2 per hip joint receives an evaluation of normal while a total score of > 18 per hip joint receives an evaluation of severe HD. This technique is further described (see Chapter 10).

While the objective method of evaluation appears to be more scientific, the original assignment of the specific parameters to be evaluated and the determination of the weight to be given to each parameter needs to be questioned for its appropriateness. If errors exist in the manner of creation of the protocol, errors will then be present in the final judgment. Also, a technique of this type forces the viewer to assign a value to each parameter even though its evaluation is compromised by film quality or patient positioning. So, while an objective system looks good on paper, it can be questioned. The results from a subjective evaluation can actually be more accurate since the viewer has the freedom to study the film as is appropriate considering its unique features. One possible value of an objective evaluation is that it provides an owner/breeder a numerical ranking of the status of the hips that can be compared with another dog. Therefore, even if the basis for the numerical assignment is incorrect, since it is used consistently, it has a value when comparing scores between dogs.

It is important as we assign numerical values to various selected parameters that are seen in dysplastic hips that we remember the warning of Schnelle (1973) that: "Pelvic deviations from perfection should be kept in proper perspective." Thus, the arbitrary assignment of a sharp line of separation between what is considered normal and what is considered abnormal can result in a division that is not accurate and can classify differences as pathologic that are actually normal variations. Forcing the hips of each dog into a specific mold can be counterproductive.

Regardless of the method of radiographic evaluation, the report can ultimately offer an evaluation of the status of the hips using terms such as: excellent, normal, near-normal, mildly dysplastic, moderately dysplastic, or severely dysplastic. Other schemes assign the degree of dysplasia as grade 1, 2, 3, or 4. These terms have slightly different meanings for the various film reviewers. They also have different meanings between the registries using different certifying schemes, regardless of attempts to correct this problem. Other registries require that the numerical values obtained from certain parameters are summarized and a total numerical value is assigned for the dog without using the words "normal" or "dysplastic." This information is of value in comparing the status of the hips between two or more dogs and can be used to determine a numerical level above which the dog is not recommended for breeding.

Certain breed clubs or certifying registries recommend which dogs are to be used in breeding on the basis of the radiographic study of the hips. This can be done using either a descriptive diagnosis or a numerical assignment.

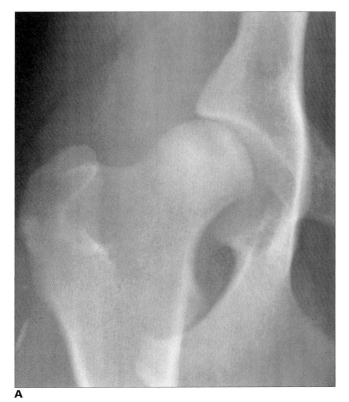 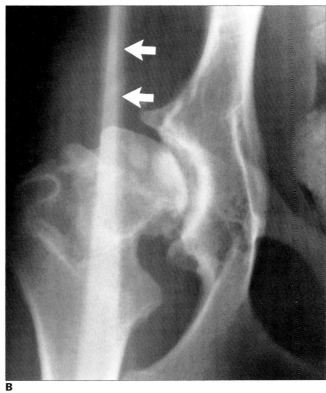

**Figure 5-32**
Radiographs of the right hip from two dogs with hip dysplasia. The earliest pattern of disease is (A) joint laxity while later (E) secondary joint disease is superimposed over the joint laxity. While position of the dog during radiographic examination and use of distraction techniques are important in identification of joint laxity in (A), the secondary changes are rather easy to detect regardless of patient positioning in (B). The heavy "white" line (arows) seen over the femur (B) is the result of a skin fold (flank fold). Appreciate the difficulty in measurement of a Norberg angle in (B).

Each of these basic systems of recording the results of the radiographic evaluation has strengths and weaknesses and it is not our intent to make a judgment on which one is best. Usually, the clinician or owner/breeder will find themselves forced into using a system by the breed club or the certifying registry with which they are associated and therefore, they will become most familiar with that system.

The radiograph continues to play an important role in diagnosis of dysplasia because it constitutes a permanent record of the status of the bony structures composing the hip joints at the time of the examination. Consensus opinions can be obtained, referral can be made to the radiographic study at a later date, and comparison can be made between studies made at different ages. However, there is always a problem with consensus opinion. The following unfortunately sounds familiar to what might be heard today: "... the veterinarian judged that there was dysplasia and consequently recommended that the dog not be used for breeding..." The second veterinarian gave the dog a clean bill of health. Obviously, a referee was needed, an "expert" who could pass final, authoritative judgment" (Freeman 1963). Hopefully, in the near future with a greater recognition and better understanding of the importance of joint laxity, the evaluation of the radiographic changes of dysplasia can become more objective.

The radiographic evaluation should be made without regard for the consequences, either for the dog or the breeder/owner. That is often not done today because of the stigma and expense attached to an evaluation of dysplastic. Unfortunately, the radiographs are often evaluated with a strong feeling as to the consequences for the dog. If the clinician reading the radiographs knows of the consequences of an evaluation indicating minimal dysplasia, a tendency exists to evaluate hips that are questionable as "near-normal" or "fair." By mixing the radiographic evaluation with a determination of the consequences for the dog or the owner's feelings, many dogs with minimal dysplasia have been "passed" and are used for breeding. In the long run, reporting a dysplastic dog to be acceptable for breeding results in continued pro-

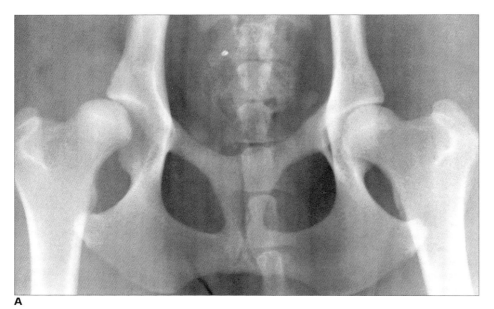

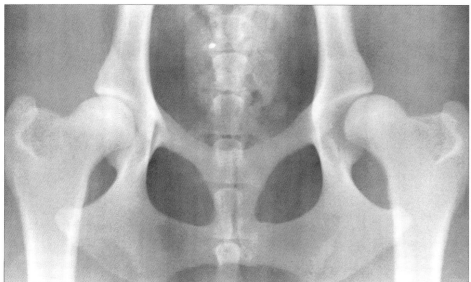

**Figure 5-33**
Two radiographs were made on the same day of a 2-year-old female Labrador Retriever in dorsal recumbency with the limbs in extension and internal rotation. On the first study (A), the right femoral head is subluxated while the left femoral head appears to be deeply seated. On the second study (B), the left femoral head is subluxated while the right femoral head appears deeply seated. A positive Ortolani sign was detected bilaterally. This inconsistency in the position of the femoral head relative to the acetabulum is not uncommon and obviously has a great influence on the evaluation of hip disease.

duction of affected litters. Instead, the radiographs should have been evaluated as "dysplastic with minimal changes," and the consequences relative to the use of that dog for breeding are based on the more honest evaluation.

## Patterns of radiographic change

Two basic patterns of change are identified on the radiograph of the dysplastic dog. The earliest pattern of change is joint laxity and we have already pointed out problems in its detection. The second pattern of change is easier to detect and its interpretation is less controversial since it includes a description of the malformed hip joint and the resulting osteoarthrosis indicative of HD.

The correct detection of secondary bony changes is not as dependent on the positioning of the dog for radiography as is the detection of joint laxity (Figure 5-32).

The commonly accepted criteria for radiological diagnosis of the secondary bony changes seen with hip dysplasia in the dog have not changed greatly from early reports (Schnelle 1954; Olsson 1962 b, 1968; Whittington, et al 1961; Riser 1962; Lawson 1963; Larsen and Corley 1971; Morgan 1972, 1974; Pharr and Morgan 1976; Ackerman and Nyland 1977; Ackerman 1982; Henry 1992). Many of the descriptions include correlations between radiographic and pathological changes as seen at necropsy. In contrast, the methods of detecting joint laxity have undergone re-evaluation and are considered to be of

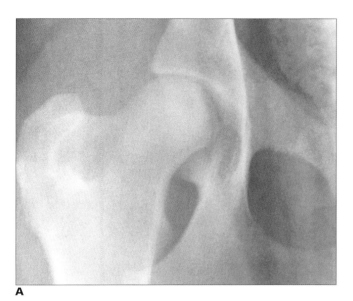 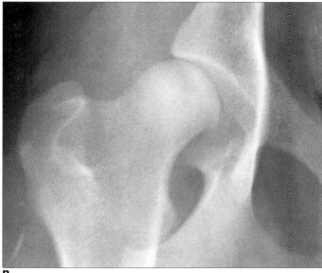

**Figure 5-34**
Radiographs made of the right hip of a 1-year-old male German Shorthaired Pointer show on the first study (A) that the femoral head is deeply seated and on the second study (B) that the femoral head is subluxated. This inconsistency illustrates the value of radiographs made with distraction of the femoral heads or the value of palpation of the hip joints at the time of radiography.

greater value today as the importance of joint laxity in the diagnosis of young dogs has increased.

## Joint laxity

Examination of the components of the hip joint is important in the determination of joint laxity. Henricson, et al (1966) stated that: "Considering all the . . . clinical and experimental evidence, joint laxity as the causal factor of hip dysplasia seems to be firmly established." Riser (1973 b) agreed that: "Radiographically the first signs of hip dysplasia are femoral head subluxation and a lag in the development of the craniodorsal acetabular rim. They are noted by the seventh week." The immediate results are those of "a stretched and thickened joint capsule" and a "teres ligament (that) is swollen and frayed." The capsule can achieve a thickness of 5 to 7 mm in an effort to restrict lateral movement of the femoral head. Many of these changes involve soft tissues and are not identified radiographically.

With early subluxation of the femoral head, Lust and Summers (1981) reported an increase in the volume of synovial fluid and an increase in the volume of the round ligament of the femoral head. These were thought to create an increased intra-articular pressure that might be the cause of the subluxation. However, the authors feel it is more likely that these changes are not causative but are secondary to early joint laxity.

Subluxation is the failure of the femoral head to sit "properly" within the acetabulum. Unfortunately, the position of the femoral head is influenced by pathologic changes within the hip joint as well as radiographic positioning of the pelvis and hind limbs (Figures 5-33, 5-34). Thus, a subluxating hip can be made to appear normal radiographically by placing the limb in external rotation and abduction. Since, radiographic detection of subluxation is subject to error, the use of measurements taken from a single routine VD view with the limbs extended is questionable. Use of compression/distraction views, comparison of routine and wedge views, or radiography combined with hip palpation are each more likely to detect subluxation and the failure to use these combinations increases the possibility for an incorrect diagnosis. (Figure 5-35).

Since the earliest radiographic changes of hip dysplasia can be subluxation of the femoral head, evaluation of the width of the joint space is of great importance. Detection of an increase in width of the joint space between the contour of the femoral head and the depth of the acetabulum indicate joint laxity but can be difficult for the novice to ascertain. The rounding of the acetabular margin is due to weight-bearing forces that shift the femoral head into contact with the dorsal acetabular margin and can serve as a more positive indicator of joint laxity.

While subjective, the most commonly used indication of an increase in the width of the joint space is the detection of incongruity between the femoral head and the

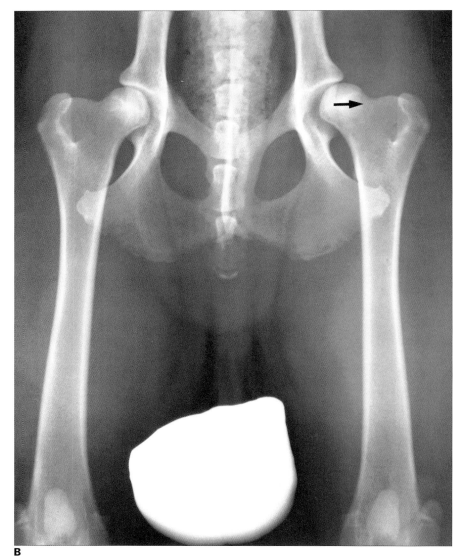

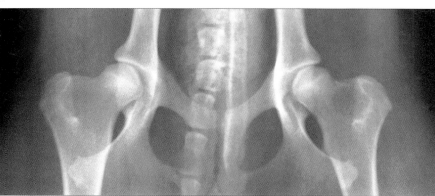

**Figure 5-35**
Two radiographs made of a 2-year-old male German Shepherd Dog using a (A) conventional VD positioning and a (B) wedge technique. The joint laxity on the left (arrow) is not fully appreciated until the distraction study is made. The radiopaque shadow between the hind limbs is made by the fulcrum device.

craniodorsal portion of the acetabular margin that results from the lateral displacement of the femoral head. This evaluation is highly dependent on the positioning of the hind limbs.

Another technique in the evaluation of joint laxity utilizes the center of the femoral head and its relative position with the dorsal rim of the acetabulum that can be seen through the femoral head. If the center of the femoral head is lateral to the dorsal rim of the acetabulum, the head is considered subluxated (Figure 5-36). The location of the center of the head can also be compared to a line drawn caudally from the craniodorsal angle of the acetabular margin parallel to the spine (Figure 5-13). If the center of the head is lateral to that line it is considered subluxated. Since positioning of the pelvis and positioning of the hind limbs influences the radiographic detection of femoral head subluxation, the presence of joint laxity can be more accurately determined using a distraction technique.

The most popular method of determining location of the femoral head as an indicator of subluxation has been measurement of the Norberg angle. This angle is formed by the intersection of a line connecting the center of the femoral heads and a line drawn from the center of the femoral head that extends through the craniodorsal margin of the acetabulum (Figure 5-14). The angle is measured on the pelvic side. It can be measured on a radiograph of a well-positioned dog in a VD view with the limbs either extended or flexed. The relationship between the center of the femoral head and the craniodorsal acetabular margin in the normal dog has been determined to be $\geq$ than 105°. As the femoral head shifts laterally the angle becomes smaller indicating joint laxity. Rounding of the diseased acetabular margin can affect the measurement and cause the angle to be smaller. Measurement of the angle can also be influenced by secondary change on the craniodorsal acetabular margin. In the older dysplastic dog, new bone deposition results in an increase in the angle, falsely causing the acetabulum to have apparent depth and the possibility exists of a false negative evaluation. However, secondary changes are in themselves indicative of a diagnosis of dysplasia negating the need for evaluation of the Norberg angle. Therefore, this measurement is most valuable in the younger dog before secondary changes have occurred and, in fact, determination of the Norberg angle becomes superfluous following the onset of secondary changes (Figure 5-31). A high degree of correlation was thought to exist between the Norberg angle in a young dog and the likelihood of future osteoarthrosis (van der Velden 1983; Banfield, et al 1996 a). However, more recently, joint laxity has been reported to be more valuable in the prediction of development of osteoarthrosis indicative of dysplasia than measurement of the Norberg angle (Smith, et al 1993), and the Norberg angle was not found to be a significant risk factor for development of osteoarthrosis either in longitudinal or cross-sectional analyses (Smith, et al 1995).

Unfortunately, the diagnosis of joint laxity is strongly influenced in all cases by the position of the hind limb during radiography. The most common error is the placement of the limbs in external rotation with abduction, which prevents detection of joint laxity. This can actually be the result of intentional effort by the radiographer to produce a radiograph with the femoral heads more deeply seated in the hope that it will be evaluated normal. Ideally, these studies should be repeated, however, time, money, and motivation do not always permit this re-examination. Some certifying registries accept radiographs made with the limbs slightly malpositioned resulting in the erroneous assignment of normal evaluations.

Other errors in positioning include pelvic obliquity caused by rotation around the longitudinal axis in which the appearance of a normal hip joint can be falsely evaluated as being subluxated as well as the joint with abnormal laxity being falsely evaluated as being normal. Hips should not be evaluated on oblique studies of this type. As the dog ages, secondary changes permit a more accurate diagnosis of the dysplastic joint even in the event of patient malpositioning. However, in the young dog, if an accurate evaluation is desired, it is safer to repeat the radiographic study than to make the diagnosis on an improperly positioned study.

Using compression/distraction techniques, it is possible to attempt to determine an index number beyond which it is possible to predict if the dog is likely to develop osteoarthrosis indicative of hip dysplasia (Smith, et al 1990). These techniques measure the range of motion of the femoral head within the acetabulum as determined by comparing a radiograph made with compression and one made with distraction. The index is determined by comparing movement of the center of the femoral head. A recent study has shown that this index can be breed dependent with a distraction index predicting greater probability for development of osteoarthrosis different in the German Shepherd Dog as compared to the Rottweiler (Popovitch, et al 1995).

### Secondary bony changes

Osteophytoses (periosteal new bone or enthesophytosis) or periarticular new bone (periarticular lipping) reflect

# 150 Hip dysplasia

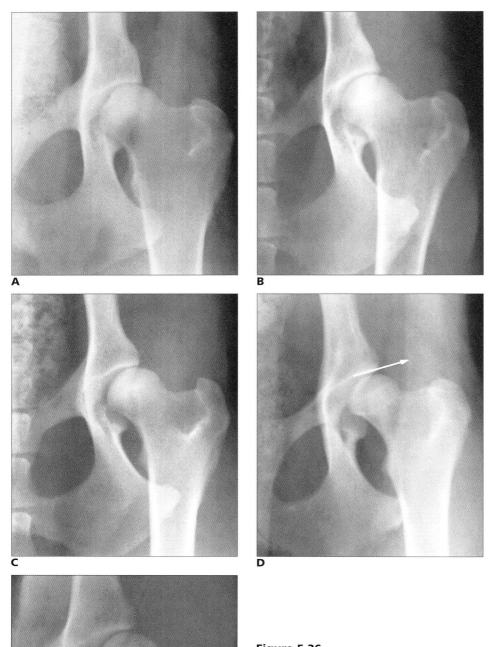

**Figure 5-36**
A series of radiographs from different dogs that illustrate progressive subluxation of the femoral head and development of the secondary changes within the acetabulum. Starting with the tight-fitting head (A), the degree of joint laxity progresses to a point of complete luxation (J). Note that in the final case, the depth of the acetabulum is filled with bone. In the evaluation of femoral head laxity, the subchondral bone within the craniodorsal portion of the acetabular rim becomes sclerotic. Note as the head rides further lateral, the acetabular cup opens and the dorsocranial margin is directed more cranially as seen on the radiographs (arrows).

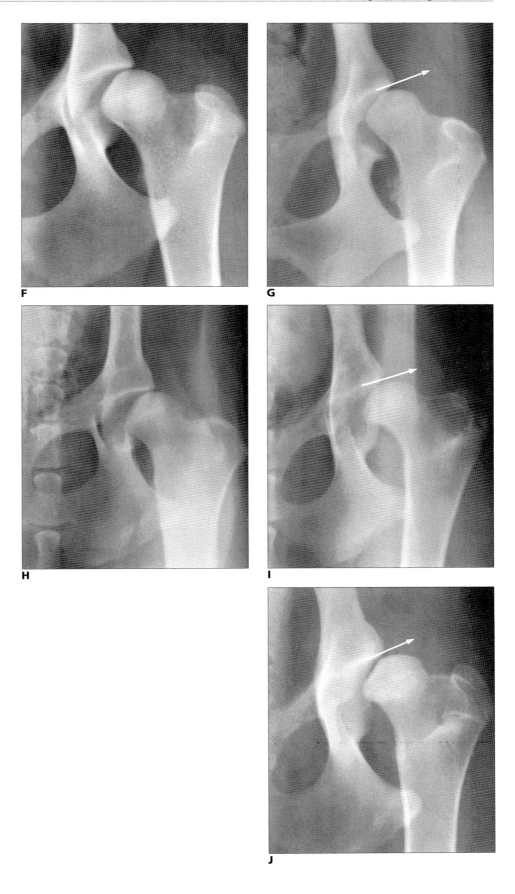

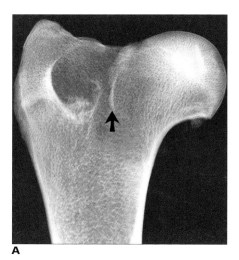 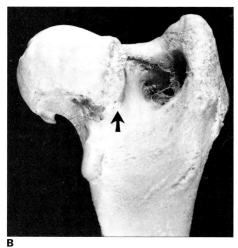

**Figure 5-37**
Radiograph and photograph of a femoral specimen show early enthesophyte formation on the caudal aspect of the femoral neck (arrows) that reflects joint laxity indicative of hip dysplasia. Note the varus deformity in this dog.

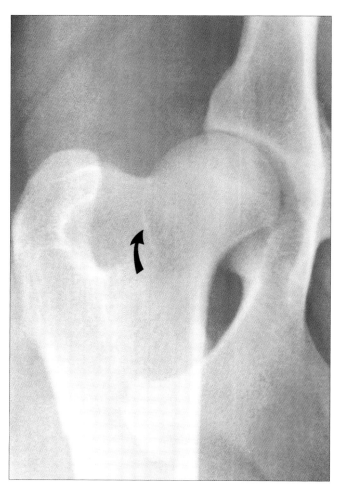

**Figure 5-38**
Radiograph of the right hip joint of a 1-year-old female German Shepherd Dog showing a minimal enthesophyte on the caudal aspect of the femoral neck (arrow) indicative of early joint laxity. If the radiograph is underexposed, this change is not identified.

the secondary bony changes occurring within the dysplastic joint. In addition to joint laxity the detection of any new bony growth is an important indicator of osteoarthrosis and thus, in most dogs an indicator of hip dysplasia. The new bone can appear as a "spur" or as a "lip" depending on how it is projected by the x-ray beam. Often the new bone is in the form of a "collar" or "ring" around the femoral neck. However, since the new bone is projected tangentially, it may appear as a bony spur. This new bone takes two forms, one is periarticular in location and has the purpose of enlarging the articular margin in a joint with laxity and is referred to as periarticular lipping. The other form of new bone is referred to as ent-hesophytosis and occurs at the site of soft tissue attachments and reflects unusual traction on these attachments due to joint instability. By knowing the normal attachments of the joint capsule, muscle tendons, and ligaments, the location of the bony prominences can be predicted.

Osteophyte formation on the caudal aspect of the femoral neck in young dogs assumes a linear pattern at the attachment of the joint capsule (Morgan 1987) and has been called the "Morgan Line" (Klimt, et al 1992). These osteophytes are visible radiographically and are the earliest bony signs of the effect of joint laxity (Figures 5-37, 5-38). The presence of the new bone suggests tension on the capsular attachment, the result of instability of the joint. The location of the osseous ridge was described previously when femurs were examined at necropsy (Ackerman and Nyland 1977, Ackerman 1982). Joint capsule attachment on the femur is 1 to 2 cm from the margin of the cartilage covering of the femoral head. An understandable hesitancy to diagnosis HD exists if this is the only radiographic change noted. However, it is thought that this sign is reliable and dogs with only this change should be: (1) classified as dysplastic, (2) examined

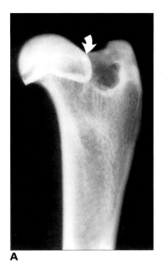 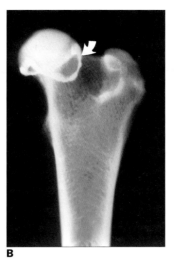 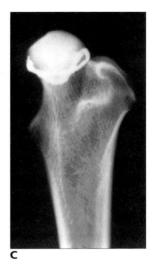

**Figure 5-39**
Radiographs of the proximal femur in different positions with a radiopaque marker on the margin of the articular surface of the femoral head indicating the site of attachment of the joint capsule. (A) With the limb in internal rotation, the marker outlines the location of the attachment of the joint capsule superimposed over the femoral neck and indicates the expected location of the enthesophyte (arrow). (B) With the limb in a position of minimal external rotation, the marker shows the attachment of the joint capsule as it shifts in position toward the femoral head and an enthesophyte at this location (arrow) is more difficult to visualize. (C) With the limb in a position of external rotation, the marker shows that the enthesophyte formed at the site of attachment of the joint capsule would not be identified. Note the fovea capitis with external rotation (B, C) giving the appearance of flattening of the head.

further radiographically using distraction or wedge techniques, or (3) palpated to obtain additional evidence of joint laxity that supports the diagnosis of hip dysplasia. Dogs with this early pattern of new bone should at least be recognized as genetically dysplastic. However, if this sign is the only indication of abnormal stress within the joint in the mature dog (>18 months of age), especially in the heavy breeds, its significance at this time in questionable.

On radiographs of the hind limbs extended, this new bone is seen as a vertically directed linear radiodensity projected through the center of the femoral neck. On radiographs made with the hind limbs in the "frog leg" position, the new bone is seen as a spur formation projected beyond the cortex on the caudolateral border of the femoral neck. If the limbs are extended, but rotated externally, projection of the femoral neck is altered so the greater trochanter is superimposed over the neck and the Morgan Line is not identified (Morgan and Stephens 1985; Klimt, et al 1992) (Figures 5-39, 5-40).

It is possible to position the limbs in such a manner that the bone forming the slope from the femoral head onto the femoral neck is projected on end causing a dense shadow to be seen at the location of physeal closure of

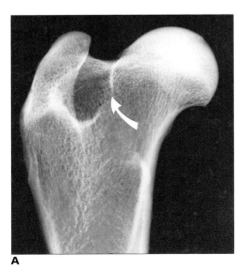 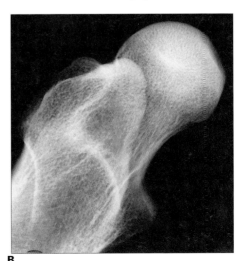

**Figure 5-40**
Radiographs of a specimen of the femoral head and neck in a dog with an enthesophyte creating a Morgan-Line on the caudal aspect of the femoral neck (arrow) that is clearly identified (A) if the limb is correctly positioned, but the ridge on the femoral neck is lost (B) on a second radiograph made with the limb in external rotation.

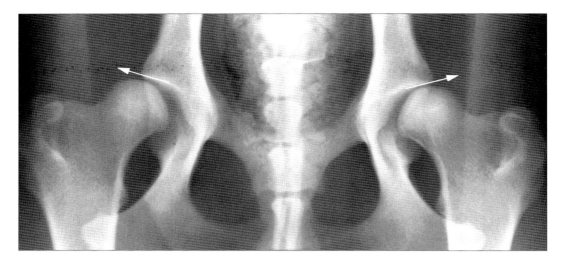

**Figure 5-41**
A radiograph of the pelvis of a 1-year-old female Labrador Retriever shows flattening of the dorsocranial margin of the acetabula (arrows) and subluxation of the femoral heads. The change in appearance of the acetabular rim indicates abnormal forces between the femoral head and the acetabular rim regardless of the position of the femoral head. Thus, the appearance of the acetabular rim can be a valuable diagnostic feature in the unstable hip in which laxity is not demonstrated because the femoral head is forced into the acetabula.

the femoral head. This transversely directed line can be incorrectly diagnosed as a ring of osteophytes around the head.

Evaluation of the acetabular margin provides an indication of the relationship between the femoral head and the acetabulum. In puppies, lesions in the cartilage of the acetabular margin are first seen between 2 to 4 months of age depending on the severity of the disease (Riser 1975). Normally, the cartilaginous margin of the acetabulum does not completely convert to bone until 8 to 9 months. This provides a period of several months in which the acetabular margin is particularly vulnerable to biomechanical forces that result from a disparity between muscle growth and skeletal growth. The delayed growth of muscle relative to skeletal growth results in a dorsolateral displacement of the femoral head and joint laxity. As the femoral head slides back-and-forth over the acetabular lip, wearing occurs and the lip is rounded. Because of the overloading forces on the lip, chondrogenesis and osteogenesis are affected with a delay in the conversion of fibrocartilage to hyaline cartilage and then to bone. This abnormal modeling results in flattening of the acetabular margin and reflects the abnormal contact between femoral head and acetabulum (Figure 5-41). Although severe modeling of the acetabular margin can be identified radiographically by 3 months of age, the more commonly occurring modeling is not seen radiographically until the dog is 6 to 9 months of age. Frost (1989) further described this effect of abnormal loading of the femoral head as it shifts toward the rim of the acetabular articular cartilage and used the term "lateralized loading." Retardation of normal downward growth of the acetabular margin results.

## Subchondral sclerosis

Dense bands of subchondral bone of equal thickness are present within the cranial acetabular margin as a result of normal contact between the weight-bearing surfaces. With a loss of congruity consequent to joint laxity and lateral displacement of the femoral head, the loading pressures are concentrated on a smaller area of the opposing articular surfaces. As a result, the pressure on the dorsocranial edge of the acetabular margin, which is the remaining contact area, is increased above that which is normal for healthy cartilaginous or bony tissue. An increase in deposition of subchondral bone results and can be referred to as bony sclerosis due to the increase in number and thickness of bony trabeculae (Prieur 1980). With a decrease in pressure on the subchondral bone of the medial acetabular surface as a result of the femoral head riding laterally, there is a loss of bone tissue with a less dense appearance radiographically. These changes in density of the subchondral bone indicate the nature of the altered contact between the femoral head and the acetabulum (Figure 5-42).

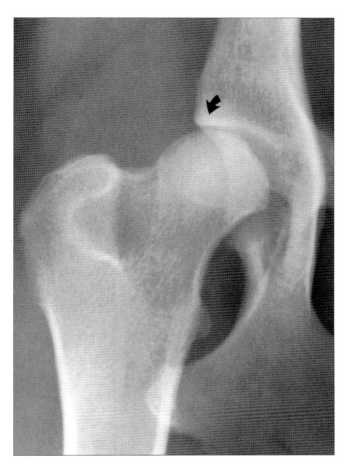

**Figure 5-42**
A radiograph of the right hip of a 1-year-old German Shepherd Dog shows minimal subluxation of the femoral head that is associated with focal sclerotic subchondral bone in the lateral aspect of the acetabular margin. Note the uneven width of the bony band at the margin with increased width and density at the site of maximum force from the femoral head (arrow). The femoral head appears flattened due to the fovea capitis.

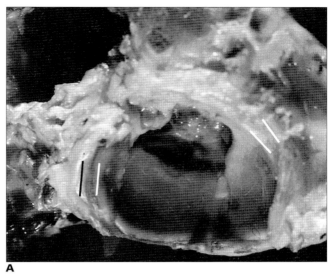

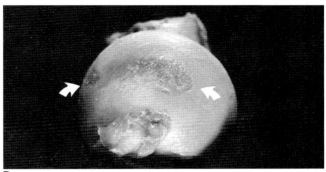

**Figure 5-43**
Photographs of the acetabulum (A) and femoral head (B) show the effect of chronic subluxation of the femoral head. Palpation of the acetabular margin reveals the presence of two lips (lines). The lips are best imagined dorsocranially and caudally on the photograph. The zone of wearing of the articular cartilage on the femoral head (arrows) indicates the site of contact between the acetabular margin and the femoral head.

## Bilabiation

If the joint laxity is prominent and occurs at an early age the effect on the cartilaginous margin is one of severe deformity characterized by a rounding of the acetabular margin. If a lesser degree of joint laxity is present and occurs at a later age, ossification of the margin occurs and secondary lipping extends the margin of the acetabulum in an attempt to stabilize the joint. Thus, the cranial acetabular margin changes from a smooth arc to one with a new margin that is characterized by a double-curved line referred to as bilabiation. This description is helpful in the understanding of the effect on the margin of the acetabulum as the femoral head shifts in position laterally (Lawson 1963). The original articular cup remains in part, while a new articular surface forms dorsolaterally and cranially on the acetabular margin. Thus, a pattern of two lips of smooth articular bone is created with the new lip just lateral to the original lip (Figure 5-43). Following bilabiation, new bone can be added to the acetabular margin as the dog tries to hold the femoral head in its new lateral position. Radiographically, the new bone appears as periarticular new bone.

Destruction of the bilabiation can result from abnormal forces created if the femoral head continues to ride against the acetabular margin. Modeling can stop at any stage of subluxation when the joint capsule provides sufficient support to stabilize the joint. Progression of bilabiation can also be terminated when the subluxation proceeds to a completely luxated head with no further contact between head and acetabulum. Change in the

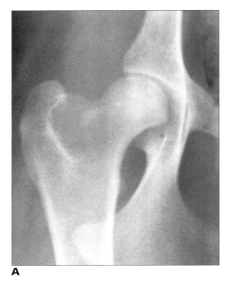 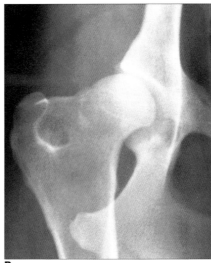 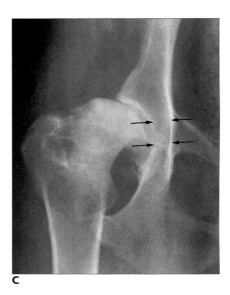

**Figure 5-44**
Radiographs of the right hip joint of three different dogs show the change in the appearance of the acetabulum as the femoral head shifts laterally. They show: (A) normal depth of the acetabulum, (B) early subluxation with only minimal new bone deposition within the depth of the acetabulum, (C) and chronic subluxation with filling of the depth of the acetabulum by new bone (arrows). With filling of the depth of the acetabulum with bone, the attachment of the round ligament is destroyed.

acetabular margin at this time is influenced by lack of bony contact and it is characterized by bone atrophy and disappearance of the dense bands of subchondral bone that previously defined the craniodorsal acetabular margin.

The persistence of the shape of the acetabulum is dependent on the tightness of the fit of the femoral head. Therefore, as the femoral head shifts laterally, the acetabular fossa fills with new bone medially and ventrally. Eventually, this deposition of new bone results in complete destruction of the site of origin of the round ligament of the femoral head and the shape of the acetabulum shifts from that of a cup to that of a shallower saucer (Figure 5-44).

## Modeling patterns

Thus, a total of four patterns indicating abnormal bone development can be seen in association with joint instability. The femoral head can subluxate and: (1) causing rounding (flattening) of the acetabular margin, (2) forming a pattern of modeling on the acetabular margin referred to as bilabiation, (3) remaining within the acetabulum with the formation of heavy osteophytes attempting to create a functional lip that holds the head in position, and (4) separate completely from the acetabulum with atrophy of the acetabular margin due to disuse. Any of these stages can be an end-point being somewhat age dependent or the patterns can be progressive within the same patient.

## Acetabular margin

The acetabular margin is normally a uniform cartilage lip with the size depending on the age of the dog. In some dogs, the presence of an ununited bony ossicle at the dorsocranial acetabular margin is seen. It was previously thought to play a role in the development of HD since it might constitute an area of weakness. It was described in eight of 35 dogs with minimal secondary osteoarthrosis who were 8 months to 6 years of age (Olsson and Audell 1978) (Figure 5-45). However, the presence of this free ossicle did not seem to alter the gross appearance of the hip joint and histologically, little difference was noted between the acetabular margin in dysplastic dogs with or without this ununited bony ossicle. At the present time, this bony ossicle is not thought to be of value in predicting femoral head subluxation and is not thought to lead to an osteoarthrosis. Additional study is needed, especially in younger dogs, to learn more of the clinical significance of this separate ossification center. In the author's experience, this ossicle is seen in larger breeds and is unrelated to the status of the hip joint.

## Ilial and ischial new bone

Dogs with severe secondary changes due to dysplasia can have deposition of smooth bone on the medial aspect of the ilium and ischium adjacent to the acetabulum that can cause increased thickness of bone as measured from

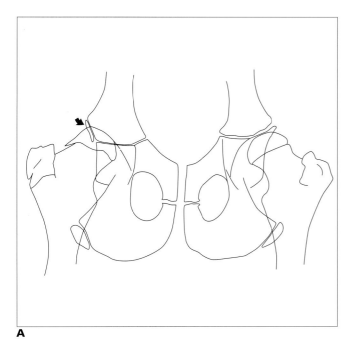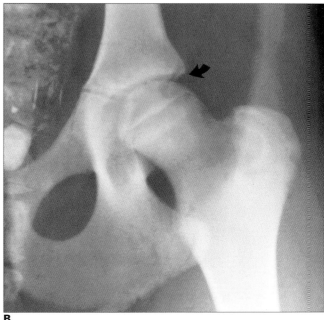

**Figure 5-45**
A drawing and a radiograph illustrate the location of a free bony ossicle within the acetabular margin. (A) A drawing of a pelvic radiograph of a 4-month-old Saint Bernard clearly illustrates the ossicle (arrow) on the margin of the right acetabulum. (B) The radiograph of the left hip of a 6-month-old dog shows the free ossicle (arrow).

the medial side of the pelvis to the depth of the acetabulum (Figure 5-46). Early, a "fluffy" halo of new bone is seen adjacent to the original cortical shadow. As the bone matures it appears to shift the cortical margin medially forming a neocortex. This reactive pattern is presumed to be a response to the lax fit of the femoral head and the alteration in pattern of stress lines through the altered hip joint. It has no known clinical significance, but is another of the secondary changes that reflect the malformed hip joint.

## Femoral head and neck

The first changes in the femoral head consist of a wearing of the articular cartilage and a thickening of the attachment of the round ligament (Figure 5-47), neither of which can be appreciated radiographically. Later changes result from subluxation and the femoral head models in response to failure of the femoral head and the acetabulum to fit normally. The progressive changes are dependent on the: (1) degree of joint laxity, (2) age the laxity began, (3) athletic activity of the dog, (4) weight of the dog, and (5) the age of the dog at the time of the radiographic examination.

Changes in the skeletally immature dog always occur more rapidly since the modeling involves the actively developing bony tissue. Thus, with subluxation of the femoral head in the puppy, changes to the femoral head can be massive with the result resembling a "melting ice cream cone." As much as 5 mm of the immature femoral head can be worn away due to the incongruous fit of the head and acetabulum with development of a varus deformity (Figure 5-48) (Riser 1973 b, 1975).

In the more slowly progressive disease, the changes within the femoral head and neck begin with the development of a slight bony ridge on the caudal aspect of the femoral neck (Morgan-Line). With persistent joint laxity, the secondary changes cause a thickening of the femoral neck. The femoral head appears to change from a spherical shape to one that is flattened with varying degrees of varus deformity. The pattern of change within the femoral head and neck parallels the pattern of change within the acetabulum (Figure 5-49). This is an important feature in understanding the pathophysiology of osteoarthrosis associated with hip dysplasia.

If the head luxates completely, no contact exists with the acetabulum and the head undergoes less modeling and, instead, appears somewhat atrophic with a minimal loss of sphericity. The smooth margin persists since no part of the acetabulum is in contact with the head to cause a design due to the abrasive action of bone on bone. Thus, the earlier and more complete is the luxation, the less

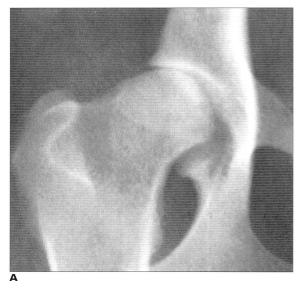

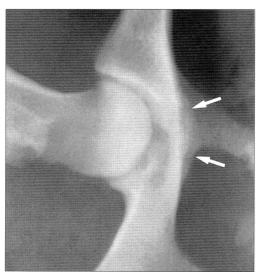

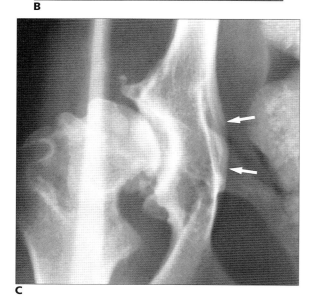

change occurs in the shape of the femoral head, however, the neck can be expected to respond to the absence of forces from the acetabulum with a resulting valgus deformity.

In larger breeds such as the Saint Bernard, noticeable subluxation can be evident as a puppy but the head tends to partially return within the acetabulum and undergoes only minimal modeling. These dogs with lax hip joints often show only minimal signs of osteoarthrosis later in life. This phenomenon is also seen in Bernese Mountain Dogs (Scartazzini 1972, Flückiger 1993). The authors have also seen this is the Pyrenean Mastiff. The existence of mature dogs with persistent joint laxity but with only minimal bony changes of osteoarthrosis suggests the concept of a physiologically near-normal joint in a dog with "genetic dysplasia" in contrast to a "clinical dysplasia." These dogs, while appearing without radiographic changes of osteoarthrosis, have hips that can be shown to readily luxated using distraction techniques. The dogs displaying this phenomenon are usually large dogs and cause a compromise in film quality because positioning for routine VD radiography is difficult and usually the limbs are positioned in external rotation and abducted. With this positioning of the limbs, minimal new bone production on the femoral neck can not be seen. Thus, changes of osteoarthrosis may actually be present, but not identified radiographically. The joint laxity indicates capsular as well as round ligament weakness and one wonders how the dog can compensate for this injury while ambulating and maintain joint stability as suggested by the presence of only a minimal osteoarthrosis.

### Inclination of the femoral neck

Inclination of the femoral neck can influence the development of the hip joint. However, several studies suggest that there is no positive correlation between the angle of inclination and the presence of hip dysplasia (Hauptman, et al 1985; Banfield, et al 1996 a). The angle of inclination is a measurement reflecting the manner of attachment of the femoral neck onto the shaft of the femur measured

**Figure 5-46**
Radiographs of the right hip of three dysplastic German Shepherd Dogs show the character of the medial cortex of the acetabulum. (A) The femoral head is minimally luxated, the femoral neck is thickened, and spurring is evident on the dorsocranial acetabular lip of a 6-year-old in which the medial cortex of the acetabulum is normal. (B) A "frog leg" view of a 2-year-old shows new bone formation on the medial cortex of the acetabulum (arrows). (C) Severe secondary modeling in a 4-year-old is associated with luxation of the femoral head and formation of a neocortex on the medial aspect of the acetabulum (arrows).

**Figure 5-47**
Photographs of femoral heads from dysplastic hip joints from different dogs show (A) early wearing of the articular cartilage as indicated by the ease in which the blood can be seen within the subchondral tissues and (B) more extensive wearing and fibrillation of the cartilage and hypertrophy of the round ligament.

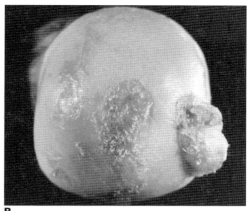

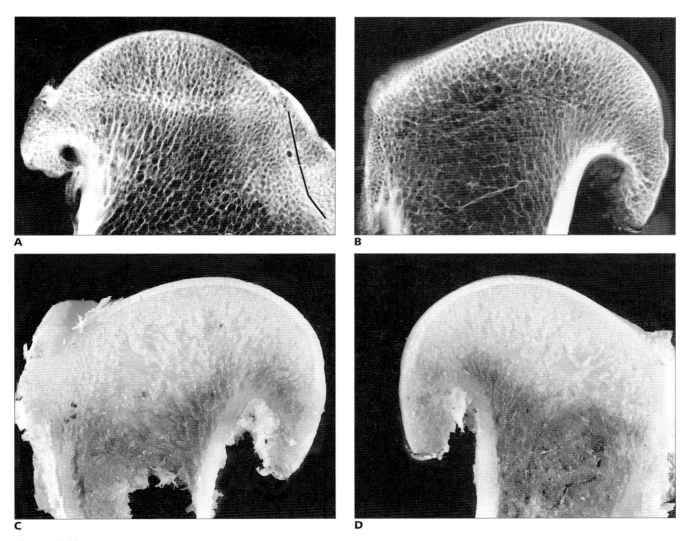

**Figure 5-48**
Radiographs (A, B) plus photographs (C, D) of slab sections taken from a severely dysplastic femoral head show modeling with the creation of the appearance of a "melting ice cream cone." Note the thickening on the dorsum of the femoral neck (A) with identification of the original cortical line (lines).

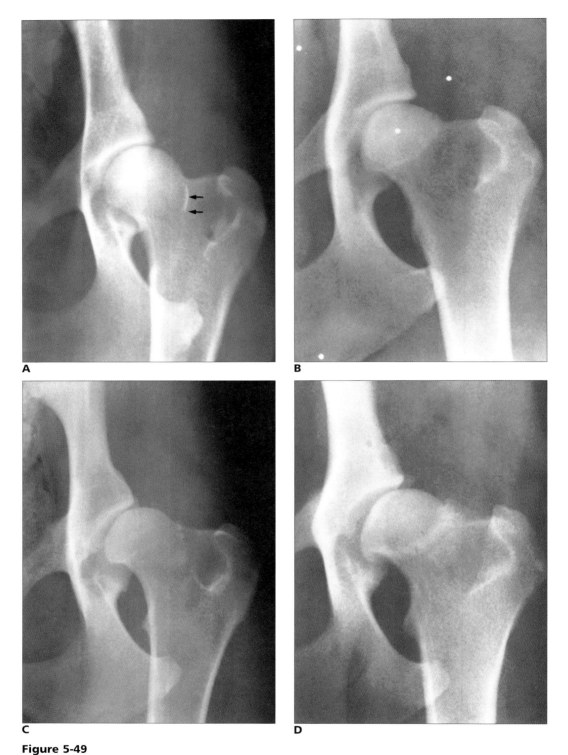

**Figure 5-49**
Radiographs of a sequence of patients illustrate a pattern of change within the femoral head and neck beginning with (A) a near normal in which there is a slight bony ridge on the caudal aspect of the femoral neck (Morgan Line) (arrows) and progresses to stages of greater subluxation leading to (D) production of a large cuff of bone on the neck and progressing to (G, H) a final flattening of both the acetabulum and femoral head. If the femoral head maintains some contact with the acetabulum, it models extensively with eventual formation of a varus deformity.

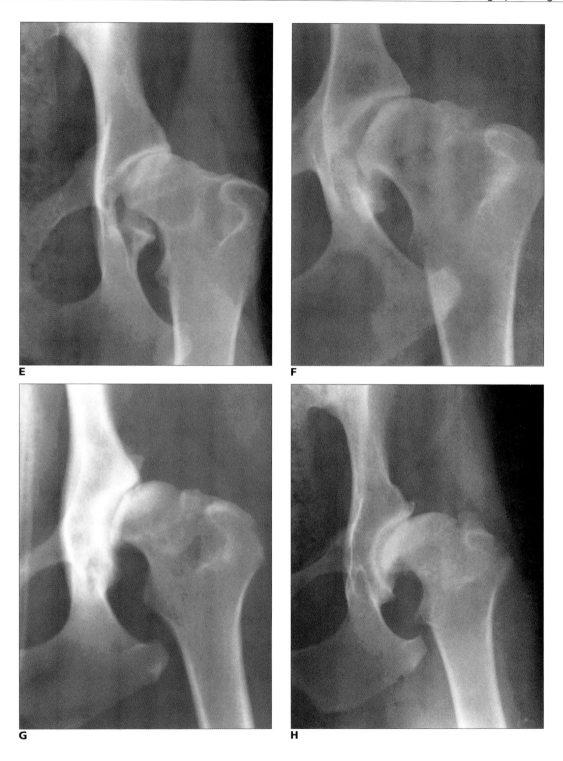

within the sagittal plane along the medial surface of the proximal femur. The angle of inclination measured on normal dogs is reported to be 146° ± 4.8° using one method of measurement and 129° ± 4.9° by a second method of measurement (Haupman, et al 1979). This range of measurements is the result of inaccurate attempts to determine the center of the short thick femoral neck in the dog and the resulting wide range of measurements. Radiographic positioning of the limb also affects the image of the neck and it is often difficult to obtain a repeatable position from which to obtain a measurement of inclination (Figure 5-50). An angle of 135° is generally accepted as the normal angle of inclination even though wide ranges of measurements have been obtained from normal dogs. A deformity in which the measurement is greater than normal is termed a "coxa valga" while a measurement that is less than normal is termed a "coxa vara."

With minimal subluxation, a wearing away of the articular surface of the femoral head and marked thickening to the neck, especially ventrally, results in a varus deformity. This can be described as an "osseous drift" of the neck. If the modeling of the femoral head and neck creates a varus deformity it may result in a better fit between the head and acetabulum (Figure 5-49 e). A surgical procedure, called a varus osteotomy, has been described that attempts to produce a similar type of correction. A dysplastic hip with a varus deformity and a decrease in angle of inclination when positioned in external rotation can be made to appear to have a more nearly normal angle of inclination as a result of this malpositioning.

In contrast to the varus deformity, a valgus deformity is also identified. This anomaly can be either true or false with some cases being secondary to HD and others unrelated to HD. An apparent valgus deformity can be due to positioning and is due to external rotation and abduction of the limb. Carlson (1967) warned of the danger of using a valgus deformity alone as a basis for diagnosing hip dysplasia because of the possibility of incorrectly interpreting change due to malposition of the limb (Figure 5-50 b). With early and complete luxation of the femoral head unrelated from hip dysplasia and due to an accident or congenital anomaly, contact between the femoral head and acetabulum is absent and a valgus deformity develops with the neck remaining relatively smooth and unchanged in thickness. Thus, a true valgus deformity can be seen with early femoral head luxation that may be due to: (1) congenital luxation, (2) early luxation with severe HD, or (3) may be due to a traumatic luxation. Other true valgus deformities can be due to: (1) an old femoral fracture with healing in external rotation of the proximal fragment or (2) a developmental abnormality of the femur associated with a lateral patellar luxation. An evaluation of the entire hind limb giving care to limb positioning usually prevents errors in interpretation of the cause of the valgus deformity.

Another error in diagnosis of a valgus deformity can result from a marked inclination of the femoral neck and an almost sagittal positioned acetabular cup that causes a true deformity that can result in an incorrectly evaluated Norberg angle in an otherwise normally developed coxofemoral joint (Prieur and Brüse 1988). These examples further point out the problems in using the evaluation of the angle of inclination as a feature in the radiographic diagnosis of dysplasia. The determination of the angle of inclination has little importance in the diagnosis of HD because secondary changes are prominent in cases with a varus deformity and a valgus deformity due to HD, is easy to detect because of the luxated femoral head, and may most likely be unrelated to HD. The valgus deformity may be created by malpositioning and a varus deformity can be obscured by malpositioning. The determination of the angle of inclination may be of major importance if surgical correction is contem-plated.

If the pattern of deformation of the femoral neck begins prior to physeal closure or skeletal maturation, the increased rate of bone turnover at this age permits modeling at a faster rate than occurs in adult bony tissue. The unclosed physeal plate permits an asymmetrical pattern of growth with the portion involved determining whether an increase or decrease in the angle of inclination is noted.

### Anteversion/retroversion

Anteversion/retroversion are terms that refer to the angle of attachment of the femoral head and neck onto the shaft of the femur and are determined by the degree of diversion from a transverse plane through the trochanteric region. The resulting angles are described as those of anteversion, normoversion, or retroversion. These angles are biomechanically important in the way in which forces are transferred from the femur to the acetabulum and determine the manner in which the femoral head articulates with the acetabulum which influences how the hind limb is placed during ambulation. Accurate determination of the angles is difficult and, therefore, they have not played an important role in diagnosis of dysplasia.

The normal angle is seen when the neck is positioned slightly cranially to the transverse plane with the angle of anteversion of 27.0° ± 6.5° as measured from radio-

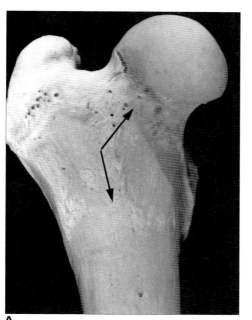 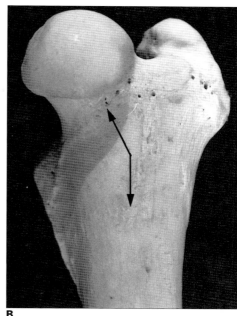

**Figure 5-50**
Photographs of the femurs from a normal dog show the effect of positioning on the perceived angle of inclination (arrows). (A) The positioning of the right femur is what would be ex-pected using a conventional VD view with internal rotation of the limb and the angle is within the normal range (130°) while (B) the positioning of the left femur is influenced by ex-ternal rotation and the angle erroneously indicates a valgus deformity (153°).

graphs (Nunamaker, et al 1973). On the lateral radiograph, this angle is seen when the cranial cortex of the femur, when extended proximally, passes near the center of the femoral head. An angle greater than this is abnormal and would be recognized on the radiograph when a line representing the cranial cortex of the femur, when extended proximally, passes caudal to the center of the femoral head. An angle formed if the neck is at right angles to the shaft of the femur is called normoversion but is physiologically abnormal. This angle is seen on the lateral radiograph when the head is positioned between the proximally extended cranial and caudal femoral cortices. Retroversion is a negative measurement indicating that the femoral neck is directed caudomedially and appears on the lateral radiograph with a portion of the femoral head projected caudal to the proximally extended caudal cortex of the femur (Figure 5-51).

Excessive anteversion has been reported to be rare and is probably of little significance as a cause of hip dysplasia (Riser and Shirer 1966, Dueland 1980). Others have reported excessive anteversion as a separate femoral hip dysplasia to be a small portion of the dysplastic population that is usually associated with dogs that have a cow-hocked and knock-kneed conformation. In the mildest form, femoral torsion is the only radiographic sign (Slocum and Slocum 1992). In a single study in July hounds, anteversion was felt to be a major mechanical factor in the development of dysplasia (Forsyth and Paschall 1963). However, more recently, the importance of both anteversion and coxa valga was shown to be slight, or even nonexistent, in the development of HD (Hauptman, et al 1985). That study clearly outlined the reasons for inaccurate measurements to be due especially to the presence of secondary osteophytes and thickening of the neck of the severely dysplastic dog. Their conclusion was that after measuring the angles of inclination as well as angles of anteversion in a large number of dogs maintained in a well-defined and controlled environment that: (1) no difference could be detected in the angle of inclination between normal and dysplastic dogs, (2) only a slight decrease in the angle of anteversion was noted in dysplastic femurs, and (3) hip angles of anteversion, retroversion, and inclination, did not play a demonstrable part in the development of HD and were not of value in early detection of dysplasia.

## Greater trochanter

The greater trochanter is positioned laterally on the proximal femur and acts as the point of insertion of the gluteal muscles and its appearance can be altered in the dysplastic dog (Riser 1973 b). The shape of the trochanter in the mature dog reflects the influence of these muscles, plus that of the piriformes that joins the caudal portion of the middle gluteus muscle, during the period of skeletal maturation. Often the proximal tip of the trochanter deviates medially suggesting increased muscular tension due to a delay in growth. This finding can reflect an effort to compensate for the discrepancy between bone and muscle growth. However, the shape of the trochanter in the mature dog can also vary with the difference being breed dependent (Figure 5-18).

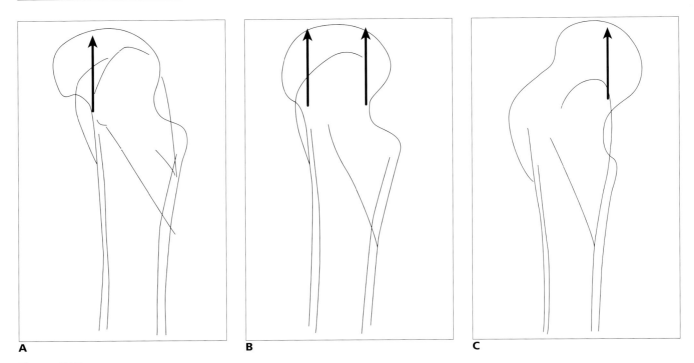

**Figure 5-51**
Drawings of the proximal femur indicating: (A) an angle of anteversion that is physiologically normal in which a line drawn along the cranial cortex when extended proximally (arrow) passes near the center of the femoral head, (B) normoversion in which the femoral head is positioned between the cranial and caudal cortex (arrows) when the lines representing the cranial and caudal cortex are extended proximally, and (C) retroversion in which a portion of the femoral head is positioned caudally to a line drawn along the caudal cortex when it is extended proximally (arrow). The femoral condyles are superimposed on the lateral radiograph to permit these measurements.

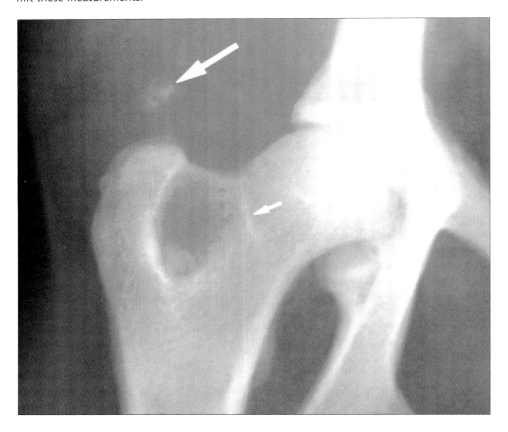

**Figure 5-52**
A ventrodorsal radiograph of the right hip of a 9-year-old male Brittany with a small calcified mass positioned within the gluteal muscles adjacent to the greater trochanter (large arrow). Its presence suggests a small avulsion fracture from the greater trochanter and supports the idea that muscle development lags behind skeletal development. Presence of the Morgan Line (small arrow) support the presence of minimal osteoarthrosis.

A small, calcified body may be positioned just proximal to the greater trochanter, first seen prior to skeletal maturation and then persisting in the mature dog. They may be noted unilaterally or bilaterally. It is tempting to assume that these soft tissue calcifications are the consequence of a small avulsion fracture from the greater trochanter at a time it was formed of softer cartilage (Figure 5-52). Their presence can support the concept that muscle development lags behind skeletal development. The same can be true of similarly appearing small calcific densities that have been identified adjacent to the lesser trochanter in the area of attachment of the iliopsoas muscle (Figure 5-53). These calcific densities near the trochanters deserve further attention since they can be supportive of the concept that hastened skeletal development causes abnormal stresses on the soft tissues on the hip joints.

In children with dysplasia, premature fusion of the proximal femoral physis can occur, thus shortening the femoral neck and flattening the femoral head. In these children, physeal and appositional growth of the trochanter can appear excessive with the differential growth having been termed "trochanteric overgrowth" in the orthopedic literature. The overgrowth results in shortening of the lever arm of the hip abductors, including that of the deep gluteal muscle, causing them to work at a less effective muscle length with decreased muscle strength (Fernbach, et al 1985). Neck lengthening procedures have been devised in man to counteract the effect of the shortened lever arm. A difference in prominence of the greater trochanter is seen in radiographs of dogs that may reflect a similar growth problem.

## Pelvic conformation

Pelvic conformation has been examined briefly in studies of dysplasia. It has always been attractive to consider the possibility of making the diagnosis of hip dysplasia by performing a measurement on a radiograph of the pelvis. The angle of the pelvic walls relative to the midsagittal plane of the body was thought to have an influence on the tendency for subluxation of the femoral heads (Olsson and Kasström 1972). Measurements of width made at the widest part of the pelvic inlet, the pelvic inlet at the level of the acetabulum, and the level of the obturator foramina form a pattern that was indicative of the plain of the pelvic walls that determined the position of the acetabulum. When the bones forming the lateral walls of the pelvis were tilting inwardly, this resulted in a slanting of the acetabular roof providing the possibility for the femoral head to subluxate laterally and dorsally. A tilting outward of the pelvic wall provided more coverage of the

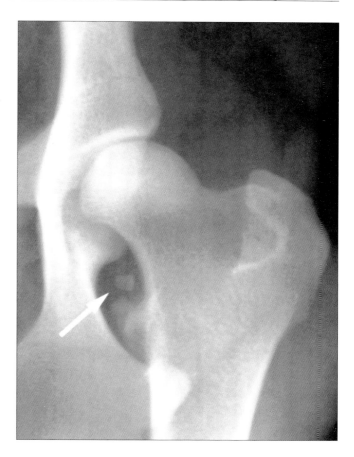

**Figure 5-53**
A ventrodorsal radiograph of the left hip of a 2-year-old female Shepherd-cross with a small calcified mass positioned within the iliopsoas muscle adjacent to the lesser trochanter (arrow). Its presence suggests a small avulsion fracture from the lesser trochanter and supports the idea that muscle development lags behind skeletal development.

head by the acetabulum and a more tightly fitting hip joint. Measurements made at 12 to 16 weeks were found to be good predictors of the eventual status of the hip joints. The greater the difference between the measurement at the pelvic inlet and the level of the acetabula, the greater is the possibility that the dog would have normal hips.

In a subsequent study, radiographs of four breeds of dogs were examined using the study described above as a model in an effort to support the concept that a pelvic measurement(s) might be of value in predicting the position of the acetabulum and thus the development of hip dysplasia. The differences between pelvic measurements in adult dogs made at the widest part of the pelvic inlet and the level of the acetabula (Figure 5-54) were found to be highly significant when comparing normal and dysplastic Saint Bernards, Labrador Retrievers, and German Shepherd Dogs, but interestingly were insignif-

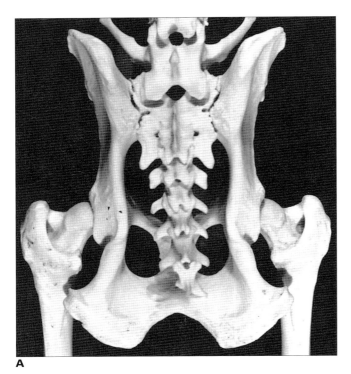 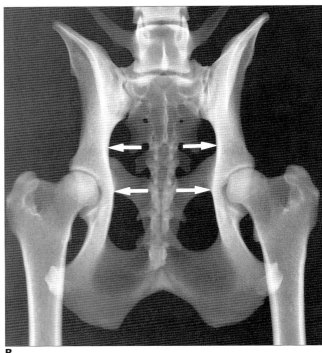

**Figure 5-54**
Photograph (A) and radiograph (B) of a pelvic specimen show the site of measurements (arrow) made in an effort to determine the nature of tilting of the acetabulum within the pelvic walls and thus, the ability of the acetabulum to hold the femoral head tightly. The greater the difference between the measurements, the greater the tendency for the hips to be normal.

icant in the Great Pyrenees breed. Thus, in the three breeds, the difference between the two measurements in a normal individual were greater than the difference between the two measurements in a dysplastic dog. No significance was noted within the breed/hip status group due to age (Morgan and Rosenblatt 1986). This study was performed in adult dogs, but it still suggests that measurements made in puppies could be a method of selection for breeding that would result in the improvement of pelvic shape that would permit a more firm placement of the femoral head within a deeper acetabular cup and thus reduce the frequency of hip dysplasia in that breed. These findings tended to support the theory of Olsson and Kasström.

A further study of pelvic measurements was made and significant differences were noted between the length and width of the pelvis, however utilization of these differences in diagnosis of hip dysplasia was difficult (Köppel 1983). Later, it was recognized that the position of the acetabulum varied in relationship to the horizontal or transverse plane of the pelvis. This change in position of the acetabulum resulted in an inward rotation of the ischiatic spine, a decrease in the pelvic diameter, and a flattened projection of the acetabulum. Thus, determination of acetabular positioning within the pelvic walls could be based on the radiographic appearance of other parameters and provide a suggestion of hip joint laxity (Prieur and Brüse 1988).

In other studies it was possible to create an increase in the stability of the hip joint through surgical procedures. The pubic symphyseal growth plates contribute substantially to the development of the pelvis and thus to the positioning of the acetabulum. Surgical pubic symphysiodesis in guinea pigs resulted in the narrowing and shortening of the pubic bones, outward rotation of the roof of the acetabula, and narrowing of the caudal aspect of the pelvis. Because of the attachment of the acetabula to the pelvis, the surgery caused the cup to rotate in such a manner that improved acetabular coverage of the femoral head resulted and enhanced hip joint stability (Mathews, et al 1996). This has been observed in other species and the results are expected to be similar in the dog. Thus, an increase in the growth of the symphyseal growth plates causes the possibility of hip joint laxity while limited growth is of value in creating the development of a joint that provides greater acetabular coverage and is more stable.

The nature of the pelvic attachment to the sacrum can be detected radiographically and can influence the effective depth of the acetabulum and thus the manner of

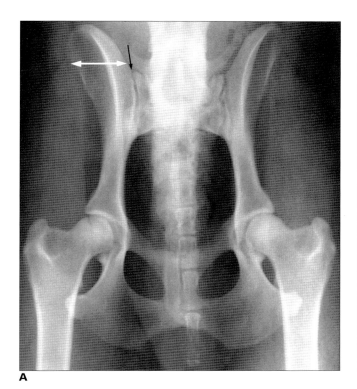 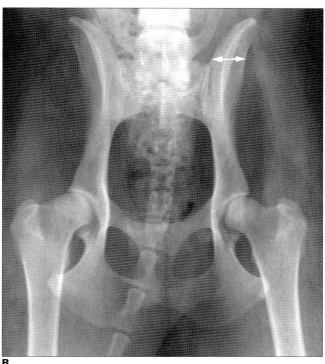

**Figure 5-55**
Radiographs of the pelvis of (A) an Australian Shepherd Dog and (B) a German Shepherd Dog, both made in an extended VD position illustrate differences in the character of the pelvic attachment to the sacrum (black arrows) and the width of the iliac wings (white arrows). These features may permit an estimation of the relative position of the acetabulum. In principle, the more vertical is the wing of the ilium, the greater is the dorsal coverage of the femoral head by the acetabulum. These features may be influenced by breed.

development of the hip joint. If the iliac wings are seen to be narrow with thin iliac crests as seen radiographically on the VD view, the acetabular roof covers a greater portion of the femoral head. If the iliac wings are wide with broad iliac crests as seen radiographically on the VD view, the dorsal acetabular roof is rolled medially and the covering of the femoral head is decreased. Changes such as these are probably not of importance in diagnosis since joint laxity and the presence of secondary changes are more accurate in the determination of the status of the hip joint (Figure 5-55). However, these findings might have value in prognosis. The appearance of the iliac wings on the radiograph also appears to be related to the appearance of the sacroiliac joints. If the iliac wings appear wide, the sacroiliac joints appear opened, while if the iliac wings appear narrow, the sacroiliac joints appear closed.

While most sacroiliac joints are symmetrical, some are asymmetrical with one joint positioned cranial to the other causing the pelvis to be angled obliquely. This can be found in dogs in which the lumbosacral vertebrae are normal in number and type. In other dogs, the pelvic attachment is more severely affected by a congenital abnormality referred to as transitional lumbosacral segments resulting in marked asymmetry of the sacroiliac joints. Deformities of this nature result in a pelvis that is obliquely positioned causing one acetabulum to be positioned more cranial with less dorsal acetabular coverage of the femoral head. The acetabulum positioned caudally provides greater coverage of the femoral head (Figure 5-56).

The frequency of asymmetry of the pelvic attachment and of transitional segments has been shown to be breed dependent. While significance between normal or dysplastic hips and the character of pelvic attachment could not be made, the severity of secondary osteoarthrosis was associated to a greater degree with asymmetrical pelvic attachment and transitional segments. Thus, the study showed that character of the dysplasia within each hip joint was somewhat dependent on the nature of the pelvic attachment (Morgan and Rosenblatt 1987).

Pelvic asymmetry can influence the course of the hip dysplasia, however, the asymmetry can also be the result of positioning during radiography. If the spinous processes of either the lumbar spine or the pelvis are seen posi-

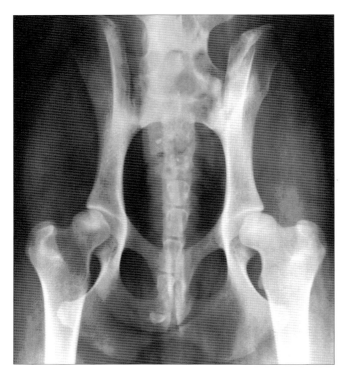

**Figure 5-56**
A radiograph of the pelvis of a 2-year-old male Australian Shepherd Dog with a lumbosacral transitional segments causing tilting and rotation of the pelvic attachment. While the sacroiliac attachment is unequal, the effect on the hip dysplasia is minimal at this time, with the changes limited to subluxation of the femoral heads. Note the difference in the level of the iliac crests and the difference in apparent thickness of the wings of the ilia that help in ascertaining the pelvis malposition. Note the separation of the spinal process on the transitional segment.

tioned centrally of the vertebral body on the VD view, the obliquity is real and indicates an error in attachment of the pelvis to the spine. If the spinous processes of both the lumbar spine and pelvis are not centered on the vertebral body, the obliquity indicates rotation of the entire body and only an error in positioning for radiography.

These studies point up differences in: (1) the character of pelvic conformation, (2) the nature of pelvic attachment to the sacrum, and (3) the character of the lumbosacral junction and their effect on the ultimate positioning of the acetabulum. Most of the patterns directly influence the tightness of the hip joint and cause subsequent hip dysplasia. Other differences only influence the manner in which the dysplasia progresses, while others appear to have no effect on the status of the hip joint. Because some of conformational patterns are genetically influenced, and most can be readily detected radiographically, it is possible to select against them. An altered acetabular position can be a most important feature in the evaluation of the hip joint and can only be determined in-

directly through the evaluation of other pelvic parameters. Thus, it will probably not become a helpful factor in radiographic determination of dysplasia.

Asymmetry of radiographic changes between the hip joints is confusing to the clinician when evaluating a dog for dysplasia because of the erroneous thought that the disease is symmetrical. While many dogs with dysplasia have radiographic changes that are bilaterally symmetrical, asymmetry occurs commonly in two patterns: (1) unilateral dysplasia with one hip affected and the other normal or (2) bilateral dysplasia with marked dissimilarity in the degree of joint laxity or secondary bony change (Figure 5-57). A frequency of unilateral dysplasia was reported in 18 of 53 dogs (34%) between 5 and 12 months of age (Lust, et al 1973), in 38 of 176 German Shepherd Dogs (21%) (Henricson, et al 1965), in 30% of a clinic population (Strande 1962), in 10% of a group of Beagle colony dogs (Morgan 1974), and 15% of a large clinic population (Morgan 1986). The frequency of asymmetry in appearance between the two dysplastic hips has been reported less often but it can approach 13% (Morgan 1986). These frequencies are based on radiographic studies made with limbs extended and do not include distraction techniques or palpation. Therefore, unilateral dysplasia, especially when characterized by unilateral or unequal joint laxity, is probably less frequent than reported.

## Grading radiographic changes

In an effort to provide more "information" to the owner/breeder concerning the severity of the disease, or the "amount of dysplasia," affecting their dog, various methods of reporting have been instituted. This need for additional information is generally based on the idea that if a dysplastic dog is to be breed, it should be a dog affected to a lesser degree since the grade is thought to reflect something of the magnitude of the disease genetically. Hutt (1967) used the quantitative expression reflecting the degree of dysplasia by making use of a grading system and found this expression to be consistent with a polygenic mode of inheritance. Thus, the more severe the dysplasia, the larger percentage of progeny expected to be dysplastic and the greater the severity of the dysplasia within each of the offspring. This was confirmed by others (Henricson, et al 1966, 1972; Olsson 1974). As with most pathologic conditions, grading the severity of the radiographic changes has been more attractive than grading the results of physical examination of the hip joint and findings on palpation have not often affected the final grade of the disease until more specific measurements of the amount of joint laxity have been advocated (Smith,

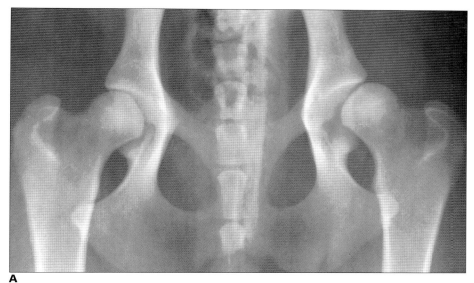
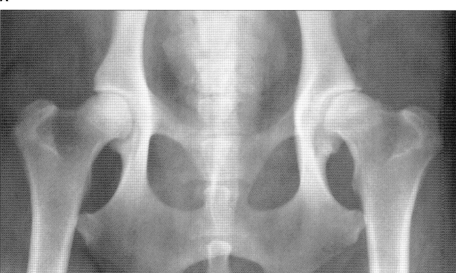
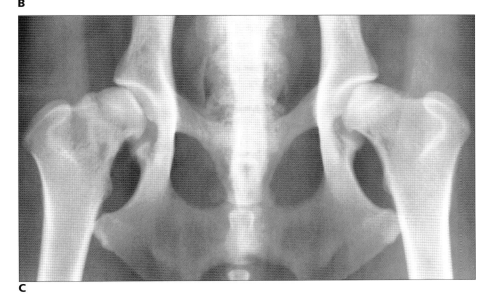

**Figures 5-57**
Asymmetry of the character of the hip joints as seen (A) in a 10-month-old male Labrador Retriever with unilateral dysplasia characterized by subluxation of the left hip, (B) in a 2-year-old male Labrador Retriever with unilateral dysplasia characterized by secondary bony changes in the left hip, and (C) in a 3-year-old male Australian Shepherd Dog with bilateral dysplasia with more severe secondary changes on the right.

et al 1990, 1993). Grading can be important to an owner/breeder if a breed club permits a dog with only minimal dysplasia (secondary changes?) (grade I) to be used for breeding. This demand for information beyond that of a simple diagnosis of dysplasia has lead to the development of several schemes for recording the extent of change within the affected hip.

However, it should be understood that the degree of joint laxity and level of secondary changes do not parallel severity of the clinical signs. In other words, a dog with a low grade of dysplasia (grade I) can show severe clinical signs while a dog with a high grade of dysplasia (grade IV) can show few if any clinical signs observable to the owner. Also, the clinical signs vary throughout the age of the dog even though the character of the secondary arthrosis remains rather constant. Thus, for the owner of a pet or owner of a dog to be used in obedience training or as a working dog, the grade of dysplasia does not predict the nature of the clinical signs the dog can be expected to demonstrate at the time of examination or later in life. A group of guide dogs, some of whom were dysplastic, were evaluated clinically and no evidence was found suggesting that hip dysplasia "caused early retirement" (Goddard and Mason 1982). A recent study of military working dogs included 116 dogs of which 57 were mildly or moderately dysplastic at the time of procurement (one was severely dysplastic). No difference was noted in the number of months worked between normal and dysplastic dogs and no clinical problems were associated with the dysplastic hips until an older age (>9 years) (Banfield, et al 1996 b).

There is no uniformly agreed-to system of grading radiographic changes of hip dysplasia that is used by all examiners. Some use subluxation as the key feature, while others rely on secondary bony modeling. Some make allowances for the age of the dog with a young dog with severe change receiving a higher grade of dysplasia than an older dog with the same level of change. This practice is based on the assumption that the osteoarthrosis is progressive and when noted in an older dog, some allowance in assignment of a grade of dysplasia is given.

Early systems by Schnelle (1954), Olsson (1957), and Whittington, et al 1961 in an AVMA Panel Report were based primarily on the fit between the femoral head and acetabulum. A later study (Riser 1962) utilized the degree of femoral head subluxation and secondary modeling in determining the grade. The pathologic changes noted on the radiograph were originally graded from one to four in increasing severity recognizing flattening of the acetabulum, subluxation of the femoral head, as well as changes within the femoral head and neck. In some schemes, grade IV was reserved only for complete luxation of the femoral head, while in others, that grade described the development of severe osteoarthrosis with or without luxation (Olsson 1962 b; Riser 1973 b; Lawson 1963; Henricson, et al 1966; Morgan 1972; Morgan and Stephens 1985).

The scientific committee of the Fédération Cynologique Internationale (FCI) proposed a classification protocol in 1978 that was finalized in 1983, to achieve uniform evaluation of radiographs and offered a scheme for an international certificate. It described criteria that makes it possible to place an animal into one of five grades of dysplasia, A through E. The grade assigned is based on the more severely effected of the two joints. This description of the grades was modified in 1991 and fits most current theories concerning the pathophysiology of dysplasia (Brass, et al 1978, 1983; Brass 1993). A description of the grading system endorsed by the FCI is included in the final chapter of this book.

Any grading based on the severity of the osteoarthrosis is influenced by a number of factors, such as the age, weight, and physical activity of the dog. The age of the dog seems to have the greatest effect since the osteoarthrosis is progressive and thus age dependent (Townsend, et al 1971). At 100 months after the original examination, dogs classified as having grade I dysplasia had progressed to a level in excess of grade II, while dogs classified as having grade II dysplasia had progressed to a level of grade III. Dogs classified normal at less than 18 months of age had a greater progression of change than those classified normal at over 18 months of age suggesting a high level of inaccuracy in the evaluation at the younger age.

The development of the osteoarthrosis is also thought to be affected by athletic activity. A sedentary dog that fails to exercise has little opportunity to maintain or develop muscle mass with a resulting persistent joint laxity. However, a regular pattern of limited exercise is thought to encourage development of good muscle mass and a tendency to provide stabilization for the lax joint. Another dog, with irregular periods of excessive activity, would be expected to not maintain as strong a muscle mass, and the osteoarthrosis would develop more quickly because of the periodic insults to the joints. This can be seen in the dog that occasionally plays Frisbee with its owner. Because of enjoyment in the game, it participates actively ignoring any pain in the hips and thus hastening the development of the osteoarthrosis. Whatever the nature of the physical activity practiced by the dog, it definitely influences the development of osteoarthrosis in either a positive or negative manner.

Obesity affects the progression of the osteoarthrosis by increasing the stress on the hip joints. The overweight dog has little interest in exercise and thus, the possibility of a positive effect from that activity is lost. The breed size also influences the progression of the osteoarthrosis and, thus, lighter weight dogs have less severe secondary changes (Pharr and Morgan 1976).

Physical activity, body weight, breed size, and age influence the resulting radiographic grading of the disease. Thus, any grade of dysplasia assigned to the dog has its greatest comparative value when it is compared with grades of members of the same breed made at the same age, preferably between 1 and 2 years of age.

## Systems of grading

A well developed evaluation system in Great Britain (Willis 1984) uses specific bony changes plus the degree of joint laxity in each hip to arrive at a numerical score for each dog rather than using only the diagnosis of normal/dysplastic. In addition, the number of scored progeny, the number of scored progeny from a scored dam, and the number of different dams are listed along with the range of scores of the progeny, the mean score for progeny, and the mean score for the dams. The range of scores and mean score for the breed and data for other sires within the breed are tabulated as well (Willis 1986, 1990). While this might appear to have minimal value in examination of the single dog, the potential breeder can readily determine the position of a given dog in that breed. Further discussion of this system is included in the final chapter.

A recent objective scheme to record numerically the nature of the dysplasia has been established in Switzerland (Flückiger 1993). It is discussed further in the final chapter.

## Breed influence on radiogaphic changes

Often it is questioned whether the radiographic changes of dysplasia vary with the breed. While the pattern of joint laxity and secondary change appear to be similar in all dogs, their development does seem to be somewhat breed dependent. While we have described a rather predictable development of hip dysplasia as seen on the radiograph, nevertheless, many variations to this pattern are seen. One pattern of presentation is characterized by subluxation of a well-formed femoral head with the acetabulum showing only minimal modeling change and is often seen in young Saint Bernards (Figure 5-58), young Labrador Retrievers, young German Shepherd Dogs, and young Great Pyrenees. In the older German Shepherd Dogs, a slightly modeled, tightly fitting femoral head with secondary bony changes is commonly seen (Figure 5-59). In older Labrador Retrievers, a subluxating femoral head is often associated with acetabular flattening (Figure 5-60). Older Saint Bernards have a dysplasia that is characterized by loose fitting femoral heads with a minimum of secondary bony changes (Morgan and Stephens 1985). Any variations from these patterns are thought to be the result of athletic activity, body weight, and age and reflect environmental influences more than breed differences. The size of the dog can influence the pattern of dysplasia as shown in a study of Beagle dogs where a slower rate of development of osteoarthrosis and less severity of secondary changes were noted (Pharr and Morgan 1976).

In which pattern do we place the changes typically seen in the hips and pelvis of an average English Bulldog? The caudal aspect of the pelvis is atrophic, the acetabula fail to develop, the femoral heads luxate, and secondary changes in the acetabula, femoral head, and neck are more of a response to the luxation and consist of coxa valga and loss in bone density (Figure 5-61). Is this hip dysplasia? Probably it should more correctly be referred to as a congenital hip luxation but it is certainly an inherited trait.

## Influence of age on diagnosis

Generally, the earliest of the changes in the young dog with HD affect only the cartilage, joint capsule, and round ligament of the femoral head which cannot be identified on a routinely positioned VD radiograph. However, joint laxity can be detected radiographically as early as 4 to 6 months of age, especially if using a method of distraction. In dogs with exceptionally severe hip dysplasia, femoral head luxation, femoral neck thickening, and a shallow acetabulum are present at 12 to 18 weeks and diagnosis based on bony changes can be made at that young age (Riser and Shirer 1966). Most examiners observe that in the general population, early diagnosis based only on radiographic changes is both difficult and unreliable before 6 months of age. This is because of the influence of the cartilage content within the pelvic bones on the radiographic appearance as well as the minimal nature of the early bony changes (Jessen 1970; Townsend, et al 1971; Henricson, et al 1972; Freudiger 1973; Pharr and Morgan 1976; Ackerman 1982).

Another method of early diagnosis centers on the concept of delayed ossification of the femoral head. All puppies in which the femoral head was not visible radiographically at 2 weeks of age developed CHD at 12 months of age. Most in whom ossification of the femoral

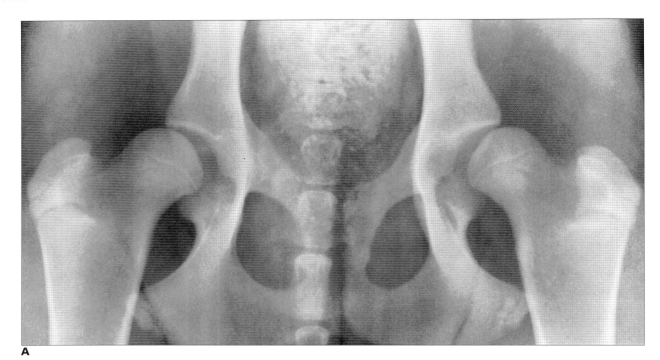

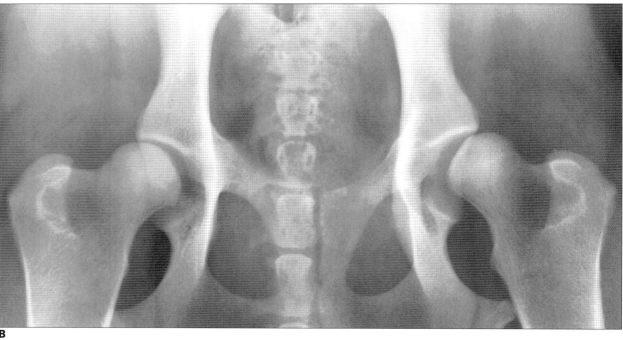

**Figure 5-58**
Radiographs of a female Saint Bernard at the age of (A) 7 months and (B) 19 months show marked joint laxity but an apparent absence of development of secondary bony changes. This pattern of dysplasia is often seen in larger breeds.

**Figure 5-59**
A radiograph of a 9-year-old female German Shepherd Dog that exhibits a malformed left femoral head and neck with minimal joint laxity. The pattern of dysplasia seen in this hip is often seen in this breed. Only a minimal enthesophyte is seen on the femoral neck on the right (arrow).

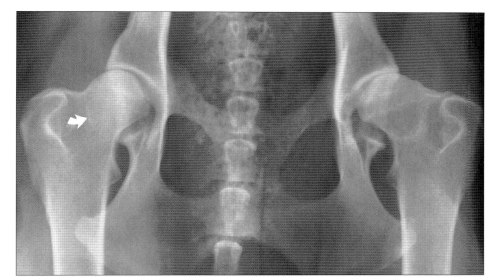

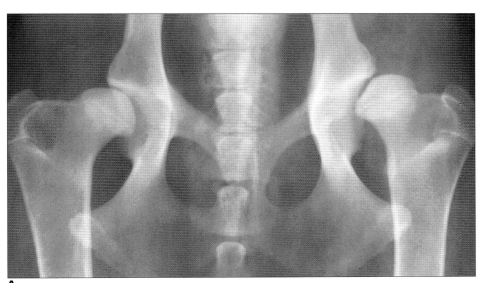

**Figure 5-60**
Radiographs of 2 Labrador Retrievers at the age of (A) 8 months and (B) 28 months show marked joint laxity with acetabular flattening. Secondary changes within the femoral heads are minimal. This pattern of dysplasia is often seen in this breed. Note that the femoral head flattening is not due to the fovea capitis but represents a true wearing of the contour of the femoral head. Changes on the left hip of the older dog are limited to joint laxity.

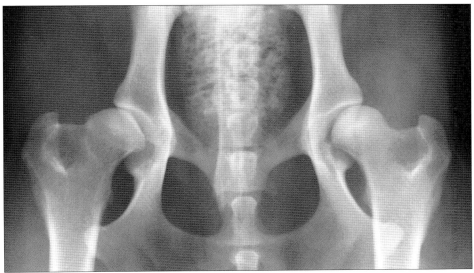

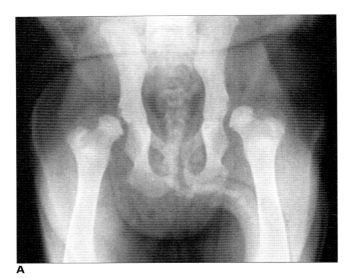
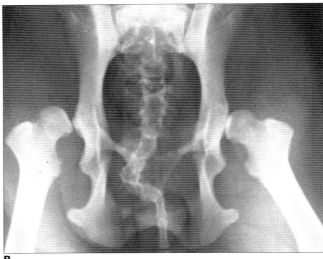

**Figure 5-61**
Radiographs of an English Bulldog at the age of (A) 6 months and (B) 8 years show a failure of development of the hip joint. A valgus deformity in the femoral neck is seen along with flattening of the acetabula and luxation of the femoral heads. Because of the separation of femoral head from the acetabulum, secondary changes are atrophic in nature rather than that of reactive new bone. This pattern of hip development is often seen in this breed.

head was evident at 2 weeks of age developed normal hip joints. It seemed as though later ossification of the femoral head provided additional time for the development of CHD (Madsen, et al 1991; Todhunter, et al 1997).

A positive correlation between the Norberg angle at 30 weeks and the eventual development of osteoarthrosis between 2 and 5 years confirms an association between early laxity of the hip joints and changes secondary to joint laxity (Kealy, et al 1997).

Early longitudinal studies strongly suggested the impossibility of accurately clearing a dog from having hip dysplasia until 1 or 2 years of age using a single conventional VD radiographic view. A study that radiographed a group of 196 dysplastic German Shepherd Dogs reported a definitive positive diagnosis in only 15.8% at 6 months, increasing to 68.9% at 12 months, 82.7% at 18 months, 95.4% at 24 months, and 97.5% at 36 months. In a similarly investigated group of 40 dysplastic Vizslas, 32.4% were diagnosed as having dysplasia at 6 months, 62.5% at 12 months, 72.5% at 18 months, 92.5% at 24 months, and 97.5% at 36 months (Jessen 1969, Jessen and Spurrell 1972 a, b). Another well controlled study of Afghan Hounds reported dysplasia diagnosed at 6 months of age in 28.5%, whereas, at 12 months of age, 67% were diagnosed positively; by 18 months of age, 90.5% were diagnosed positively, and 100% were diagnosed as dysplastic by 36 months (Ackerman 1982). All of these studies were made with VD positioning with the limb extended at a time when the importance of joint laxity was not as well appreciated and therefore the radiographs were probably evaluated in a conservative manner. Freudiger, et al (1973) found that preliminary radiography made prior to the animal reaching the age of 12 months produced an accuracy of diagnosis of 80.3%.

Most of these studies used a radiograph made at an older age to compare with the earlier study in determining the accuracy of the earlier study. In contrast, recent data from the OFA compared early evaluations (>24 months) with those made at least 24 months later and reported that the overall reliability of the radiographic evaluation on the first study for 25 breeds was 88.9% (Corley 1992). A more recent study from the OFA suggested that reliability of preliminary evaluations increased significantly as age at the time of preliminary evaluation increased, regardless of whether dogs received a preliminary evaluation of normal phenotype or disease (Corley, et al 1997). A recent study of military working dogs showed progression of normal to a minimal grade of dysplasia in some dogs, however, the change was such that no dogs normal at 24 months of age progressed to a moderate or severe dysplasia (Banfield, et al 1996 a). One study found a change in radiographic evaluation of 20% of the dogs between studies made at 5 and 12 months of age, but felt that preliminary examination remained a valuable procedure for potential breeding dogs (Freudiger 1973).

Additional data are available from Swedish studies concerning the detection of dysplasia in German Shepherd Dogs at 12 months and 24 to 36 months of age. This is not a longitudinal study on the same dog, but is the result of evaluations of different populations based on the age at the time of examination. At the onset of their studies the frequency of dysplasia (40%) was almost the same for both age groups (Norberg 1962). In a later report of a different population of dogs, 43% were dysplastic if less than 12 months of age while 38% were dysplastic between 24 to 36 months of age. This suggests that dysplastic puppies were being removed from the population prior to examination. The largest material came later and reflected improved diagnostic skill. The frequency of dysplasia under 12 months of age was 33%, while 34% were dysplastic between 24 and 36 months of age (Audell 1972, 1973). This last study should be considered the standard of examination today and shows that little difference exists in evaluation at the younger age.

From a summary of these studies, it appears that accuracy of radiographic diagnosis made from a single VD extended view increases until by 2 years of age the accuracy is probably > 90%. These findings were strongly influenced by willingness or hesitancy to judge minimal radiographic changes as being indicative of dysplasia. Thus, the studies can falsely suggest that radiographic diagnosis of dysplasia characterized by minimal radiographic changes can not be made until 2 years of age. While some of the studies ignored the importance of joint laxity, others did not recognize early osteophytosis, such as the "Morgan Line" on the caudal aspect of the femoral neck. Distraction testing or use of a wedge technique would have changed the results of these studies markedly.

The use of compression/distraction studies has shown that it is possible to successfully evaluate puppies at a younger age. Indices obtained in 4 months old dogs compared favorably with those obtained later at 6, 12, and 24 months of age (Smith, et al 1993). However, studies in 2-month-old puppies were not sufficiently reliable to use in a predictive sense (Smith 1994). This offers the breeder the possibility of earlier evaluation of the hips than used with conventional VD extension views.

The owner/breeder often demands an early ruling on the status of the hips and this has influenced schemes for dysplasia control to evaluate radiographs at as early an age as possible. A partial solution to a definitive evaluation of radiographs at an early age is to permit their review and divide the results into three groups: (1) questionable studies that require a second evaluation at a later date, (2) normal studies that require a second evaluation at a later date, and (3) dysplastic studies that can be evaluated as dysplastic on the basis of the early study. It is the authors' experience that of those dogs in which radiographic findings are questionable at a young age, most are judged dysplastic when re-examined. Unfortunately, those dogs thought to be normal at a young age should not receive a final judgment on a routine VD study but should be re-evaluated as a 1-year-old. A scheme of this type permits detection of obvious dysplasia at an early age and avoids having to maintain those dogs awaiting a judgment on the status of the hips at an older age. It does however, require an increase in cost of evaluation since studies are performed twice in the normal or suspect population. The use of distraction techniques can change this system markedly.

In an effort to reach some form of a compromise that enables breeders to obtain an evaluation at the earliest practical age, the scientific committee of the FCI recommended the minimum age for certification at 1 year for most breeds but selected a minimum of 1 $1/2$ years of age for giant breeds (eg, Saint Bernard, Pyrenees Mountain Dog, Newfoundland, Mastiff, Great Dane, Bull Mastiff) (Brass and Paatsama 1983). The program administered by the OFA in the United States recommends dogs be certified at a minimum of 2 years of age and the Wind-Morgan program for Labrador Retrievers in the United States recommends a minimum of 1 year of age.

A potential problem exists in the radiographic evaluation of the older dog because of the possibility of misinterpreting the etiology of an osteoarthrosis noted on the radiograph. Six years of age has been suggested as the upper limit for radiographic evaluation of hip dysplasia because degenerative changes due to aging (primary joint disease) can be incorrectly interpreted as being associated with secondary changes the result of hip dysplasia (Lawson 1968).

## Differential radiographic diagnosis

Certain diseases have radiographic features in common with those seen in hip dysplasia, such as congenital hip luxation, aseptic necrosis of the femoral head, capital physeal fracture, infectious arthritis, primary osteoarthrosis, and healed fractures. In some, the primary changes of the disease resemble those seen with dysplasia, while in others, the secondary changes are the same as those seen with dysplasia.

Some dogs have disease in the hip joint that closely resembles hip dysplasia radiographically and pathologically. These are referred to as phenocopies that are a non-hereditary disease causing an alteration in the phenotype that mimics an inherited disease. It is possible for phenocopies to be induced by specific environmental conditions. For example, estradiol can be used to retard growth

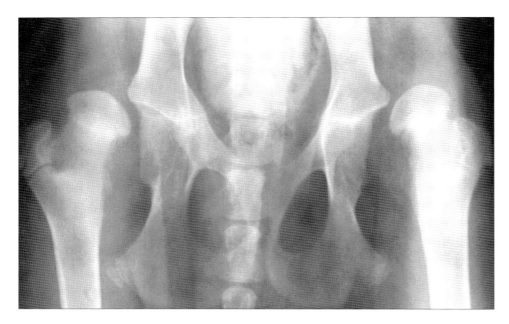

**Figure 5-62**
A ventrodorsal radiograph of the pelvis in a 4-month-old Great Pyrenees with luxation of the femoral heads. Note the marked valgus deformity and the shallow acetabula that are more typical of a congenital luxation than of HD. The caudal aspect of the pelvis is atrophic and underdeveloped because of disuse of the hind limbs.

of cartilage in the femoral head and thus induce structural changes in the hip joint similar to that seen in dysplasia (Pierce and Bridges 1967; Gustafsson 1968; Gustafsson, et al 1972). It is also possible to improperly immobilize a hind limb in a young dog by casting and cause disease of the hip mimicking dysplasia (Schoenecker, et al 1984). While phenocopies are important clinically in the affected dog, they cannot genetically transmit the defect to their offspring and therefore, they are unimportant in regard to control of the hip dysplasia within a breed. They uncommonly cause a problem in diagnosis. Certain phenocopies are discussed below.

## Hip luxation

Hip luxation can be congenital, traumatic, or developmental. With a congenital luxation of the hip, the femoral head is completely luxated prior to, or shortly after birth, and the hip joint fails to develop in a normal manner (Figures 5-61, 5-62). The femoral head becomes atrophic with a marked coxa valga of the femoral neck. The acetabulum becomes flattened because of the absence of normal forces of weight bearing. Because of failure of the femoral head to seat into the acetabulum, the sclerotic strip of subchondral bone fails to form. Secondary periarticular changes that are commonly noted in HD as the bony response to joint instability do not develop since there is no contact between the femoral head and the acetabulum. The caudal aspect of the pelvis becomes atrophic because there is minimal weight bearing through the hip joint. Clinical signs including a mechanical lameness that can mimic that noted in dysplasia. The major radiographic differences not seen in hip dysplasia are the absence of modeling changes and the finding of bone atrophy and the valgus deformity of the femoral neck. This pattern of hip disease is often identified in the English Bulldog.

Experimental dislocation of the hips in young dog was shown to produce changes in the hips similar to those seen in dysplasia (Smith, et al 1958; Smith, et al 1963). In addition, a hip dislocation occurring in young dogs as a result of neuromuscular or musculoskeletal abnormalities could lead to the development of joint disease and an appearance similar to that seen in congenital hip luxation.

Traumatic luxation of the femoral head can result in craniodorsal position of the femoral head as it lies against the body of the ilium where a pseudarthrosis develops. These changes do not mimic those seen in hip dysplasia. Fractures of the femoral shaft when not adequately treated can result in a persistent external rotation of the shaft of the femur and cranial anteversion of the head and neck and often result in malunion of the fracture, a marked valgus deformity, subluxation, and a resulting osteoarthrosis of the hip joints that could mimic that seen with hip dysplasia. However, a complete examination of the femoral shaft clearly shows the true cause of the hip lesion, the malunion fracture.

## Aseptic necrosis of the femoral head

Aseptic necrosis of the femoral head occurs as a spontaneous disease in smaller breeds of dog that are typically unaffected with hip dysplasia. While the chronic disease can resemble hip dysplasia, the occurrence in the smaller

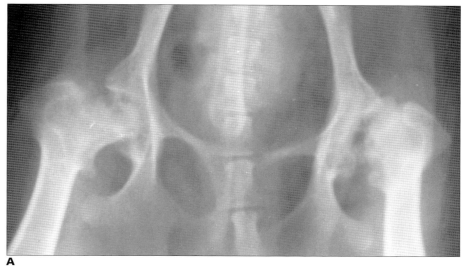

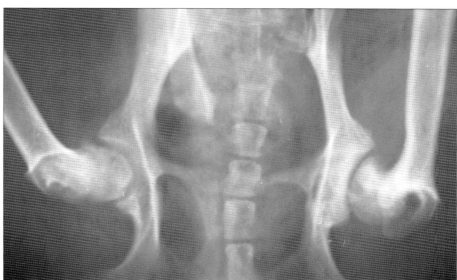

**Figure 5-63**
Radiographs of the pelvis of a 3-year-old male Miniature Poodle made (A) with the limbs in extension and (B) in flexion. The severe changes in the hip joints involve the acetabula, femoral heads, and femoral necks and are secondary to repair of aseptic necrosis of the femoral heads. The osteoarthrosis as seen on the right more closely resembles that seen in hip dysplasia. Only the breed and clinical signs are different.

breeds makes the diagnosis of hip dysplasia less likely (Olsson 1958). While the disease is usually bilateral on histological examination, the radiographic changes often are asymmetrical leaving the impression that one hip is normal (Ljunggren 1967). The first change is atypical of anything seen in HD and is a loss of metaphyseal bone density probably due to disuse. Next, an uneven pattern of bone density is noted within the femoral head indicative of bone necrosis. In some dogs, the modeling within the femoral head is indicative of bone death, osteolysis, and new bone deposition (creeping substitution) and can result in separation of a segment of subchondral bone (Figure 5-64). This flap can be identified on the radiograph and is diagnostic of aseptic necrosis. A pattern of secondary change consisting of flattening of the femoral head (Figure 5-65) minimal joint laxity and flattening of the acetabulum occurs (Figure 5-63). These secondary changes result from collapse of the femoral head and the replacement of dead bone with living bone tissue. Even though the disease is slowly progressive, the pain is rather acute in onset and can resemble that noted in a patient with chronic hip dysplasia who had suffered an acute injury to the hip joint(s).

Another form of necrosis of the femoral head is steroid induced, has bilateral involvement, and is usually noted in larger dogs who have been on long-standing steroid therapy (Figure 5-66). This is an uncommon response to what is assumed to be the widespread use of steroids for skin diseases in the dog. The changes seen in steroid induced bone necrosis seem to exclusively involve the femoral head and leave the acetabulum undisturbed until later in the course of the disease. The first changes in the previously normal joint are collapse of the joint space

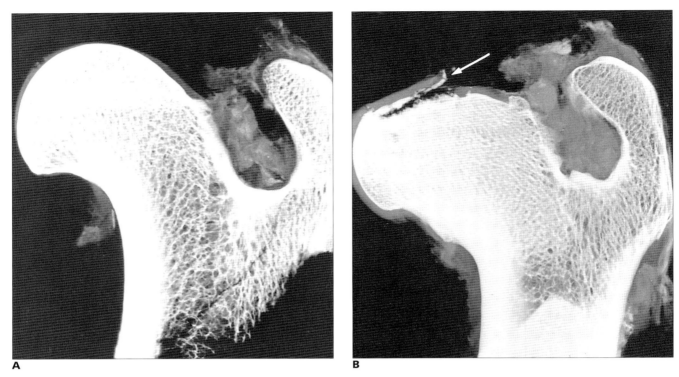

**Figure 5-64**
Radiographs of slabs of bone tissue from a (A) normal femoral head and (B) a femoral head with aseptic necrosis. The flap of subchondral bone with overlying articular cartilage (arrow) is seen along with thickening of the trabeculae in the affected head. Thickening of the femoral neck is a secondary change.

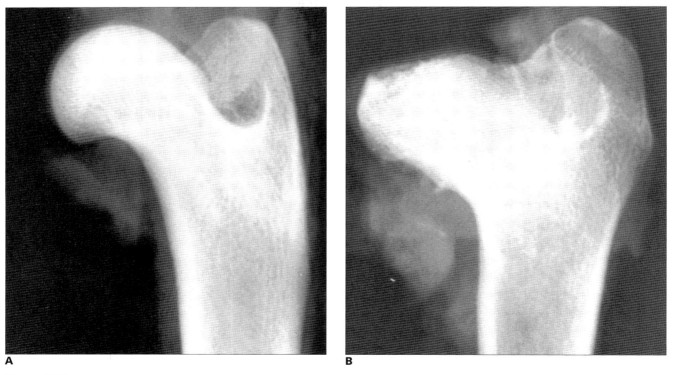

**Figure 5-65**
Radiographs of specimens of a (A) normal femoral head and (B) a femoral head with aseptic necrosis. The marked change in shape of the femoral head and neck is seen. This modeling has an appearance somewhat similar to that seen is hip dysplasia.

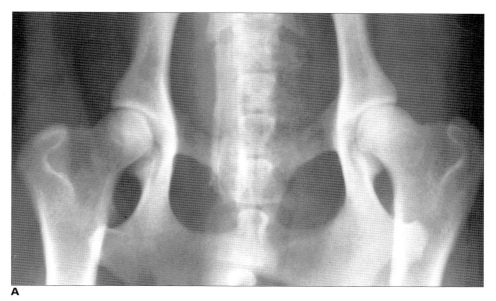
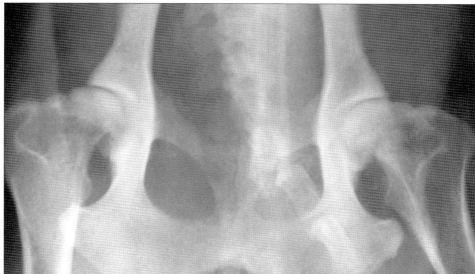

**Figure 5-66**
Ventrodorsal radiographs of the pelvis of a male Shepherd-cross made at 10 years of age (A) and at 13 years of age (B). The previously normal hip joints changed remarkably between the two studies with collapse of the femoral heads and secondary changes consisting of thickening of the femoral necks. These changes are secondary to death of the bone in the femoral heads probably associated with chronic steroid therapy. Change in the acetabula is minimal at this time.

often not appreciated radiographically. Next, the head collapses within a normal acetabulum and appears to have an increased density probably the result of collapse of the trabeculae and deposition of new bone on the ischemic cancellous bone. This can be somewhat suggestive of the modeling that occurs as part of the secondary bony change in dysplasia, however, the delay of acetabular modeling should make the clinician suspicious that it is not a dysplasia induced osteoarthrosis. The changes of this form of necrosis when superimposed over a dysplastic joint are impossible to interpret and are misdiagnosed.

### Acute fracture

Capital physeal fractures can occur unilaterally and be due to trauma. When they occur bilaterally in the younger dog they cause acute pain and lameness and are often associated with hypothyroidism. The disease when seen acutely is without change in the femoral heads and acetabula and is recognized by the displacement of the femoral heads. Later, loss of bone tissue within the metaphyses is indicative of healing at the fracture site. However, if the disease is not radiographed for several days, impaction of the heads onto the femoral necks can occur. This results in a varus deformity of the neck as can be seen with hip dysplasia (Figure 5-67). Often bony healing occurs if the head remains impacted onto the femoral neck. This cre-

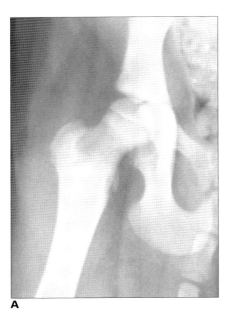 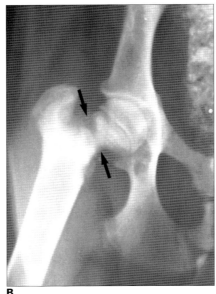 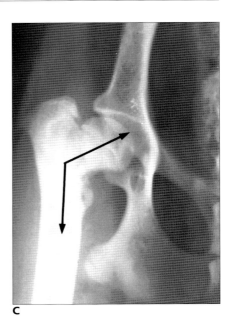

**Figure 5-67**
Radiographs of the right hip of a 6-month-old dog with a physeal fracture of the femoral neck. (A) A radiograph made at the time of injury with the limb in extension reduces the fracture so it is not identified. (B) A radiograph made 1 week later clearly shows osteolysis at the fracture site (arrows). The density of the femoral head remains normal because of its avascular nature. (C) Impaction of the fragments during healing causes a varus deformity (arrows). This patient will develop a severe osteoarthrosis that will resemble that seen in HD.

ates a lesion with an appearance similar to that seen with hip dysplasia. However, if the femoral heads remain separated from the femoral necks, the heads remain avascular and unchanged in density and shape while resorption of the bone in the femoral necks occurs rather quickly. This appearance is dissimilar to that seen in hip dysplasia.

Fractures may also involve the dysplastic hip causing problems in diagnosis. Identification of radiolucent fracture lines makes diagnosis relatively straightforward. However, if the fracture involves a femoral head in a joint affected by dysplasia, the diagnosis is complicated. If the lesion is not identified until healing has begun, the fracture lines are not identified because of the covering provided by the secondary callus (Figure 5-68). Clinical signs in these dogs are confusing because the acute signs from the trauma are superimposed over the chronic lameness due to the hip dysplasia and they may not be recognized.

### Healed fracture of the femoral head or acetabulum

A traumatic fracture involving the hip joint often results in an interruption of the articular surface involving the acetabulum. Malalignment of the articular fragments when healed can cause a secondary osteoarthrosis with modeling changes suggestive of hip dysplasia (Figures 5-69, 5-70). Although the appearance of the injured hip following healing is like that seen in severe hip dysplasia, the unilateral occurrence and the malposition of the fragments points to changes secondary to trauma. Clinical signs are usually markedly different from those seen in dysplasia, being acute at the time of the injury with the dog completely non-weight-bearing on the affected limb for some days. However, not all owners are observant of their pets and the acute onset may have been missed. Perhaps only the chronic pain and lameness were observed and that could easily resemble that seen with hip dysplasia.

### Infectious arthritis in the older dog

Although infectious arthritis is uncommon in the dog it can occur in the older dog, due to hematogenous spread of infection to the hip joint, often from chronic bladder or prostatic infection (Figure 5-71). If the infection is superimposed over secondary changes of dysplasia, the early radiographs can indicate only an osteoarthrosis secondary to dysplasia. However, with time, the destructive nature of the infectious process becomes prominent and permits a more accurate diagnosis.

Clinically, the dog probably has some signs of chronic pain and lameness associated with the long-standing dys-

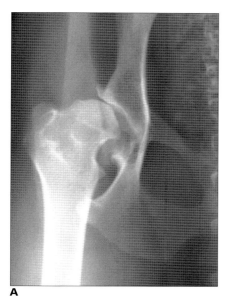 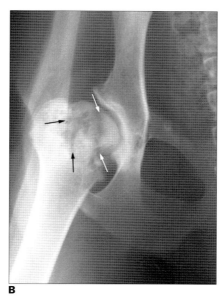 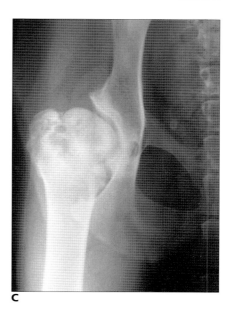

**Figure 5-68**
Radiographs of the right hip of a female Shepherd-cross. (A) A radiograph at 4 years of age shows extensive osteoarthrosis secondary to hip dysplasia. (B) A radiograph at 8 years of age following trauma shows radiolucent fracture lines (arrows) through the dysplastic femoral head and neck. (C) A radiograph 4 months after the trauma shows healing of the fracture with further modeling of the femoral head, neck, and acetabulum. Following fracture healing, it would not be possible to determine the role of the trauma in the appearance of the hip joint.

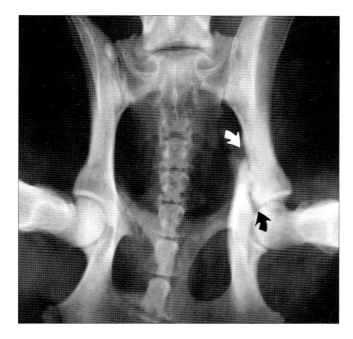

**Figure 5-69**
A ventrodorsal radiograph of the pelvis with a chronic, healing fracture extending into the left acetabulum (arrows). In addition there are fractures of the right pubis and right ischium. The changes associated with the injury at this time are unlike those seen with dysplasia, but with healing, the acetabulum could develop an appearance similar to that seen with a severe secondary osteoarthrosis. At that time the appearance could be confused with a unilateral osteoarthrosis due to HD.

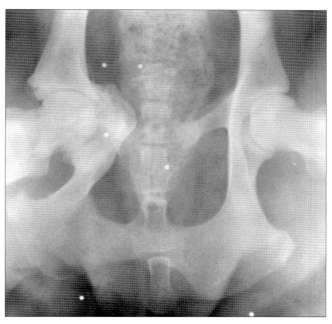

**Figure 5-70**
A ventrodorsal radiograph of the pelvis of a mature female Australian Shepherd Dog that had a mass palpated by rectal examination on the right side of the pelvic inlet. The radiographic changes are those of a malunion acetabular fracture of the right hip joint. The nature of the malunion prevented the dog having a complete range of motion of the limb. Note that the femoral head remains well-formed and spherical, not expected in a patient with hip dysplasia. The marked changes are noted within the acetabulum while the femoral head remains relatively unscathed.

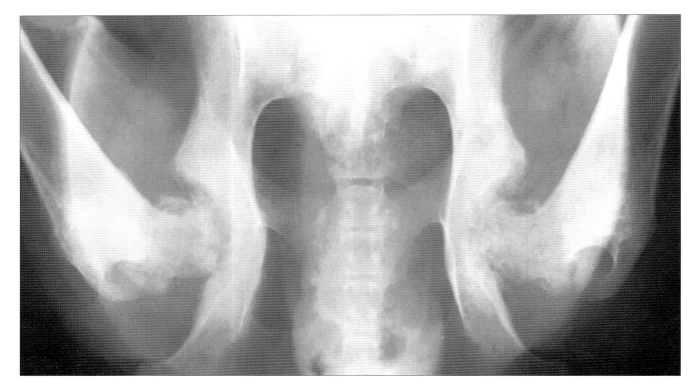
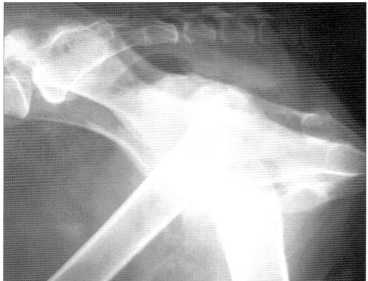
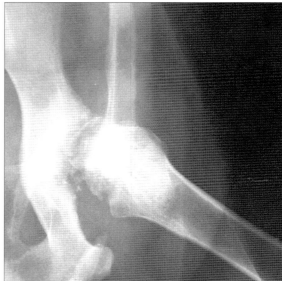

**Figure 5-71**
Multiple radiographs of the hip joints of a male Shepherd-cross with chronic prostatic infection and secondary hematogenous infectious arthritis of both hip joints. Note the marked destruction of the articular surfaces on both the femoral heads and the acetabula that are typical for an inflammatory process. In hip dysplasia, the disease is noninflammatory and the articular surfaces "grind" together and form polished surfaces (eburnation). In an infectious, inflammatory joint disease, the lysis and destruction of the articular surfaces plus the formation of less-dense, "fluffy-like" periosteal new bone are unique radiographic findings. It is not possible in this dog to determine what was the status of the hip joints prior to the onset of the infectious disease.

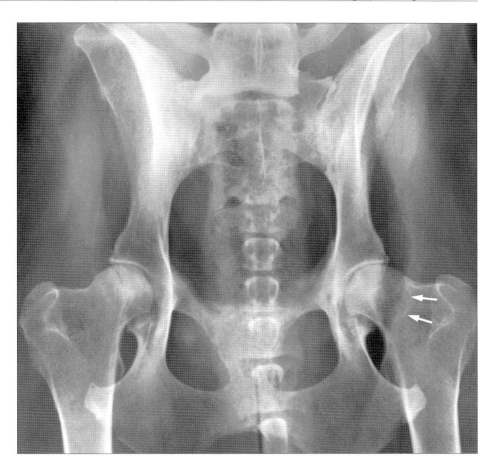

**Figure 5-72**
A ventrodorsal radiograph of the pelvis of a mature Shepherd-cross shows collapse of the joint spaces typical of that seen in primary joint disease. Note that the femoral heads are well formed and the acetabula are deep. Minimal enthesophyte formation is present on the left femoral neck (arrows). All bones are osteopenic associated with disuse and the age of the patient.

plasia. The presence of infection causes an acute inflammatory process that is painful and can cause the dog to become acutely three-legged lame. Still, the signs can be thought to be only due to dysplasia and secondary osteoarthrosis, since a dog with dysplasia can often suffer trauma and become acutely lame and non-weight-bearing. It behooves the clinician to be on the alert for the possibility of an infection superimposed over the dysplastic joint. A diagnostic joint tap is imperative to confirm the diagnosis and to establish the most effective form of treatment. Changes in the hemogram usually do not accompany infection of this nature and the dog often remains non-febrile.

## Primary osteoarthrosis

Primary osteoarthrosis is usually not a clinical entity but is probably present in all joints to a certain degree as the dog ages. This was confirmed in a colony of Beagle dogs in which the dogs often reached an age of 16 to 18 years at the time of death. Primary osteoarthrosis occurred in the hip joints and was characterized by wear-and-tear of the articular cartilage with eventual collapse of the joint space leading to minimal reactive periarticular new bone.

However, joint laxity and modeling of the head and acetabulum, both of which characterize dysplasia, are absent with primary joint disease. The clinical signs with primary osteoarthrosis are not well described, but are probably minimal, and may be the result of a chronic synovitis. The clinical signs associated with primary osteoarthrosis can change following trauma and the previously minimal clinical signs can become more acutely severe.

In fact, the pattern of radiographic change noted in primary joint disease due only to "wear and tear" is markedly different from that seen with secondary joint disease associated with HD. The shape of the femoral head and acetabulum remains essentially unchanged with narrowing of the joint space being the primary finding along with uniform subchondral sclerosis and generalized osteopenia (Figure 5-72).

Secondary joint disease can also follow a traumatic injury such as an acetabular fracture or be present following infectious arthritis of the hip joint and can more closely resemble changes found with HD. In any regard, the older the dog at the time of evaluation of the hip joints, the greater is the possibility of disagreement relative to the cause of the secondary osteoarthrosis. This is especially a problem in the dog with unilateral dysplasia. However, the issue of interpretation of change in the older dog is probably a greater problem in the minds of the owner / breeder than in the minds of the clinician evaluating the radiographs.

## Treatment

No management regime or treatment of the individual dog with hip dysplasia will restore normal function to a dysplastic hip. However, it is expected that some measure of relief can be provided to any dog that is weakened by dysplasia. With sensible care by the veterinarian and owner, many affected dogs live reasonably normal lives and function as happy companions. In the discussion of treatment it is important to separate what is recommended for the immature puppy from treatment recommended for the older, mature dog. Remember that no matter the nature of the treatment, the lessening of clinical signs, or the increased ability of the dog to perform better after treatment, the genetic makeup of the dog is not altered, it still has dysplasia that can be transmitted to any offspring. Ideally, every dog treated for dysplasia should be castrated or spayed.

Treatment is divided into three major divisions; conservative, medical, and surgical (Table 5-7). Conservative treatment centers on the maintenance of the dog through careful control of the dog's activities, surroundings, and diet. Medical treatment employs certain medicaments to control pain. Surgical procedures have various goals and their use is age dependent. No matter the drug or surgical treatment used, they should be combined with conservative treatment which consists of weight and exercise control. Conservative and medical treatments can be attempted in a dog of any age and with any degree of dysplasia and are usually considered first because of the relative ease of use. Certain of the surgical procedures are best performed in the younger dog prior to development of the secondary osteoarthrosis in an effort to minimize that process, while others can be used as salvage procedures in the older dog. Methods of therapy have been reviewed (Rettenmaier and Constantenescu 1991, Remedios and Fries 1995, Tomlinson and McLaughlin Jr 1996 b).

### Table 5-7: Treatment of hip dysplasia

I. Conservative

II. Medical

III. Surgical

### Conservative treatment in the immature dog

The progression of secondary osteoarthrosis in the immature dog with hip dysplasia can be controlled with conservative management (Table 5-8). It is important that the owner understand this because it strongly suggests that actions taken early in the life of the dog can influence the progression of clinical signs. Exercise at a young age can be regulated, understanding that excess athletic activity can cause further injury to the hip. Ideally, treatment at a young age should consist of persistent abduction of the hind limbs resulting in the femoral head being deeply seated in the acetabulum. This is regularly performed in babies with dysplasia through the use of double diapers. Unfortunately, the only actions available to minimize the effect of joint laxity in the puppy are to control weight and delay the rate of body growth through strict diet control. This enables the musculoskeletal system to develop more slowly.

### Table 5-8: Conservative treatment for hip dysplasia control in the puppy

I. Limit exercise and utilize non-weightbearing tasks (eg, swimming)

II. Force the dog to sit to attempt abduction of the limb

III. Control body weight

IV. Control growth rate

### Conservative treatment in the mature dog

Much can be done to alleviate pain in the mature dog with osteoarthrosis secondary to HD short of medical or surgical treatment (Johnson 1992) (Table 5-9). Adequate rest for dogs with osteoarthrosis is important for several reasons. Excessive use of damaged joints, regardless of etiology can aggravate clinical signs and can accelerate destruction of the articular surfaces. Thus, it is important to avoid overexertion of the dysplastic hip through rough play or long exercise. It can be difficult to control exercise since the dogs so often are eager to please their owners that they easily overexert themselves. After warning of the problems of over exercise, it is just as important to prevent the dogs from becoming invalids. Controlled exercise is important in the maintenance of muscle tone and delays contracture of periarticular soft tissues that results in limited movement of the joints. Controlled exercise can consist of defined periods of walking with the owner interspersed with short periods of play. Swimming is especially recommended. The dog needs to be closely observed during these times of walking to determine signs of pain or discomfort that suggest that the exercise is too vigorous. The owner needs to understand that often their dog can be so willing to please, and the time in walking with the owner can be so enjoyable, that the dog overexerts itself.

**Table 5-9: Conservative treatment for hip dysplasia control in the mature dog with osteoarthrosis secondary to hip dysplasia**

I. Exercise should:
    A. Be regular
    B. Be moderate
    C. Include swimming when possible
    D. Avoid excesses
II. Prevent obesity
III. Provide warm environment

Weight Control is important since increased body weight places greater stress on the vulnerable joint(s). Avoid slippery surfaces since falling can cause painful injury to the affected hip. Provide a good surface on which the dog can move, for example, choose the wet sand that is hard packed when walking on the beach rather than have the dog walk in the loose dry sand. Insure that the dog has a warm, dry place in which to sleep. When conservative treatment is not sufficient to keep the dog comfortable, medical treatment can be used (Pedersen, et al 1982).

One of the best studies on the long-term results of conservative management evaluated a group of dogs for a 10-year period. The 68 dogs were immature at the time of first examination when all had clinical subluxation and radiographic evidence of minimal hip dysplasia. Of this group, 76% were successfully managed in a manner that they had only minimal gait abnormalities despite the progression of radiological evidence of moderate or severe osteoarthrosis (Barr, et al 1987). Another group of military working dogs whose lives differed markedly from the typical clinical patient was studied throughout their lives. These dogs worked one or two 8-hour shifts each week, were put through strenuous training daily, and were maintained in excellent physical condition. Of the 116 dogs, 57 had mild or moderate hip dysplasia and yet none had problems in performance throughout their working lives due to the condition of the hips until an old age (<9 years) (Banfield, et al 1996b).

## Medical treatment

**Table 5-10: Drugs used for relief of pain in dogs with hip dysplasia**

1. Aspirin
2. Phenylbutazone
3. Meclofenamic acid
4. Carprofen
5. Polysulfated glycosaminoglycan
6. Naproxen
7. Flunixin meglumide
8. Ibuprofen

A variety of analgesic and non-steroidal anti-inflammatory drugs (NSAIDs) are recommended for use in controlling attendant pain and lameness in dogs with hip dysplasia (Fox and Johnson 1997) (Table 5-10). Remember that the drugs are only administered to achieve pain relief and there is no reversal of the joint disease. In fact, the dog with less pain after medication can tend to overuse the hip joint and cause a more rapid progression of the osteoarthrosis. Thus, despite administration of drugs, owners need to exert control over both physical activity and body weight.

Certain medicines can cause problems following administration. Some of the common NSAIDs such as aspirin, phenylbutazone, and meclofenamic acid can cause vomiting and ulceration of the stomach or duodenum and thus should not be used in a susceptible dog (Boulay 1986). Most dogs, however, tolerate buffered aspirin (Ascriptin). Dosages of: (1) 25 mg/kg every 8 hours, or (2) 25 to 50 mg/kg divided into three daily doses are usually well tolerated and can afford good relief (Booth 1977). A lesser dose of 10 to 20 mg/kg every 12 hours can be sufficient for some dogs (Johnson 1992).

Aspirin is the world's most extensively used drug and the most commonly used anti-inflammatory drug in dogs. The recommended dosage in dogs is 10 to 40 mg/kg PO every 8 hours. Adverse effects are common including gastric ulceration. It is questionable if buffered or enteric-coated aspirin decreases the risk of gastrointestinal hemorrhage and ulceration (Fox and Johnson 1997).

In addition to aspirin, there are several other drugs that are considerably more expensive, have their own unique side effects, but are not necessarily more effective. These drugs should be used only if aspirin is proven to be ineffective. Phenylbutazone can be effective in certain dogs that do not respond to aspirin. However, in addition to intestinal side effects, it can cause bone marrow depression, thus the hemogram should be monitored with chronic use. For long term use in dogs, the dosage is

40 mg/kg divided three times a day for the first 48 hours, then adjusted to 10 to15 mg/kg every 8 hours (Booth 1977, Johnson 1992). Others use much lower dosages. The total daily dosage should not exceed 80 mg regardless of the size of the dog to avoid bone marrow suppression (Johnson 1992).

A new drug with good potential is carprofen (RIMA-DYL® Pfizer Animal Health, NY) and has been shown to be well tolerated and to be highly effective with most dogs responding positively when treated. It is a NSAID and inhibits cyclooxygenase (a prostaglandin synthetase), blocking production of prostaglandins, and provides analgesic, anti-inflammatory, and antipyretic activities. It is administered at a dosage of 2 mg/kg every 12 hours. It is recommended that carprofen, like other drugs, should not be administered in conjunction with other medications until further information is available regarding potential drug interactions (Vasseur 1992; Vasseur, et al 1995; Fox and Johnson 1997). This drug has gained much of the analgesia market in the UK since the time it has been available in that region and has received favorable comments.

Meclofenamic acid, a NSAID of the fenamate class has the potential for gastrointestinal damage, yet may be considered when other drugs with less potential risk have been tried unsuccessfully. The drug is administered orally and the dosage should not exceed 1.1 mg/kg divided into two or three daily doses for 7 to 10 days. The dose is then reduced to a divided dosage of 0.5 mg/kg for the next 4 to 7 days and then decreased to a single dosage of 0.5 mg/kg per day for a maintenance level. It is approved for use in dogs but is currently available only in equine granules (Johnson 1992).

Prednisolone or prednisone are stronger and more effective drugs that can also be used to relieve the pain associated with HD and are given at an initial oral dosage of 2 mg/kg once daily for several days, followed by a chronic maintenance dose that should not exceed 1 mg/kg every other day. However, corticosteroids can actually hasten degeneration of the cartilage by delaying normal cartilage repair and encouraging the dog to over-exercise because of the lessening of pain. So, what is gained in the short term can be lost in the long term. For this reason, corticosteroids should be restricted to advanced cases that are totally unresponsive to more conventional therapy. When used in end-stage osteoarthrosis unresponsive to other drugs, prednisone can be given orally at 1 mg/kg twice a day for 3 days, then reduced to 0.5 mg/kg twice a day for 3 days, then 0.5 mg/kg once a day for 3 days, and then 0.5 mg/kg once every other day (Tomlinson and McLaughlin Jr 1996 b). Intra-articular injections of steroids should be avoided (Pedersen, et al 1982).

Some clinicians have used naproxen, flunixin meglumine, or ibuprofen, all of which have been approved for use in people and horses, in treating the pain associated with hip dysplasia. However, all of these drugs have been reported to cause serious complications in dogs including gastric ulceration (Daehler 1986).

Another group of drugs that can have application in the medical treatment of hip dysplasia are polysuflated glycosaminoglycans (PSGAG) made up mainly of chondroitin sulfate extracts which protects the articular cartilage by slowing the degenerative process. It is a natural substance found in the chemical composition of articular cartilage and uniquely inhibits the effects of lysosomal enzymes, the synthesis of prostaglandins and interleukins, and the release of free radicals. The drug is only approved currently for equine use. Studies indicate that systemic treatment results in concentrations of the drug in articular cartilage and its use is associated with positive therapeutic effects. Others suggest that any differences noted following use of the drug (Adequan) are not statistically significant (Lust, et al 1992). A double blind clinical study using PSGAG to treat dogs with chronic advanced hip dysplasia showed no beneficial effect (DeHaan, et al 1994). The drug is also sold under the name Arteparon (Hannan, et al 1987). While this drug can provide some protection to articular cartilage, it should be understood that in advanced joint disease associated with hip dysplasia, little, if any, articular cartilage remains to be protected, thus, the value of the drug can be questioned.

Whenever chronic drug therapy is initiated, owners should be made aware of the fact that the control of signs is only partial and can never be complete. In fact, the dog can feel better with the drug therapy and wants to overuse the joints resulting in more rapid progression of the secondary osteoarthrosis. Drug therapy is usually attempted to learn of the effects on the patient who is not responding to weight and exercise control and prior to the election of a surgical procedure. While drug therapy is utilized in patients of all ages, it is especially valuable in the older dog in whom a surgical procedure can be considered inappropriate because of age, cost or pain and discomfort associated with the surgery.

## Surgical treatment

No surgical treatment will restore totally normal function to a dysplastic hip; however, it is usual that some measure of pain relief and improved hip configuration can be offered to any dog with HD. Often stabilization of the hip joint using reconstructive osteotomies is a most effective method of dealing with the severely dysplastic hip in young dogs. The use of surgical treatment involves a greater commitment of time in nursing by the owner, implies a greater cost, and is performed with some pain and discomfort to the dog. Surgery includes use of an anesthetic which, while commonly used in medicine, is not without risk. For these reasons, this form of therapy needs to be undertaken only following a lengthy discussion with the owner of the procedure and the expected results. Many owners are not pleased with surgical results simply because of not having a good understanding of the expected results. When the surgical technique and anticipated outcome is well understood, most owners are satisfied with the outcome (Table 5-11). In the discussion of surgical treatment, it is important to separate treatment recommended for the immature dog from the treatment recommended for the older, mature dog.

**Table 5-11: Factors to review with the owner prior to surgery**

I. Need for a second opinion relative to
   A. Necessity of surgery
   B. Type of surgery

II. Cost of the surgery and hospitalization

III. Length of hospitalization

IV. Length of recovery time
   A. Required nursing
      1. Who will perform nursing?
      2. Time required for nursing
   B. Where will recovery take place?
   C. Is kenneling required?

V. Physical therapy
   A. Time required
   B. Who will perform?

VI. Anticipated use of the dog following surgery
   A. Are expectations realistic?
   B. How will surgery influence use of dog?

VII. Age of dog at the time of treatment
   A. Life expectancy

VIII. Effect of surgery on personality of the dog

IV. Possibility of surgical complication
   A. Infection
   B. Loosening of implant
   C. Fracture of implant
   D. Femoral head luxation

## Surgical treatment in the immature dog

Before considering a surgical procedure, a careful physical and radiological examination is required to ensure that the exact cause of the pain and lameness is hip dysplasia. In addition, a thorough examination of the patient is necessary to make certain that no other congenital/developmental lesion is present such as elbow dysplasia that might require subsequent treatment. The concurrence of developmental diseases was recognized early (Seer and Hurov 1969, Sprinkle and Krook 1970) (see Chapter 9). The puppy is painful because of the early subluxation of the femoral head and the stretching or tearing of the joint capsule and the round ligament of the femoral head along with the microfractures of the acetabular margin due to the trauma caused by the femoral head riding on this margin (Riser 1975). Since it appears that contracture of the pectineus muscle, in part, causes the femoral head to ride dorsally on the acetabular margin, surgical procedures directed toward this muscle or its tendon have been described (Table 5-12). They are grouped together and called tension relief procedures. These are palliative procedures and do not alter the course of the disease. A procedure that attempts to correct the joint instability is a triple pelvic osteotomy (TPO) and this can be considered both a preventive and corrective procedure relative to the joint instability. A different preventive surgical procedure can be used in giant breeds in which the principle abnormality is anteversion and valgus deformity of the femoral head and neck. Neurectomy of the articular capsule has also been suggested in conjunction with pectineal myectomy and iliopsoas tenectomy as a symptomatic treatment (Ballinari, et al 1995).

**Table 5-12: Surgical treatment for dysplasia in the immature dog (6-15 months)**

I. Pectineus tendon surgery
   A. Tenectomy
   B. Tenotomy

II. Pectineus muscle surgery
   A. Myectomy
   B. Myotomy

III. Triple pelvic osteotomy
   A. With femoral neck lengthening
   B. Without femoral neck lengthening

IV. Intertrochanteric derotational varus osteotomy

## Tension relief procedures

The first surgical procedure described in the treatment of hip dysplasia was that of severance of the pectineus muscle insertion in 4 weeks and 8 weeks old dogs. The pectineal muscle is an adductor of the femur and the original idea was that its transection would allow for abduction of the femur and thus better seating of the femoral head into the acetabulum. Transection of the pectineal muscle or tendon is quite effective in decreasing the pain of the acute hip dysplasia, which occurs around the age of 6 months. Early on, good results were reported (Bardens and Harwick 1968).

This treatment is somewhat similar to the post-natal multiple diaper treatment of infants with congenital dysplasia. This treatment in children usually leads to a normal development of the hip because weight-bearing forces as yet play no role in the disease and hip development in children takes years to develop fully. In the dog, however, by the time hip dysplasia becomes noticeable, weight-bearing forces have already been at work for many weeks and the hip joint is more than halfway in the process of ossification. These surgical procedures in the dog, although they relieve pain, have little effect on the course of the disease, and the osteoarthrosis and acetabular deformity continue to progress (Wallace, et al 1970; Lust, et al 1972 a,b).

The decrease in discomfort is probably in part due to the relaxing effect of the procedure on the joint capsule, but the marked decrease in pain has not been completely understood. As mentioned before, the acute phase of hip dysplasia becomes gradually less painful as the joint capsule thickens and the hip becomes more stable, even if subluxated. The apparent continued effect of the surgery on the comfort of the animal is most likely due to the stabilizing effect of the osteoarthrosis and not due to the surgical procedure. Thus, this procedure can make the transition from a very painful unstable joint to a less painful stable one more comfortable. Weight of the patient does not seem to influence the surgical results and both male and female benefit equally from the surgery (Wallace, et al 1972).

When this procedure is done in the mature dog with obvious osteoarthrosis, the decrease in pain is marginal and short-lived and therefore not recommended. A major reason for recommending this procedure is in cases where the degree of subluxation is severe enough that a pelvic osteotomy is inadvisable or as an alternative treatment for owners who have a problem spending the larger sum of money necessary to pay for a TPO. In other patients, the tension relieving procedure enables the animal to be reasonably comfortable until it is mature enough to become a candidate for a total hip replacement.

Tension relieving procedures can vary in a technical manner and include the transection of the pectineus muscle or tendon (myectomy, tenectomy) with or without the removal of a portion of the muscle or tendon (myotomy, tenotomy) from the distal end. The removal of a portion of the tendon or muscle prevents reunion of the severed ends. Both limbs can be operated at the same time. Care must be taken to avoid surgically severing the closely positioned femoral artery and vein. If partial or complete pectineus myectomy or myotomy is performed, hemorrhage and subsequent seroma formation can be a complication (Wallace, et al 1972, Wallace 1992). A partial myotomy has been performed by some (Bowen, et al 1972). A later modification to the surgery included transecting the tendon at the muscular junction and suturing the cut end back onto the belly of the pectineus muscle. This eliminated any fibrotic reattachment of the severed ends of the tendon and greatly decreased seroma formation (Wallace 1992).

A high success rate (90%) has been reported using these tension-relieving procedures with relief from pain noted to begin within 24 to 72 hours post surgical and lasting for periods of up to 6 months. In the evaluation of the surgical results, it is important to recognize that even with a reduction in the pain, the gait can remain abnormal and secondary joint disease can continue to develop, although hopefully at a reduced rate (Wallace 1971; Wallace, et al 1972). The duration of the success of the procedure is often difficult to evaluate because of the nature of the disease in the untreated dog that progresses in many cases to a fairly stable and comfortable joint by the age of 15 months. Therefore, predicting how long lasting is the effect of the surgery is difficult. Some studies have reported no difference radiographically or pathologically between operated and non-operated sides in bilaterally affected puppies (Cardinet, et al 1974 a, b) even though improvement in the clinical status of dogs is generally thought to exist. This suggests the possibility for a major misunderstanding on the part of the owner and clinician in the thought that these procedures can reverse the progression of the osteoarthrosis or that the level of osteoarthrosis is directly related to the clinical signs noted. It also points out that trying to compare the level of discomfort in the dog and the degree of osteoarthrosis at the age of 15 months is deceptive and certainly the two are not parallel.

These tension-relieving procedures are not without controversy (Rubin, et al 1979) and while individual investigators advocate them wholeheartedly (Wallace, et al

1972), others are more reserved in their recommendations (Nunamaker and Newton 1975). Vaughn and Clayton-Jones (1975) treated 100 dysplastic dogs, diagnosed by radiography and palpation, by complete myectomy with an improvement noted in 80% but only 35% ever achieved a high level of recovery. After a time, a fibrous band replaced the muscle. All dogs became progressively worse radiographically indicating joint incongruity remained. Some, but not all, dogs improved clinically immediately after surgery. Others reported that simultaneous sectioning of the adductor magnus muscle provided more relief than if the pectineus muscle was sectioned alone (Nunamaker and Newton 1975).

Certain dog club show rules can specify that a dog can be disqualified if its appearance has been changed by artificial means other than those recognized by the standard of the breed. Therefore, it is possible that dogs which have undergone tension relieving procedures can not be exhibited in the show ring (Crawford and Pharr 1975). While this limitation has been recognized for many years, it seems to be conveniently ignored in many instances.

Even if the surgery does not alter the course of the disease, tension-relieving procedures are recommended. In the final analysis, the authors feel that this form of surgery has a definite position in the management of the dysplastic puppy. First, in many dogs obvious relief of the acute pain of early hip dysplasia is noted and the dog can comfortably reach the stage of greater joint stability due to the progressive osteoarthrosis. The surgery is relatively easy, appears to cause little pain to the dog, and the dog is willing to actively use the limb on the first day after the surgery. The surgical procedure is less expensive than alternative procedures such as a triple pelvic osteotomy. The tension relieving procedures allow the dog with severe dysplasia to achieve a relatively comfortable state until they are old enough to become a candidate for a total hip replacement (Table 5-13). The main complication of the surgery is seroma formation, therefore, it is advised to restrict the dog's physical activity for one week following the surgery.

## Triple pelvic osteotomy

Stabilization of the hip joint using reconstructive osteotomies is an effective method of treating the severely dysplastic hip in the young dog. Surgical repositioning of the entire acetabulum by pelvic osteotomy has been advocated in younger patients with subluxating hips, prior to the development of osteoarthrosis in an effort to create a more normal relationship between the acetabular roof and the femoral head. A first report utilized three osteotomies that separated the acetabulum (Brinker 1966). Later, a double pelvic osteotomy was described utilizing a step-wise cut in the ileum and an osteotomy of the ischium into the obturator foramen. A trochanteric osteotomy was used in conjunction with the pelvic osteotomy (Hohn and Janes 1969). Later a triple pelvic osteotomy was described with an ischial osteotomy just caudal to the acetabulum close to the hip joint, a pubic osteotomy, and an ilial osteotomy performed in a step-wise fashion. This was performed in addition to a trochanteric osteotomy (Schrader 1981). Another technique described using two pubic osteotomies in which the entire pubic ramus was removed and was used later as a graft medial to the ilial osteotomy. The ischial cut was made with a Gigli wire and the ilial cut was made perpendicular to a preplaced Steinman pin placed along the shaft of the ilium. A spike of bone was removed from the caudal ilial fragment to avoid irritation to the gluteal muscles following the outward rotation of the acetabular fragment (Slocum and Devine 1986, Slocum and Slocum 1992). In all techniques, the triple osteotomy freed a fragment containing the acetabulum that was rotated outward in such a manner that the acetabulum more completely covered the femoral head. In the case of the step-wise ilial osteotomy, the stabilization was obtained by means of a lag screw and cerclage wire. In the case of a vertical ilial osteotomy, various plates were used in stabilization (Hohn and Janes 1969, Henry and Wadsworth 1975, Schrader 1981, 1986, Slocum and Devine 1986). The procedure requires considerable surgical skill and thus can have limited application. The early procedures only partially corrected the subluxation of the femoral head but they did impede the rate of progression of the osteoarthrosis (Hohn and Janes 1969, Brinker 1971, Henry and Wadsworth 1975). The basic principles of the procedure including the cutting of the pelvis cranial, medial, and caudal to the acetabulum are shown schematically (Figure 5-73). In addition, an incision is made in the sacrotuberous ligament at its caudal attachment to allow for axial rotation of the acetabular segment.

**Table 5-13: Tension relieving procedures in young dogs**

**I.** Surgery
    A. Relatively easy procedures
    B. Cause little pain

**II.** Results
    A. Use of limb immediately following surgery
    B. Relief of acute pain

**III.** Relatively inexpensive

**IV.** Permits time to consider a more extensive surgical procedure

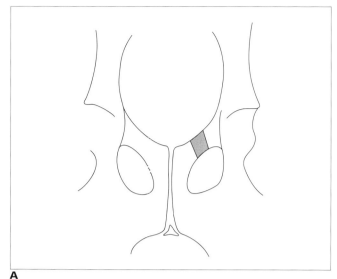

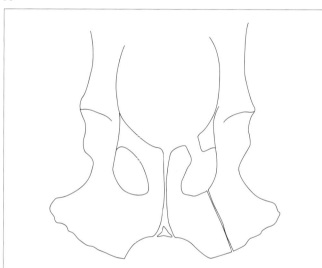

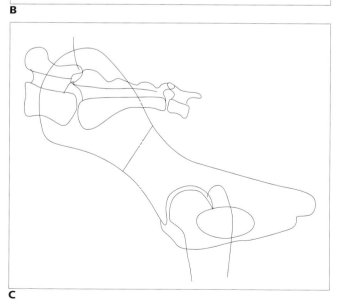

**Table 5-14: Selection of a suitable candidate for triple pelvic osteotomy**

**I.** Age
  A. Best results if operated between 5 and 9 months of age
    1. Osteoarthrosis is minimal
    2. Modeling potential after the surgery
      a. Is great
      b. Helps to create an appropriate acetabular cup
  B. Results less likely to be successful in older dogs
    1. Osteoarthrosis is more progressive
    2. Modeling potential of the hip joint postsurgically
      a. Is minimal
      b. May fail to create an appropriate acetabular cup

**II.** Level of osteoarthrosis
  A. Best results if osteoarthrosis minimal
  B. Results less likely to be successful if osteoarthrosis extensive with
    1. Loss of dorsal acetabular rim
    2. Acetabular filling
    3. Dorsal femoral neck enthesophytes

**III.** Nature of joint instability
  A. Surgery likely to be successful in a hip with minimal subluxation
  B. Surgery less likely to be successful in a hip with complete luxation

Certain factors need be considered in determining a suitable candidate for an osteotomy (Table 5-14). Consideration of the progress of osteoarthrosis, the degree of femoral head luxation, and the percentage of femoral head coverage were not associated with subsequent hip function (Rasmussen, et al 1998).

The decision to perform a TPO is often made when the dog is 6 or 7 months of age. Often the dog at this age has clinical sign of hip dysplasia but the signs may not be severe and the dog may be ambulatory at the time of examination. Thus, the decision to perform a rather complicated surgical procedure is made at a time the dog may even have minimal clinical signs. The decision is made in surgery. Therefore, the surgeon has to predict how the dog is going to respond to the hip dysplasia by using

**Figure 5-73**
Drawings show the general placement of the three osteotomy sites that are commonly used to free a portion of the pelvis containing the acetabulum in preparation for placement of an ilial bone plate to achieve a triple pelvic osteotomy, (A) the pubic ostectomy, (B) the ischial ostectomy, and (C) the ilial ostectomy.

clinical signs and radiographic changes as predictors. It is thought that the greater the joint laxity with the femoral head resting against the dorsal rim of the acetabulum, the greater is the indication for surgery. Often the owner participates in the decision to perform a TPO when they wish to remove the uncertainty relative to the pet being clinically happy by agreeing to a surgical procedure with little or no discomfort. Still, it is a little like playing "god."

This surgical procedure is much more complicated than the tension relieving procedures. Whereas, those surgeries involve only the soft tissues, a pelvic osteotomy involves surgery on the bone. The purpose of this surgery is to counteract the combined effects of joint instability and insufficient acetabular coverage of the femoral head due to a shallow acetabulum. It is designed to prevent the more crippling osteoarthrosis by producing a stable joint. It is best performed in dogs 5 months to 9 months of age when osteoarthrosis is minimal and some modeling potential of the newly aligned acetabulum is still present. Some positive results, however, have been obtained in animals as old as 18 months if the osteoarthrosis is mild. Regardless of age at which surgery is performed, the joint will not become perfect and, in fact, the osteoarthrosis still is progressive, but to a much lesser degree than otherwise would have occurred.

Age at which the surgery is performed influences the end result. In the younger patient, the partial cartilaginous head and acetabulum can more easily adapt through modeling to their altered position. When the joint is more ossified as in an older dog, this modeling is both delayed and somewhat limited and the success of the surgery can be less pronounced with development of a more severe osteoarthrosis. However, if the surgery is performed prior to 6 months of age, the holding power of the screws in the soft bone is less than in the mature dog. This can increase the possibility of loosening of the plate especially if the dog is allowed to be active post-surgically. Recently, the age at surgery was reported to be significantly related to the degree of osteoarthrosis as seen on follow-up radiographs, with the development of osteoarthrosis being much greater if the surgery was performed at 6 months of age as compared to performing the surgery at 12 months of age (Rassmussen, et al 1998).

The pre-existing osteoarthrosis has been suggested to influence the clinical outcome following surgery. However, a recent study suggests that dogs with early stages of osteoarthrosis are thought to be suitable candidates for TPO and that pre-existing osteoarthrosis did not result in poorer radiographic and clinical outcome (Rassmussen, et al 1998).

The surgical procedure consists in cutting the bones surrounding the acetabulum, ie, the ilium, the ischium, and the pubis, so that the acetabulum is freed and can be rotated over the top of the femoral head to increase its dorsal weight-bearing coverage. Three surgical approaches are required. The pubis is approached through an incision over the origin of the pectineus muscle and the abdominal wall muscles are elevated from the pubis and a section of the pubis is excised (Figure 5-73 a). This section of bone can provide a graft to be used around the ilial plate. The ischium is approached by a second incision and it is cut using a power saw or a Gigli wire (Figure 5-73 b). It is possible to make this osteotomy immediately caudal to acetabulum. The third approach is made over the body of the ilium where it is osteotomized immediately caudal to the sacrum (Figure 5-73 c). The acetabular segment is now completely free. Following the osteotomies and rotation of the acetabular fragment, the ilial osteotomy site is stabilized with a specially designed cranial pelvic osteotomy plate with a preformed angle of 20° or 30° (Slocum Enterprises, Eugene, OR) or an ASIF DC plate that has been contoured to the adjusted shape of the ilial body and rotated to the predetermined angle (Figure 5-74). The ischial and pubic osteotomy sites are not usually stabilized other than indirectly by the ilial plate; however, some surgeons may place a wire to join the ischial fragments. If joint laxity seems to be excessive following fixation of the acetabular fragment, it may be necessary to imbricate the joint capsule and/or shift the greater trochanter distally to achieve joint stability. Thus, the surgery is extensive and the outcome is dependent on the skill of the surgeon and the avoidance of possible problems in post-operative recovery by the patient.

The degree of rotation necessary to cover the femoral head adequately is estimated from radiographs, from measuring the angles of reduction of the femoral head into the acetabulum as detected when performing an Ortolani procedure, and from direct observation during surgery. The best candidates for the surgery are those where a 20° to 30° rotation of the acetabulum is adequate for obtaining joint stability. If joint stability is not obtained following a 30° rotation of the acetabulum, it is not advisable to proceed to a 45° rotation since extension and abduction of the femur following surgery are compromised by the impinging of the femoral neck on the dorsal acetabular rim and the dog has an unsightly gait. If joint stability is not obtained at 30° rotation, it is advisable to add a femoral neck lengthening procedure to the pelvic osteotomy (Slocum and Devine 1986). This procedure re-establishes stable hip biomechanics without the necessity for over-rotation of the acetabular segment. The femoral neck lengthening procedure reduces the amount

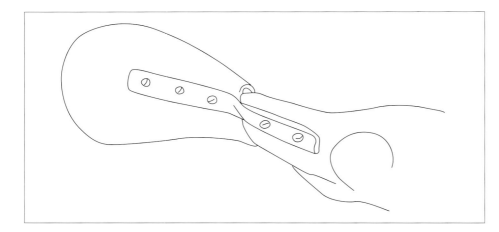

**Figure 5-74**
Drawing of the pelvis showing placement of an individually prepared DC bone plate across the iliac ostectomy site to stabilize the free acetabular fragment that has been rotated laterally in a triple pelvic osteotomy.

of acetabular segment rotation by 10° allowing for increased hip abduction.

Owners need to be advised that recovery can be slow and painful, and that the dog requires confinement with limited exercise for 3 weeks. Because most patients are young, this can require caging or kenneling for this period. The dog's confinement prevents the main complication of the surgery, which is loosening of the ilial plate that is especially likely to occur in very young dogs of the soft character of the bone at that age. However, healing of the osteotomy sites is more rapid in the younger dog.

Complications are classified into three major categories. Case selection errors include: (1) unrecognized fracture of the acetabular rim, (2) filling of the acetabulum, and (3) excessive femoral neck enthesophyte formation. The requirement for over-rotation of the acetabular segment results in pain owing to interference between the femoral neck and the dorsal rim of the acetabulum. Technical errors include: (1) trapping of the sciatic or obturator nerve or damaging the cranial gluteal nerve, (2) mechanical interference between the femurs if the entire pubic ramus is not removed, (3) impingement of pubic bone on the urethra if the lateral pubic osteotomy is not performed at the lateral margin of the obturator foramen, (4) failure of the ischial osteotomy wire to hold in the apophysis of a young dog, (5) failure to obtain good holding of the two dorsal screws of the cranial plate segment in small dogs, (6) failure to direct the ilial osteotomy perpendicular to the guide pin, and (7) failure to remove the spike of bone projecting from the dorsal acetabular segment. Narrowing of the pelvic canal can follow the repositioning of the acetabular segment if the procedure is performed bilaterally and cause problems in defecation. This error has been overcome by use of the specially designed pelvic osteotomy plate. Lack of client and animal compliance prior to bone healing may result in failure of a pelvic osteotomy procedure (Slocum and Slocum 1992).

The owner can expect that the surgical procedure will provide the dog with a hip that is better aligned and stable with a slower rate of progression of the osteoarthrosis. However, in many dogs, the gait is more abducted. Joint disease still progresses because the procedure fails to produce a perfectly congruent joint. In the authors' experience, no dogs treated by a TPO, that have had an uncomplicated recovery, have responded so poorly to the surgery that they have required an added surgery in the form of a total hip replacement at a later date.

### Intertrochanteric derotational varus osteotomy

Intertrochanteric derotational varus osteotomy is intended to correct a valgus deformity and anteversion that is sometimes associated with hip dysplasia. The surgery improves the hip biomechanics and reduces discomfort by re-establishing or improving the congruity of the acetabular and femoral joint surfaces and, thus, improves the stability and quality of joint motion (Brinker 1971, Paatsama and Jussila 1974, Nunamaker and Newton 1975, Prieur and Scartazzini 1980, Piermattei 1982 a, Prieur 1987, Walker and Prieur 1987). Surgical correction attempts to place the femoral head and neck in a more normal position relative to the acetabulum and attempts to force the subluxating femoral head deeply into the acetabular cup. This causes a medial shifting of contact areas of joint surfaces and induces functional modeling of the femoral head and acetabulum. This type of surgical technique is best used in dogs with a near normal acetabular cup. An acceptable congruity of articular surfaces can be re-established. Stability can be improved by changing the angle of the femoral neck to a varus position and by decreasing the angle of anteversion. Thus, the results of the surgery can be enhanced if performed early when there is maximum bone turnover, which occurs during osseous development, so the modeling can create the best hip joint possible (Braden, et al 1990). This surgery is not of value in the patient with a flattened acetabular cup.

In the intertrochanteric derotational varus osteotomy, the femoral neck is cut between the trochanter minor and trochanter major and the femoral head and neck are rotated caudally with a slight varus position. The osteotomy site is stabilized with a specially designed hookplate. The technique of intertrochanteric derotational varus osteotomy is well described (Nunamaker 1974, Walker and Prieur 1987). Aftercare of the patient is similar to that required for pelvic osteotomy.

In some giant breeds, the valgus and anteversion of the femoral head and neck may be present causing a lameness in a dog in which a normal acetabular cup is present. Some feel this is another form of hip dysplasia. The authors, however, recognize this as a separate developmental disease. This surgical procedure can be used successfully in these patients.

## Neck lengthening or intertrochanteric lateralization of the proximal femur

This procedure is designed to increase the force by which surrounding muscle groups push the femoral head medially into the center of the acetabulum. The surgery consists in incompletely dividing, or splitting, the proximal femur into a medial and lateral half. The vertically directed osteotomy within the proximal femur extends over a length of 6 to 8 cm. The lateral half consists of the greater trochanter, the third trochanter, and sites of the insertions of the middle and deep gluteal muscles cranially on the greater trochanter and the sites of insertion of internal and external obturator, gemelli, and quadratus femoris muscles on the trochanteric fossa. The medial half consists of the lesser trochanter and the head and neck of the femur. A space is created between the medial and lateral halves of the proximal femur that is maintained by means of: (1) plastic inserts, (2) spacing screws, or (3) cortical and cancellous bone graft (Slocum and Slocum 1993; Stoll, et al 1995; Brown 1996).

This procedure can be compared to tensing a bow with an arrow in position. The pelvis including the acetabulum is the bow and the muscles are the string cranial and caudal to the arrow stretched from the pelvis to the lateral half of the femur. The lateralized proximal femur, the spacing, and neck of the femur are the arrow shaft with the femoral head as the arrow being driven into the acetabulum.

The surgery can also be accomplished by starting the cut vertically and splitting the proximal femur. The osteotomy is then turned laterally and breaks through the lateral cortex distal to the greater trochanter. A screw is inserted into the femoral neck with the head left protruding. A lag screw is placed distally to reposition the bony fragment, however, the fragment containing the greater trochanter remains spaced because of the screw head resulting in lateralization of the trochanteric segment (Brown 1997).

These procedures are often used in conjunction with a triple pelvic osteotomy where subluxation remains following application of a 20° or 30° osteotomy plate.

## Greater trochanteric repositioning

Greater trochanteric repositioning is an orthopedic procedure designed to correct the biomechanical consequences of hip joint laxity and is accomplished by moving the greater trochanter and its attached muscles laterally and distally. This technique is biomechanically sound if the gluteal muscles as well as the muscles of the small pelvic association remain attached to the greater trochanter after its separation. In practice, the cut is often made incorrectly so that only the gluteal muscles remain attached and the stabilizing effect of the repositioned trochanter is minimal.

## Acetabuloplasty

Acetabuloplasty, or shelf arthroplasty, attempts to overcome or improve the relationship of the acetabulum with reference to the femoral head by causing a lateral or outward rotation of the dorsal acetabular margin by positioning bone grafts to increase the angle of the acetabular roof. This causes formation of a deeper cup that accommodates the femoral head and prevents luxation (Brinker, et al 1968, Brinker 1971). Best results are obtained when some lipping of the acetabular roof remains. The surgical techniques that have been used have not provided consistently good results for this procedure to be considered valuable in treatment of dysplasia at this time (Oakes, et al 1996).

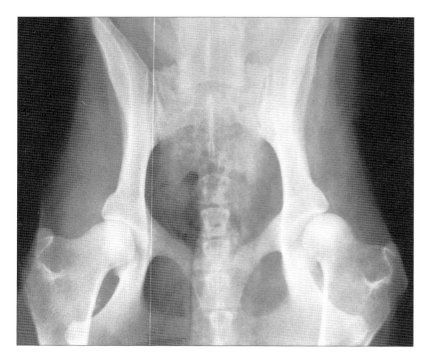 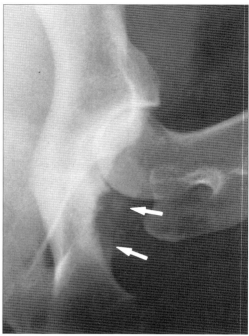

**Figure 5-75**
Pelvic radiographs in a female mature dog with pain in the left hip thought to be associated with hip dysplasia. Unilteral soft tissue atrophy was prominent. The radiographs demonstrate minimal joint laxity on the left, however, the flexed view permits closer examination of the left ischium and identification of an unsuspected primary bone tumor (arrows).

## Surgical treatment in the mature dog

In the mature dog, where weight reduction and the use of analgesics are no longer satisfactory in controlling pain, the animal can be a candidate for a salvage procedure such as either a femoral head and neck excision or a total hip replacement (Table 5-15).

**Table 5-15: Surgical treatment for dysplasia in the mature dog (>15 months)**

I. Femoral head and neck excision arthroplasty

II. Total hip arthroplasty

Prior to selecting a surgical procedure in the older dog, a thorough physical examination is necessary to ensure that the pain and/or lameness is due entirely to the disease within the hip joints. Often stifle joint disease or lumbosacral disc disease can be the cause for part or all of the clinical signs. Neurological conditions can be present in the older dog in the form of a degenerative myelopathy, chronic cord compression from a protruding disc, or a tumor in the spinal canal. Failure to recognize the specific cause of the pain can lead to an inappropriate treatment. Surgical treatment that centers on the hip joints in such a patient obviously can not provide the degree of relief expected (Figure 5-75).

## Femoral head and neck ostectomy (excision arthroplasty)

Dogs with intractable hip pain due to hip dysplasia who are relatively light in weight with a fairly stoic personality and with limited muscle atrophy of the hind quarters are the best candidates for excision of the femoral head and neck. The procedure leads to formation of a false joint (pseudoarthrosis) within the soft tissues lateral and dorsal to the acetabulum with some restoration of limb function despite shortening of the operated limb. The owner should understand that the gait will not be normal and the final range of motion of the limb is restricted with some loss of extension and abduction. This is especially important if the owner anticipates a particular athletic performance. The prognosis and alternative treatments must be made clear to the owner prior to surgery (Table 5-16). Still, the procedure is recommended because excision of the femoral head and neck removes the bone to bone contact that causes a part of the pain (Figure 5-76).

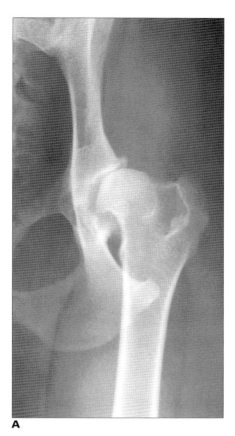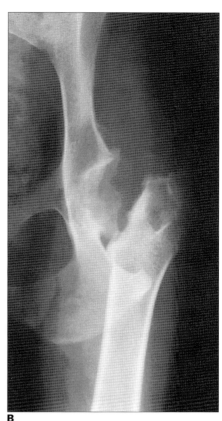

**Figure 5-76**
Radiographs of the left hip of an 8-year-old female Shepherd-cross (A) preoperative and (B) postoperative. The secondary osteoarthrosis associated with hip dysplasia was painful and lead to a decision to perform excision of the femoral head and neck.

**Table 5-16: Factors to consider in selection of femoral head and neck ostectomy**

I. Owner expectations

II. Nature of patient
    A. Weight >20 kg have less satisfactory results
    B. Obese
        1. Have more difficulty with rehabilitation
        2. Have more postoperative nursing problems
            a. Pressure sores
            b. Urine scalds
    C. Coexisting orthopedic disease may effect recovery

III. Chronicity of hip joint arthrosis
    A. Influences post-operative recovery
        1. Muscle atrophy
        2. Fibrosis limiting motion of the hip joint
    B. Interposition of soft tissue between acetabulum and cut surface of the femur at the time of surgery may be necessary

IV. Owner compliance
    A. May require 6 to 12 months of therapy to achieve optimal results

Because smaller dogs form more functional joints (Gendreau and Cawley 1977), the procedure is primarily useful in those breeds. The authors feel that acceptable functional results are usually not obtained in dogs larger than a Labrador Retriever and in all dogs with considerable joint motion restriction because of the thickening of the joint capsule, muscle atrophy, and muscle fibrosis. However, others have reported that many large dogs do benefit from the surgery (Olsson, et al 1969, Gendreau and Cawley 1977). Reports of femoral head ostectomies indicate that they are effective in the relief of pain in many dogs (Ormrod 1961; Spruell 1961; Jenny 1963; Piermattei 1965, 1982 b; Strande 1968; Olsson, et al 1969; Duff and Campbell 1977; Gendreau and Cawley 1977; Berzon, et al 1980; Bonneau and Bretton 1981). It is advisable prior to surgery to attempt weight reduction if the dog is obese. Swimming would be a good selection of exercise both to reduce weight and increase muscle mass.

The goal of the excision is to create a "false" joint with formation of a cartilage-like cover on the stump of the neck and a comfortable range of motion in regards to flexion and extension of the hind limb. The key to reach that goal is early use of the limb after the surgery. Considerable physiotherapy is required to encourage development of the false joint. Dogs with prolonged hip lameness and dogs more ready to curtail their activity because of pain are reluctant to engage in the required therapy and the desired limb motion is not obtained.

Physical therapy should begin within a few days after the surgery and consists in walking the dog slowly on a leash and praising it when the operated limb is put down and is bearing some weight. A slow walk encourages use of the operated limb more than when moving at a faster walk or at a trot. At the faster gaits, the dog simply becomes three-legged and fails to use the operated limb. Passive flexion and extension is also recommended if the dog allows it. After the skin incision has healed, slow walking upstairs and swimming are both excellent forms of physical therapy. Hopefully with correct patient selection, proper surgery, and good postoperative nursing care, the animal should willingly use the limb in 4 to 5 weeks after the surgery. Others report more rapid pain relief and earlier use of the limb (Olsson, et al 1969). With the gradual lessening of the pain, the excursion of the limb becomes greater, helping the false joint to develop. At 4 to 6 months, no further increase in limb excursion is expected.

The dog compensates for the limb shortening by tilting the pelvis and extending the stifle joint on the operated limb (Ormrod 1961; Spruell 1961; Strande 1968; Olsson, et al 1969; Brinker 1971). Near-painless motion can be restored and some dogs surprisingly return to an active physical life (Olsson, et al 1969). The usual course of the excision surgery as the dog ages is a gradual decrease in the degree of limb excursion, due to fibrosis around the "false" joint, but this can take many years to occur.

Patients have had both femoral heads removed and have learned to ambulate satisfactorily. Often two separate surgical procedures are recommended rather than performing both femoral head ostectomies at the same time. Others suggest that the surgery can be performed on both hips at the same time (Olsson, et al 1969). The authors suggest that 6 to 10 weeks should lapse before performing surgery on the opposite limb.

The clinician needs to review with the owner what is required of them following surgery. Often an owner is dissatisfied with the time required of them in post-operative care because of a failure to understand the large role that they play in the ultimate success of the surgery. The clinician needs to discuss much in addition to the cost of the surgical procedure (Table 5-17). If the owner does not understand this obligation, the surgical results may be inadequate in their mind. This is especially true in femoral head excision arthroplasty.

**Table 5-17: Average costs of surgical procedures for one hip (US dollars)**

Pectineal myotomy or tenotomy: $100-200
Intertrochanteric lateralization: $500-700
Femoral head and neck excision: $500-700
Total hip replacement: $2000-3000
Triple pelvic osteotomy: $1500-3000

## Total hip replacement (total hip arthroplasty)

Because both femoral head and acetabulum contribute to the osteoarthrosis causing pain, the most attractive treatment today is total hip arthroplasty (THA) with the removal of both diseased parts (Brinker 1971; Dueland 1975; Biggert 1978; Lewis and Jones 1980; Olmstead and Hohn 1980; Olmstead, et al 1981, 1983; Turner 1982; Olmstead 1987; Massat and Vasseur 1994). The first unipolar arthroplasty was called a Brown prosthesis and was described in 1953. Next, the Gorman prosthesis, which was the first total hip, was reported in 1957. Later came the widely used Richard's Canine II prosthesis in 1974. Further work was done to create the porous-coated anatomic (PCA) systems. While some models are cemented, others are cementless. The history of THA has been reviewed (Montgomery, et al 1992).

Total hip replacement is generally recommended for large dogs, in which femoral head and neck excision is expected to be less successful. A careful examination of the surgical candidate is required to insure that other disease conditions are not present that would compromise the total hip replacement. The range of pain-free motion after this type of surgical procedure can be nearly the same as in a normal hip joint. The life expectancy of the patient sometimes determines the appropriateness of a total hip replacement.

The intention of this surgical procedure is removal of the femoral head and neck and replacing them with a prosthetic implant. The prosthetic components consist usually of a plastic acetabular cup and a femoral component consisting of a plastic head fitted onto a metal neck and shaft. The procedure requires proper preparation of the acetabular bed and the femoral medullary canal for the prosthetic components. In addition to proper component selection, accurate alignment of the prosthetic components is essential. The shaft is placed firmly into the marrow cavity of the proximal femur and cemented to the host bone by means of polymethylmethacrylate. Post-operative care consists of strict confinement for 2 weeks, followed by limited activity for 2 weeks, and then gradual return to normal activities. Some recommend that the dog's activity is restricted to leash walking for 4 to 6 weeks.

Although used in people for more than 30 years, dislocation, infection at the bone-cement and cement-implant interfaces and implant loosening have been common complications both in people and in dogs. Because results in the dog are not always entirely satisfactory, radiographic evaluation of the prosthesis should be scheduled routinely to detect any problem as early as possible (Konde, et al 1982). These problems include: (1) implant malposition, (2) implant loosening, (3) luxation, (4) migration of the prosthesis, (5) actual mechanical breakdown of the prosthesis (Figure 5-77, page 198, 199), (6) femoral fracture at the end of the prosthesis, or (7) secondary infection in the form of osteomyelitis or infectious arthritis (Table 5-18). Improvements in implant design, implant materials, and surgical technique have resulted in decreased complications and in increased acceptance of the procedure in dogs.

Barring complications, the acceptance of the prosthesis by the dog is excellent with pain free hip motion (Table 5-18). Satisfactory results were reported in more than 90% of total hip replacements (Olmstead, et al 1983; Olmstead 1995). However, there remains a possibility of late loosening of the implant after between 5 and 7 years thus necessitating a second surgery. Aseptic loosening of the femoral implant occurs more commonly if contact exists between the distal stem tip and the endosteal surface of the femoral cortex. This can be noted on the radiographs obtained after the surgery. Another radiographic sign is a radiolucent line between the prosthesis and the polymethylmethacrylate (Edwards, et al 1997). The selection of candidates that are 7 years of age or older avoids the problem of a second surgery because of the shortened expected life span of the dog.

**Table 5-18: Complications following total hip replacement**

**I.** Implant
  A. Malposition
  B. Loosening
  C. Luxation
**II.** Prosthesis
  A. May migrate
  B. May undergo a mechanical breakdown
**III.** Femoral fracture
**IV.** Secondary infection

# Prognosis

No surgical treatment will totally restore normal function to a dysplastic hip, however, it is usual that some measure of pain relief and improved hip configuration can be offered to any dog with HD. In addition to the type of surgery performed, which is dictated by the status of the hip joint and the age of the dog, the following are important in influencing the outcome of the surgery: (1) Age of the patient is important because the surgical procedure, anesthesia, and recovery are handled better in general by a younger patient. (2) Temperament of the dog also influences the response to the surgery and especially to any special after-care that is required. The more eager and athletic dog may better handle problems following surgery and be more willing to undergo required physiotherapy. (3) The physical condition of the dog is important. Obesity increases the risk of anesthesia, increases the difficulty of the surgical procedure, and often slows recovery. A dog with muscle atrophy prior to surgery may be slower in regaining use of the hind limbs making a rapid return to athletic activity questionable. Lighter weight dogs have a better prognosis in the case of femoral head ostectomy. (4) A primary consideration should also be the experience of the surgeon selected and a second opinion may not be amiss if more than one type of surgery is to be considered. (5) The aftercare of the patient is extremely important in influencing the prognosis of surgical treatment for hip dysplasia. This encompasses the immediate post-operative care that probably takes place in the clinic or hospital. During this time, good nursing care prevents urine burns, decubital ulcers, and wound dehiscence. Physiotherapy influences the prognosis following some procedures more than others. The availability of an exercise pool can make a great difference in the dog's return to a healthy, active life. The owner's willingness to return the dog for periodic clinical examinations is important in the early detection of any post-operative problem at a stage when the problem can be handled easily. Failure to return for these examinations may compromise the success of the surgery.

A special point can be made concerning the prognosis of a working dog: top performance should not be expected for any dog that is operated on for hip dysplasia. Regardless of the variety of factors that influence the prognosis of surgical treatment of hip dysplasia, the authors have made an effort to provide some guidelines for the owner (Table 5-19).

# Heritability

Since dysplasia of the hip joint is one of the inherited developmental diseases in the dog, it is important that

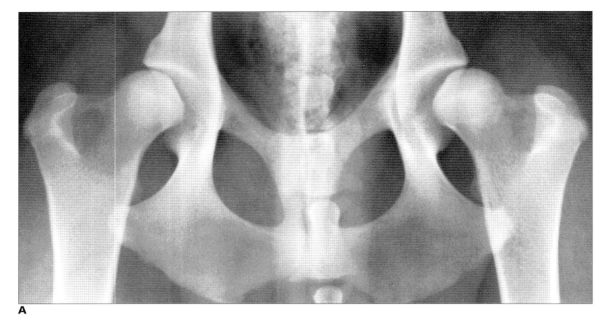
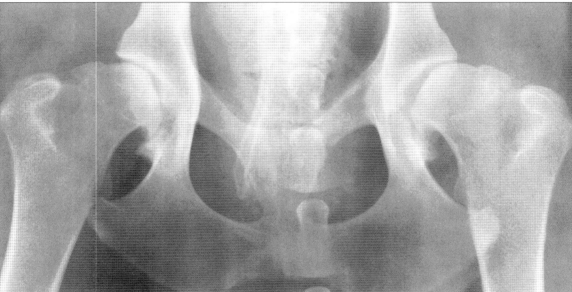

**Figure 5-77**
Pelvic radiographs of a male Shepherd, (A) at 2 years of age show joint laxity indicative of dysplasia, (B) at 5 years of age show the secondary osteoarthrosis to have become severe and the dog was painful and lame, (C) postoperatively show the total hip replacement shortly after it was performed, and (D) later after the dog was allowed unrestricted excercise show the stem to have broken free from the head. The radiopaque material around the prothesis is the polymethylmethacrylate cement (arrows).

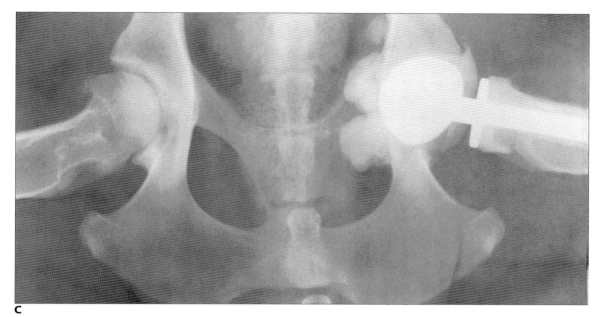

C

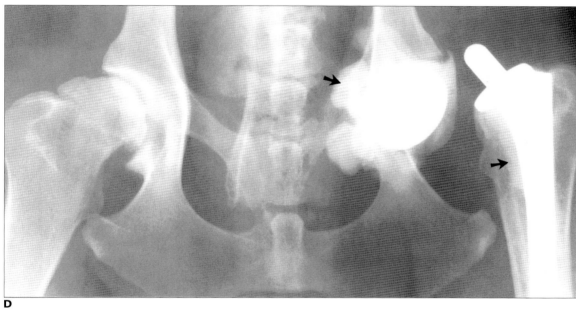

D

**Table 5-19: Factors influencing prognosis following surgical treatment of hip dysplasia**

I. Tension relieving procedures
    A. Good prognosis in relieving pain
    B. No effect on joint stability and progression of osteoarthrosis

II. Triple pelvic osteotomy
    A. Good prognosis if only 20° to 30° rotation required
        1. Increases stability of joint
        2. Delays progression of osteoarthrosis
        3. Limits ultimate severity of osteoarthrosis
        4. Good pain relief
    B. Poor prognosis if greater than 30° rotation required
        1. Limits abduction
        2. Produces awkward gait
        3. Pain relief more guarded
        4. Degree of joint congruity is limited
        5. Progressive osteoarthrosis more likely to be severe

III. Femoral head and neck excision
    A. Good prognosis
        1. < 20kg body weight
        2. Eager, athletic dog
        3. Mild to moderate muscle atrophy and fibrosis
        4. Proper physiotherapy
    B. Poor prognosis
        1. Body weight
            a. > 20 kg (not advised)
            b. Overweight for breed
            c. Large breed
        2. Low pain tolerance
        3. Extensive muscle atrophy and fibrosis
        4. Physiotherapy lacking

IV. Total hip replacement - good prognosis

---

clinicians be able to advise clients in the selection of dogs for breeding. As an inherited disease, hip dysplasia is transmitted to offspring by genetic factors. Therefore, if a dog does not have the genes for dysplasia it cannot have dysplasia and cannot transmit the disease to its offspring. On the other hand, if a dog has all or some of the genes for dysplasia: (1) the disease may not express itself and the dog is phenotypically normal or (2) the dog displays varying degrees of dysplasia. The growth rate, muscle mass, and exercise level are only some of the factors that influence how the dysplasia is manifested in a given dog. Thus, the level of disease expressed is partially dependent on the number or type of genes present and partially on environmental components (Lust and Farrell 1977).

It is of interest to search the early literature for suggestions of what were the thoughts at that time concerning heritability of dysplasia in dogs. Konde (1947) suggested that "the breeding of two so affected dogs will accentuate the fault in the offspring." Huffman (1955) showed the condition to have existed in five generations of German Shepherd Dogs and stated that it "does definitely indicate that the subluxation is a hereditary trait with the male playing a dominant part in the transmission of the offspring of this condition." These are probably only a few of the many reports in the world veterinary literature at that time.

CHD was reported between 1955 to 1959 to be a disease with statistically significant evidence of an hereditary nature and recommendation were made that selection can be made against the trait (Grounds, et al 1955; Schales 1956, 1957; Berg 1957; McClave 1957; Henricson and Olsson 1959; Snavely 1959; Carlson 1961; Brooymans-Schallenberg 1983). The disease was considered a quantitatively inherited trait (ie, it is influenced by many different genes). Early studies reporting the hereditary aspects of hip dysplasia suggested that the mode of inheritance was in accordance with that of an autosomal dominant trait caused by a gene with incomplete penetrance (about 60%) and of varying expressivity (Olsson 1962 a; Börnfors, et al 1964; Henricson, et al 1965; Henricson, et al 1966). The terms "quantitative," "additive," and "multifactorial" were used to describe the pattern of inheritance and like "polygenic," they referred to the fact that the trait was controlled by more than one gene. The breeder should understand that the genetic influence is sufficiently strong that with selected breeding, the frequency of the disease can be significantly altered. Among the polygenic traits for hip dysplasia are genetic traits for rate of growth and body weight. In addition, these are both influenced by environmental factors. This was determined to be true if the dog is phenotypically sound and is only genetically dysplastic or if the dog is a cripple from the affects of the dysplasia (Kealy, et al 1997).

Heritability is defined as the ratio between the additive genetic variance and the total phenotypic variance (genetic variance plus environmental variance). The genetic component is measured by the heritability estimate (HE) which can be defined as "the variation in the observable or measurable properties of a disease (the phenotype) which are directly transmitted to the offspring by the genes." As such, heritability can vary between different populations of dogs depending on the amount of inbreeding and differences in environmental factors. Estimates of inheritance for CHD vary according to different workers, with the higher heritability estimate indicating the greater is the control over the disease by transmissible genetic effects.

If the heritability estimate is 0.0 (0.0%) that means that the trait has no genetic component while an estimate of 1.0 (100%) means that the expression of the trait is totally genetic. It is possible to incorrectly interpret an estimate of 0.3, for example, to mean that 30% of the dogs have dysplasia of an inherited type and 70% of the dogs have dysplasia due to environmental factors. Instead, an estimate of 0.3 indicates that 30% of the observed changes are due to genetic factors and 70% of the changes are due to environmental factors. Thus, the heritability estimate measures how much of the phenotypic variation in a population is of a genetic origin.

The importance in the level of the heritability estimate is that if the estimate is 0.2 or above, it is generally accepted that the frequency of the trait can be controlled using genetic principles in breeding. All studies of hip dysplasia suggest that genetic selection should be effective against the disease (Padgett, et al 1990; Swenson, et al 1997). The estimates of heritability have ranged from a low of 0.2 to 0.3 (Henricson, et al 1972; Leighton, et al 1977; Leighton, et al 1994) to 0.4 to 0.5 based on radiographic evaluation of the hip joints of 2,404 dogs (Hedhammer, et al 1979). A recent report "found an heredity of 0.6 for HD in the Labrador Retriever breed after the evaluation of 17,000 radiographs" (Audell 1992). Interestingly, the pattern of inheritance of hip dysplasia appeared to be the same in the rarely affected Afghan Hounds as that reported in other breeds (Ackerman 1982). Regardless of the level of estimate of heritability, all of these values clearly place hip dysplasia as a disease in which frequency can be influenced by selective breeding.

Considerable variation exists between breeds studied for the frequency of dysplasia. The difference in the percentage of dogs affected by the various grades assigned from radiographic examination is in good agreement with the expected results from polygenic inheritance. It can be expected that dogs will have different degrees of severity of the problem, distributed according to a normal curve (Swenson 1987). This variation is more easily seen in examination of data from the UK, where the mean of scores assigned following radiographic evaluation ranges in the different breeds from 2.9 to 45.2. The German Shepherd Dog has a range of scores of 0 to 106 with a mean score of 18.64; the Golden Retriever has a range of scores of 0 to 106 with a mean score of 19.60; the Pyrenean Mountain Dog has a range of scores of 0 to 94 with a mean score of 12.58; and the Labrador Retriever has a range of scores of 0 to 104 with a mean score of 16.20 (Willis 1997 b).

There is a possibility that the bitch might exert a greater influence than the male on the incidence of dysplasia in the offspring. The early environment, uterine or pre-weaning, might have a negative influence on the development of the dysplasia (Swenson 1987). This maternal effect was shown in studies of the German Shepherd Dog in which normal males were bred with dysplastic females with a resulting 43% affected progeny. When dysplastic males were breed with normal females, the progeny was 33% affected (Swenson 1989; Swenson, et al 1997). Others feel that the scores of dams tend to be more or less random and close to the breed mean score and are not reliable in predicting (Willis 1997 a).

The above suggests that it is not advisable to use a dog for breeding with discernible hip dysplasia, whether detected by palpation, radiography, or a distraction technique. However, phenotype is not always the most accurate reflection of the genotype. A dog with mild hip dysplasia noted radiographically, but coming from a relatively dysplasia-free genetic family background, can be more properly selected for breeding instead of a phenotypically dysplasia-free dog which comes from a family background with a high incidence of dysplasia. Thus, for any advise concerning the selection of a dog for breeding to be accurate, it must be based on a knowledge of the status of the hips of full-siblings, half-siblings, and progeny. This concept has been tested in an attempt to improve dogs available for training as guides for blind people through the use of an estimated breeding value based on paternal half-siblings, maternal half-siblings, and offspring, and has lowered the number of dysplastic German Shepherd Dogs from 55% to 24% and the number of dysplastic Labrador Retrievers from 30% to 10% in less than five generations of selection (Leighton, et al 1994; Leighton 1997). Even using just the status of the individual dog, there are examples of a decrease in frequency of HD in smaller populations. One is in Israel where the frequency of positive German Shepherd Dogs decreased from 75.5% in 1971 to 34% in 1994 and the frequency of positive Boxer in which the breeding policy was less demanding decreased from near 80% in 1970s to around 50% in 1990's (Mazriar, et al 1998).

If the degree of heritability is high enough, why is there no change in the prevalence of HD noted over the past three decades in the US or other countries (Flückiger, et al 1995)? Some of the reasons offered are that the dog breeders in the US are a constantly changing group and require periodic re-education as to the problem of HD and its transmission. This re-education apparently has not occurred. Another possibility is that breeders are persisting in the use of known dysplastic dogs. Finally, little inducement exists in the United States to control the disease such as a restriction to the registering of puppies from breeding of dysplastic dogs (Feldman 1974). This failure to control the disease can be also due to the disappointment and frustration on the part of the breeder that follows the breeding of phenotypically normal sire and dam and discovering that a percentage of the puppies are dysplastic. This problem has been well known. To further understand the frustration associated with selection of breeding stock, it is helpful to know that when breeding German Shepherd Dogs that are radiographically normal 28% of the offspring are expected to be dysplastic, while breeding dogs with minimal dysplasia is expected to produce 44% dysplastic offspring. A similar pattern is noted with Labradors. When breeding dogs that are radiographically normal, regardless of breed, 17% of the offspring are expected to be dysplastic, while breeding dogs with minimal dysplasia is expected to produce 29% dysplastic offspring (Swenson 1987, 1989). The frequency of dysplasia in offspring from breeding affected sire and dam is almost the same as the frequency of dysplasia in offspring from breeding sire and dam that are of an unknown status.

To reduce the frequency of hip dysplasia, it is necessary to know the background of any potential breeding stock to make decisions that would lower the frequency of dysplasia in the offspring. This knowledge includes the status of the parents, littermates, and previous offspring (Swenson 1987; Swenson, et al 1997). The authors feel that this information has not been sufficiently broadcast to owners and breeders alike in the US. In summary, the diagnosis of hip dysplasia should not only be based on phenotype of an individual dog but also on the phenotype of littermates, half-siblings, and progeny in order to gain knowledge of genotype of the potential breeding animal.

Considering this apparent failure to attach importance to the heritability of the disease, it is interesting that the dog fanciers continue to pursue diagnosis of this disease radiographically.

# References

ACKERMAN N. Hip dysplasia in the Afghan Hound. Vet Rad 23:88-97,1982.

ACKERMAN N, NYLAND T. Radiographic diagnosis of canine hip dysplasia. Cal Vet 31:9-15,1977.

ALBRECHT G, ARNOLD P. Standing radiography of the hip joint. Mh Vet Med 27:542-545,1972.

ARNOCZKY SP, TORZILLI PA. Biomechanical analysis of forces acting about the canine hip. Am J Vet Res 42:1581-1585,1981.

ARONSON E, KRAUS KH, SMITH J. The effect of anesthesia on the radiographic appearance of the coxofemoral joints. Vet Rad 32:2-5,1991.

AUDELL L, GUSTAFSSON P-O. The acetabular bone in caine hip dysplasia. A radiographic study. JAM Vet Rad SOC 1:6-10,1973

AUDELL L. Personal communication,1972.

AUDELL L. Personal communication,1973.

AUDELL L. Personal correspondence,1992.

BADERTSCHER II RR. "The half-axial position: Improved radiographic visualization of subluxation in canine hip dysplasia," Thesis, University of Georgia College of Veterinary Medicine 1977.

BAILEY CS, MORGAN JP. Diseases of the spinal cord. In: Textbook of Veterinary Internal Medicine: Diseases of the Dog and Cat. 2nd ed. Ed SJ Ettinger, W B Saunders Philadelphia PA 1983, pp532-607.

BALLINARI U, MONTAVON PM, HUBER E, WEISS R. Die Pectineusmyektomie, Iliopsoastenotomie und Neurektomie der Gelenkkapsel (PIN) als symptomatische Therapie bei der Coxarthrose des Hundes. Schweiz Arch Tierheilk 137:251-257,1995.

BANFIELD CM, BARTELS JE, HUDSON JA, WRIGHT JC, HATHCOCK JT, MONTGOMERY RD. A retrospective study of canine h ip dysplasia in 116 military working dogs. Part I Angle measurement and Orthopedic Foundation for Animal (OFA) grading. JAAHA 32:413-422,1996a.

BANFIELD CM, BARTELS JE, HUDSON JA, WRIGHT JC, MONTGOMERY RD, HATHCOCK JT. A retrospective study of canine hip dysplasia in 116 military working dogs. Part II Clinical signs and performance data. JAAHA 32:423-430,1996b.

BARDENS JW. Palpation for the detection of joint laxity. Proc Canine Hip Dysplasia Symposium St. Louis, MO 205-109,1972a.

BARDENS JW. Palpation for the detection of dysplasia and wedge technique for pelvic radiolgraphy. Proc 39th Annual AAHA Meeting 468-471,1972b.

BARDENS JW, HARDWICK H. New observations on the diagnosis and cause of hip dysplasia. VM/SAC 63:238-245,1968.

BARLOW TG. Early diagnosis and treatment of congenital dislocation of the hip. J Bone Jt Surg 44B:292-301,1962.

BARR ARS, DENNY HR, GIBBS C. Clinical hip dysplasia in growing dogs: The long-term results of conservative management. J small Anim Pract 28:,243-252,1987.

BELLKOFF SM, PADGETT G, SOUTAS-LITTLE RW. Development of a device to measure canine coxofemoral joint laxity. VCOT 1:31-36,1989.

BERG E. Die angeborene Hüftgelenksdysplasie beim Hund. Deutsche tierärztl Wchnschr 64:509,1957.

BERZON JL, HOWARD PE, COVELL SJ, et al. A retrospective study of the efficacy of femoral head and neck excisions in 94 dogs and cats. J Vet Surg 9:88-92,1980.

BIGGERT JF. Prosthetic joints. Vet Clin N Am 8:538-550,1978.

BONNEAU NH, BRETTON L. Excision arthroplasty of the femoral head. Canine Pract 8(2):13-25,1981

BOOTH NH. Nonnarcotic analgesics. In. Veterinary Pharmacology and Therapeutics 4th ed Ed. LM Jones NH Booth LE McDonald IowaState University Press Ames 1977. P351.

BOULAY JP. Effect of cimetidine on aspirin-indiced gastric hemorrhage in dogs. AJVR 47:1744-1746.1986.

BOWEN JM, LEWIS RE, KNELLER SK, WILSON RC, ARNOLD RA. Progression of hip dysplasia in German Shepherd Dogs after unilateral pectineal myotomy. JAVMA 161:899-904,1972.

BRADEN TD, PRIEUR WD, KANEENE JB. Clinical evaluation of intertrochanteric osteotomy for treatment of dogs with early-stage hip dysplasia: 37 cases (1980-1987). JAVMA 196:337-341,1990.

BRASS W, FREUDIGER U, MÜLER LF, PAATSAMA S, VAN DER VELDON NA, VAN DE WATERING CC. Bericht der Hüftgelenksdysplasie-Kommission. Kleintierpraxis 23:169-180,1978.

BRASS W. Hüftgelenksdysplasie und ellbogenerkrankung im Visier der Fédération Cynologique Internationale.1. Kleintierpraxis 38,194,1993.

BRASS W, PAATSAMA S. Hüftgelenkdyspasie - Internationales Zertifikat und Beurteilung von Röntgenaufnahmen - FCI, Helsinke 1983.

BRINKER WO, FLO G, CROSS JF. Acetabuloplasty as a corrective surgical procedure in selected cases on congenital hip dysplasia in the dog. Sci Proc 35th Ann Meet AAHA 260-262,1968.

BRINKER WO. Corrective osteotomy procedures for treatment of canine hip dysplasia. Vet Clin North Am 1:467-477,1971.

BROOYMANS-SCHALLENBERG JHC. Diagnosis of canine hip dysplasia and selection against the trait. Vet Quart 5:8-10,1983.

BROWN G, Personal communication,1996.

BROWN G. Personal communication,1997.

BÖRNFORS S, PÅLSSON K, SKUDE G. Hereditary aspects of hip dysplasia in German Shepherd Dogs. JAVMA 145:15-20,1964.

CARDINET III GH, GUFFY MM, WALLACE LJ. Canine hip dysplasia: effects of pectineal tenotomy on the coxofemoral joints of German Shepherd Dogs. JAVMAS 164:591-598,1974.

CARDINET III GH, GUFFY MM, WALLACE LJ. Canine hip dysplasia: effects of pectineal myectomy on the coxofemoral joints of Greyhound and German Shepherd Dogs. JAVMA 165:529-532,1974.

CARDINET III GH, GUFFY MM, WALLACE LJ, LABEN RC. Canine hip dysplasia in German Shepherd Dog-Greyhound crossbreeds. JAVMA 182: 393-395,1983.

CARDINET III GH, KASS PH, WALLACE LJ, GUFFY MM. Association between pelvic muscle mass and canine hip dysplasia. JAVMA 210:1466-1473, 1997.

CARLSON WD. Veterinary Radiology 1st ed, Lea & Febiger Philadelphia 1961, p330.

CARLSON WD. Veterinary Radiology 2nd ed, Lea & Febiger Philadelphia 1967, p429.

CHARLMAN JA, BUTLER HC. Coxofemoral joint laxity and the Ortolani sign. JAAHA 21:671-676,1985.

CHRISTOPH HJ, ARNOLD P, WENZEL DU, ALBRECHT G. Hip joint examination of Dingos (Canis dingo), Arctic foxes (Alopex lagopus), and foxes (Vulpes vulpes). Monatsh Veterinaermec 24:784-786,1969.

CORLEY EA. Radiographic evaluation of the canine coxo-femoral joints. Proc Am Anim Hosp Assoc Annual Meeting: 276-281,1968.

CORLEY EA. Hip dysplasia; a monograph for dog breeders and owners. OFA, Columbia Mo 1983.

CORLEY EA. Hip dysplasia; a report from the orthopedic foundation for animals. Seminars in Vet Med and Surg (SA)2:141-151,1987.

CORLEY EA. Role of the Orthopedic Foundation for Animals in the control of canine hip dysplasia. Vet Clin of NA (SAP). 22:579-593,1992.

CORLEY EA, HOGAN PM. Trends in hip dysplasia control: analysis of radiographs submitted to the orthopedic foundation for animals, 1974 to 1984. JAVMA 187:805-809,1985.

CORLEY EA, KELLER GG, LATTIMER JC, ELLERSIECK MR. Reliability of early radiographic evaluations for canine hip dysplasia obtained from the standard ventrodorsal radiographic projection. JAVMA 211:1142-1146,1997.

CRAWFORD RD, PHARR JW. Recommendations on canine hip dysplasia - diagnosis, treatment and genetic selection. Can Vet J 16:308-309,1975.

DAEHLER MH. Transmural pyloric perforation associated with naproxen administration in the dog. JAVMA 189:694-695,1986.

DEHAAN JJ, et al. Evaluation of polysuflated glycosaminoglycan for the treatment of hip dysplasia in dogs. Vet Surg 23:177-181,1994.

DUELAND R. Total hip arthroplasty. in Current Techniques in Small Animal Surgery, M.J.Bojrab editor, Lea & Febiger Philadelphia 1975, pp 448-450.

DUELAND DJ. Femoral torsion and its possible relationship to canine hip dysplasia (abstr). Vet Surg 9:48,1980.

DUFF R, CAMPBELL JR, Long-term results of excision arthroplasty of the canine hip. Vet Rec 101:181-184,1977.

EDWARDS MR, EGGER RL, SCHWARZ PD. Aseptic loosening of the femoral implant after cemented total hip arthroplasty in dogs: 11 cases in 10 dogs (1991-1995). JAVMA 211:580-586,1997.

FARROW CS, BACK RT. Radiographic evaluation of nonanesthetized and nonsedated dogs for hip dysplasia. JAVMA 194:524-526,1989.

FELDMANN BM. Letter to the editor. JAVMA 165:876-877,1974.

FERNBACH SK, POZNANSKI AK, KELIKIAN AS, TACHJDIAN MO, MARZANO MJ. Greater trochanteric overgrowth: development and surgical correction. Radiol 154:661-664,1985.

FLÜCKIGER M. The standardized analysis of radiographs for hip dysplasia in dogs. Objectifying a subjective process. Kleintierpraxis 38:693-702,1993.

FLÜCKIGER M, LANG J, BINDER H, BUSATO A, BOOS J. Die Bekämpfung der Hüftgelenksdysplasie in der Schweiz. Ein Rückblick auf die vergangenen 24 Jahre. Schweiz Arch für Tierheilk 137; 243-250,1995.

FLÜCKIGER M. Personal communication,1997.

FORSYTH HF, PASCHALL HA. A study of congenital hip dysplasia in dogs. J B & Jt Surg 45A:1781-1782,1963.

FOX SM, JOHNSON SA. Use of carprofen for the treatment of pain and inflammation in dogs. JAVMA 210: 1493-1498,1997.

FREEMAN A. The dysplasia dilemma. JAVMA 142:643-645,1963.

FREUDIGER U. Vor Röntgen zur Beurteilung der Hüftgelenks-Dysplasie. Schweizer Arch Tierheilk 115:507-515,1973.

FREUDIGER U, SCHÄRER U, BUSER J-C, MÜHLEBACH R. Die Resultate der Hüftgelenksdysplasie-Bekämpfung beim D. Schäferhund in der Zeit von 1965 bis 1972. Schweiz Arch Tierheilkd 115:169-173,1973.

FROST HM. Pathogenesis of congenital hip dysplasia (CDH). A proposal. VCOT1:1-10,1989.

FRY TR, CLARK DM. Canine hip dysplasia: Clinical signs and physical diagnosis. Vet Clin NA Sm Anim Pract. 22:551-558,1992.

GENDREAU C, CAWLEY AJ. Excision of the femoral head and neck: The long term results of 35 operations. JAAHA 13:605-608,1977

GIARDINA JF, MACCARTHY AW Jr. Evaluation of a technique for early determination of predysplastic dogs: Hip palpation. Vet Med/SA Clin 66:878-882,1971.

GODDARD ME, MASON TA. The genetics and early prediction of hip dysplasia. Aust Vet J 58:1-4, 1982.

GOLDMAN M. Skeletal mineralization in The Beagle ed by A.C.Andersen, ISU Press Ames Iowa p.216-225,1970.

GROUNDS OV, HAGEROORN Al, HOFFMAN RA. Hereditary subluxation. J. Canine Genetics January 1955.

GUSTAFSSON P.-O. Hip dysplasia in the Greyhound. A study of estrdiol induced skeletal changes. J Am Vet Radiol Soc 9:47-56,1968.

GUSTAFSSON P.-O, KASSTRÖM H, OLSSON S-E, SUZUKI K. Growth and remodeling of the hip joint and proximal femur in adolescent dogs - An investigatin with special reference to hip dysplasia and estradiol induced changes. Acta Rad Suppl 319:3-5,1972.

HANNAN H, GHOSH P, BELLENGER C, TAYLOR T. Systemic administration of glycosaminoglycan polysulfate (Artepron) provides partial protection of articular cartilage from damage produced by meniscectomy in the canine. J Orthop Res 5:47-59,1987.

HASSINGER KA, SMITH GK, CONZEMIUS MG, SAUNDERS HM, HILL CM, GREGOR TD. Effect of the oestrus cycle on coxofemoral joint laxity. VCOT 10:69-74,1997.

HAUPTMAN J, PRIEUR WD, BUTLER HC. The angle of inclination of the canine femoral head and neck. Vet Surg 8:74-77,1979.

HAUPTMAN J, CARDINET III GH, MORGAN JP, GUFFY MM, WALLACE LJ. Angles of inclination and anteversion in hip dysplasia in the dog. AJVR 46:2033-2036,1985.

HEDHAMMER Å, WU F, KROOK L, SCHRYVER HF, DELAHAUNTA A, WHALEN JP, KALLFELZ FA, NUNEZ EA, HINTZ HF, SHEFFY BE, RYAN GD. Overnutrition and skeletal disease. An experimental study in growing Great Dane Dogs. Cornell Vet 64 (Suppl 5) 1974.

HEDHAMMER Å, OLSSON S-E, ANDERSSON S-Å, PERSSON L, PETTERSSON L, OLAUSSON A, SUNDGREN P-E. Canine hip dysplasia: Study of heritability in 401 litters of German Shepherd Dogs. JAVMA 174: 1012-1016,1979.

HENRICSON B, OLSSON S-E. Hereditary acetabular dysplasia in German Shepherd Dogs. JAVMA 135:207-210,1959.

HENRICSON B, NORBERG I, OLSSON S-E. Hüftgelenksdysplasie eim Hund. Nord Vet-Med 17: 118-131,1965.

HENRICSON B, NORBERG I, OLSSON S-E. On the etiology and pathogenesis of hip dysplasia: a comparative review. J small Anim Pract 7:673-688,1966.

HENRICSON B, LJUNGGREN G, OLSSON S-E. Canine hip dysplasia in Sweden: Incidence and genetics. Acta Rad Suppl 319, 175-180,1972.

HENRY GA. Radiographic development of canine hip dysplasia. Vet Clin NA Small Anim Pract 22:559-578,1992.

HENRY JD Jr, PARK RD. Wedge technique for demonstration of coxofemoral joint laxity in the canine. Proc Canine Hip Dysplasia Symposium St. Louis, MO 117-126,1972.

HENRY WB, Wadsworth PL. Pelvic osteotomy in the treatment of canine hip dysplasia. JAAHA 11:636-643,1975.

HEYMAN SJ, SMITH GK, COFONE MA. A biomechanical study of the effect of coxofemoral positioning on passive hip joint laxity in dogs. AJVR 54:210-215, 1993.

HOHN RB, JANES JM. Pelvic osteotomy in the treatment of canine hip dysplasia. Clin Orthop 62:70-78,1969.

HUFFMAN C. Congenital dislocation of the coxofemoral articulation in the dog. Rocky Mt Vet. 20-27,1955.

HUTT FB. Genetic selection to reduce the incidence of hip dysplasia in dogs. JAVMA 151:1041-1048,1967.

IHEMELANDU EC, CARDINET III GH, GUFFY MM, WALLACE LJ. Canine hip dysplasia: Differences in pectineal muscles of healthy and dysplastic German Shepherd Dogs when two months old. AJVR 44:411-416,1983.

JENNY J. Resection of the femoral head in developmental hip disorders in dogs. Proceedings Meeting of the AVMA pp170-171,1963.

JESSEN CR. Hereditary aspects of canine hip dysplasia in the German Shepherd and Viszla breeds. Ph.D. Thesis. University of Minnesota, Minneapolis,1969.

JESSEN CR. Age of animal at definitive diagnosis of canine hip dysplasia. Veterinary Medicine Reporter, University of Minnesota Institute of Agriculture, College of Veterinary Medicine, 25:1, January 1970.

JESSEN CR, SPURRELL FA. Radiographic detection of canine hip dysplasia in known age groups. Proc Canine Hip Dysplasia Symposium St. Louis, MO 93-100, 1972 a.

JESSEN CR, SPURRELL FA. Heritability of canine hip dysplasia. Proc Canine Hip Dysplasia Symposium. St. Louis, MO 53-61,1972.

JOHNSON SA. Conservative and medical management of hip dysplasia. Vet Clin North Am Sm Aninm Pract 22:595-606,1992.

KASSTRÖM H. Nutrition, weight gain and development of hip dysplasia. An experimental investigation in growing dogs with special reference to the effect of feeding intensity. Acta Radiol (Suppl) 344:135-179,1975.

KEALY RD, OLSSON S-E, MONTI KL, LAWLER DF, Biery DN, HELMS RW, LUST G, SMITH GK. Effects of limited food consumption on the incidence of hip dysplasia in growing dogs. JAVMA 201:857-863,1992.

KEALY RD, LAWLER DF, BALLAM JM, LUST G, SMITH GK, BIERY DN, OLSSON S-E. Five-year longitudinal study on limited food consumption and development of osteoarthritis in coxofemoral joints of dogs. JAVMA 210,222-225,1997.

KELLER GG, CORLEY EA. The effect of anesthesia on coxofemoral joint subluxation. Personnal communication.1990.

KELLER GG, BOUCHARD G, FAGIN B, LATTIMER JC, ELLERSIECK MR. Influence of the estrous cycle on coxofemoral joint subluxation. Canine Practice 18: Jan/Feb 19-22,1993.

KLIMT U, TELLHELM B, FRITSCH R. Die Bedeutung der "Morgan-Linie" für dei Untersuchung auf HD beim Hund. Kleintierpraxis 37:211-217,1992.

KONDE WN. Congenital subluxation of the coxofemoral joint in the German Shepherd Dog. N.A. Vet 28:595-599,1947.

KONDE LJ, OLMSTEAD ML, HOHN RB. Radiographic evaluation of total hip replacement in the dog. Vet Rad 23:98-106,1982.

KÖPPEL E. Pelvic proportions in some breeds of dog in radiographs, a contribution to hip dysplasia. Wiener Tierärzt Monat 70:360-369.1983.

LAFOND E, SMITH GK, GREGOR TP, MCKELVIE PJ, SHOFER FS. Synovial fluid cavitation during distraction radiography of the coxofemoral joint in dogs. JAVMA 210:1294-1297,1997.

LARSEN JS, CORLEY EA. Radiographic evaluations in a canine hip dysplasia control program. JAVMA 159:989-992,1971.

LARSEN JS, CORLEY EA. Prevalence of hip dysplasia according to radiographic evaluation amoung 36 breeds of dogs. Proc Canine Hip Dysplasia Symposium. St. Louis MO 101-104,1972.

LAWSON DD. The radiographic diagnosis of hip dysplasia in the dog. Vet Rec 75: 445-456,1963.

LAWSON DD. Hip dysplasia in the dog Vet Rec 83:655 -656,1968.

LEIGHTON EA, LINN JM, WILLHAM RL, CASTLEBERRY MW. A genetic study of canine hip dysplasia. Am J Vet Res 38: 241-244,1977.

LEIGHTON EA, MCNEIL M, BIERY DN, PATTERSON DF. Results from four generations of selection to reduce the incidence of canine hip dysplasia in both German Shepherd Dogs and Labrador Retrievers at The Seeing Eye, Inc. presented at the meeting of the Int Vet Rad Assoc, Philadelphia, Aug 1-6, 1994.

LEIGHTON EA. Genetics of canine hip dysplasia. JAVMA 210:1474-1479,1997.

LEWIS RH, JONES Jr JP. A clinical study of canine total hip arthroplasty. ACVS 9:20-23,1980

LJUNGGREN G. Legg-Perthes disease in the dog. Acta Orthop Scand, Supple 95,1967.

LUST G, BEILMAN WT, RENDANO VT. A relationship between degree of laxity and synovial fluid volume in coxofemoral joints of dogs predisposed for hip dysplasia. Am J Vet Res 41:55-60,1980.

LUST G, FARRELL PW. Hip dysplasia in dogs: The interplay of genotype and environment. Cornell Vet 67:447-466;1977.

LUST G, CRAIG PH, ROSS Jr GE, GEARY JC. Studies on pectineus muscles in canine hip dysplasia. Cornell Vet 62:628-645,1972a.

LUST G, CRAIG PH, GEARY JC, ROSS Jr GE. Changes in pelvic muscle tissues associated with hip dysplasia in dogs. Am J Vet Res 33:1097-1108,1972b.

LUST G, GEARY JC, SHEFFY BE. Development of hip dysplasia in dogs. Am J Vet Res 34: 87-91,1973.

LUST G, SUMMERS BA. Early, asymptomatic stage of degenerative joint disease in canine hip joints. Am J Vet Res 42:1849-1855 1981.

LUST G, RENDANO VT, SUMMERS BA. Canine hip dysplasia: Concepts and diagnosis. JAVMA 187:638-640,1985.

LUST G, WILLIAMS AJ, BURTON-WURSTER N, PIJANOWSKI GJ, BECK KA, RUBIN G, SMITH GK. Joint laxity and its association with hip dysplasia in Labrador Retrievers. Am J Vet Res 54:1990-1999,1993.

LUST G, WILLIAMS AJ, BURTON-WURSTER N, BECK KA, RUBIN G. Effects of intramuscular administration of glycosaminoglycan polysulfates on signs of incipient hip dysplasia in growing pups. Am J Vet Res 53:1836-1843,1992.

MADSEN JS, REIMANN I, SVALASTOGA E. Delayed ossification of the femoral head in dogs with hip dysplasia. J Sm Anim Pract 32:351-354,1991.

MADSEN JS, SVALASTOGA E. Effects of anaesthesia and stress on the radiographic evaluation of the coxofemoral joint. J Sm Anim Pract 32:64-68,1991.

MASSAT BJ, VASSEUR PB. Clinical and radiographic results of total hip arthroplasty in dogs: 96 cases (1986-1992). JAVMA 205:448-454,1994.

MATHEWS DG, STOVER SM, KASS PH. Effect of pubic symphysiodesis on acetabular rotation and pelvic development in guinea pigs. Am J Vet Res 57:1427-1433, 1996.

MAZRIAR C, BARGAI U, WANER T. Hip dysplasia of dogs in Israel: Current status and assessment of the efficacy of 25 years of the control scheme. Israel J of Vet Med 53:69-72,1998.

MCCLAVE PL. Elimination of coxofemoral dysplasia from a breeding kennel. Vet Med 52:241-243,1957.

MICHELE AA. The iliopsoas muscle. Its importance in disorders of the hip and spine. Clinical symposia. 1962 pp67-101.

MONTGOMERY RD, MILTON JL, PERNELL R, ABERMAN HM. Total hip arthroplasty for tretment of canine hip dysplasia. VCNA 22:703-719,1992.

MORGAN JP. Congenital abnormalities of the vertebral column of the dog. J Am Vet Rad Soc 9:21-29,1968.

MORGAN JP. Radiographic diagnosis of hip dysplasia in skeletally mature dogs. Proc Canine Hip Dysplasia Symposium St. Louis, MO 78-92,1972.

MORGAN JP. Hip dysplasia in the beagle: a radiographic study. JAVMA 164:496-498,1974.

MORGAN JP. Canine hip dysplasia - Asymmetry of change. Cal Vet March/April 17-20,1986.

MORGAN JP. Canine hip dysplasia - Significance of early bony spurring. Vet Rad 28:2-5,1987.

MORGAN JP. Transitional lumbosacral vertebral segments in the dog: A radiographic study. J small Animal Pract 1999 In press.

MORGAN JP, ROSENBLATT L. Canine hip dysplasia. The pelvic inlet parameter in diagnosis. Cal Vet Can/June 15-18,1986.

MORGAN JP, ROSENBLATT L. Canine hip dysplasia. Significance of pelvic and sacral attachment. Cal Vet Jan/Feb 12-16,1987.

MORGAN JP, BAILEY CS. Cauda Equina syndrome in the dog: Radiographic evaluation. J sm Anim Pract 31:69-77,1990.

MORGAN JP, STEPHENS AM. Radiographic diagnosis and control of canine hip dysplasia. ISU Press Ames 1985.

MORGAN SJ. The pathology of canine hip dysplasia. Vet Clin North Amer/ SAC 22:541-550,1992.

MORGAN SJ. Pathologic alterations in canine hip dysplasia. JAVMA 210:1446-1450,1997.

MÅNSSON J, NORBERG I. Höftledsdysplasi hos hund. Medlemsbl för Sv Vetförb 12:330-339,1961.

MÜLLER LF, SAAR C. Eine Anleitung zur Röntgen-Diagnose der Hüftgelenksdysplasie. Keintierpraxis 11:33-42,1966.

NORBERG I. Höftledsdysplasi hos hund. Hundsport 69: 13-15,1961.

NORBERG I. Höftledsdysplasi hos hund. Hundsport 70: 16,1962.

NORBERG I. Höftledsdysplasi hos hund. Nord Med 69:246,1963.

NUNAMAKER DM. Surgical correction of large femoral anteversion angles in the dog. JAVMA 165:1061-1064.1974.

NUNAMAKER DM, BIERY DN, NEWTON CD. Femoral neck anteversion in the dog: Its radiographic measurement. JAVRS 14:45-48.1973.

NUNAMAKER DM, NEWTON CD. Canine hip disorders, in Bojrab MJ (ed): Current Techniques in Small Animal Surgery. Philadelphia, Lea & Febiger, 1975, pp 436-442.

OAKES MG, LEWIS DD, ELKINS AD, HOSGOOD G, DIAL SM, OLIVER J. Evaluation of shelf arthroplasty as a treatment for hip dysplasia in dogs. JAVMA 208:1838-1845,1996.

OLMSTEAD ML. Total hip replacement in the dog. Semin Vet Med Surg (Small Anim) 2:131-140,1987.

OLMSTEAD ML. Canine cemented total hip replacements: State of the art. J sm Anim Pract. 36:395-399,1995.

OLMSTEAD ML, HOHN RB. Ergebnisse mit der Hüfttotalprothese bei 103 klinischen Fällen an der Ohio State University. Klin Prax 25:407-415,1980.

OLMSTEAD ML, HOHN RB, TURNER TM. Technique for canine total hip replacement. Vet Surg 10:44-50,1981.

OLMSTEAD ML, HOHN RB, TURNER TM. A five-year study of 221 total hip replacements in the dog. JAVMA 183:191-194,1983.

OLSON RC. Physical evaluation and selection of military dogs. JAVMA 159: 1444-1446,1971.

OLSSON S-E. Missbildad höftled — ett problem i schäferrasen. Hundsport 65:8,1957.

OLSSON S-E. Acetabulumdysplasi och Legg-Perthes' sjukdom, två aktuella höftledssjukdomar hos hund. VIII Nord. veterinärmötet 1958. Sektion F, rapport 10,1958.

OLSSON S-E. The control of canine hip dysplasia in the scandinavian countries. Adv in Sm Anim Pract 3:112-116,1962a.

OLSSON S-E. Roentgen examination of the hip joints of German Shepherd dogs. Adv Small Anim Pract 3:117-120,1962b.

OLSSON S-E. Höftledsdysplasia på tillbakagång. Hundsport 71:16-19,1963.

OLSSON S-E. Höftledsdysplasi hos hund. Svensk Veterinärtidning 23:1-10,1968.

OLSSON S-E. What to do about hip dysplasia. Pure-bred Dogs American Kennel Gazette 91:44-46,1974.

OLSSON S-E, AUDELL L. Development and of the canine acetabular rim. A study with special reference to hip dysplasia and the radiographic appoearance of a separate "ossicle" at the acetabular rim. Symposium on Osteoarthrosis and Canine Hip Dysplasia. Helsinki July 29-30 978.

OLSSON S-E, FIGAROLA F, SUZUKI K. Femoral head excision arthroplasty. Clin Orthop 62:104-112,1969.

OLSSON S-E, KASSTRÖM H. Etiology and pathogenesis on canine hip dysplasia. Introduction of a new concept. Proc Canine Hip Dysplasia Symposium St. Louis, MO 1-52,1972.

ORMROD AN. Treatment of hip lamenesses in the dog by excision of the femoral head. Vet Rec 73:576-577,1961.

ORTOLANI M. Un segno poco noto e sua importanza per la diagnosi proce-ce de prelussazione congenita dell'anca. Pediatria (Napoli) 45:129,1937.

PAATSAMA S, JUSSILA J. Healing process after intertrochanteric osteotomy in canine hip dysplasia: An experimental study. J Am Vet Rad Soc 15:61-65,1974.

PADGETT GA, MOSTOSKY UV, FERRIS T. Hip dysplasia - A persistent plague - Can it be controlled?.1990.

PEDERSEN NC, POOL RC, MORGAN JP. Joint disease of dogs and cats. In: Ettinger SJ (ed). Textbook of Veterinary Internal Medicine, 2nd ed. Philadelphia: WB Saunders Company 1982:2229-2230,1982.

PIERMATTEI DL. Femoral head ostectomy in the dog: Indications, technique and results in ten cases. An Hosp 1:180-188,1965.

PIERMATTEI DL. Intertrochanteric osteotomy. Proceedings AAHA Annual Meeting, p 303.1982a.

PIERMATTEI DL. Excision arthroplasty. Proceedings AAHA Annual Meeting, p 305. 1982b.

PETROVIC B, DRAGANOVIC B, TADIC M, MISIC B. Hip dysplasia in the Yugoslasvian sheep dog - "Sarplaninac". Acta Rad Suppl 319, 181-182,1972.

PHARR JW, MORGAN JP. Hip dysplasia in Australian shepherd dogs. JAAHA 12:439-445,1976.

PIERCE KR, BRIDGES CH. The role of estrogens in the pathogenesis of canine hip dysplasia. Metabolism of exogenous estrogens. J sm Anim Prac 8:383-389,1967.

POPOVITCH CA, SMITH GK, GREGOR TP, Shofer FS. Comparison of susceptibility for hip dysplasia between Rottweilers and German Shepherd Dogs. JAVMA 206:648-650,1995.

PREU KP, BLAUROCK H, GALLE O. Zue Hüftgelenksdysplasie beim Beagle-Hund. Berl. München Tierärztl Wschr 88:211-215,1975.

PRIESTER WA, MULVIHILL JJ. Canine hip dysplasia: Relative risk by sex, size and breed and comparative aspects. JAVMA 160: 735-739,1972.

PRIEUR WD. Coxosteoarthrosis in the dog. Part l: Normal and abnormal biomechanics of the hip joint. Vet Surg 9:145-149,1980.

PRIEUR WD. Intertrochanteric osteotomy in the dog: theoretical consideration and operative technique. J sm Anim Pract 28:3-20.1987.

PRIEUR WD, SCARTAZZINI R. Die Grundlagen und Ergebnisse der intertrochanteren Variationsosteotomie bei Hüftdysplasie. Klein Prax 25:393-404,1980.

PRIEUR WD, BRÜSE S. Zum Problem der flachen Pfanne beim Hund. Kleintierpraxis, 33:253-260,1988.

RASMUSSEN LM, KRAMEK BA, LIPOWITZ AJ. Preoperative variables affecting long-term outcome of triple pelvic osteotomy for treatment of naturally developing hip dysplasia in dogs. JAVMA 213:80-85,1998.

REMEDIOA AM, FRIES CL. Treatment of canine hip dysplasia: A review. Can Vet J 36:503-509,1995.

RENDANO VT, RYAN G. Canine hip dysplasia evaluation. Vet Rad 26:170-186,1985.

RETTENMAIER JL, CONSTANTINESCU GM. Canine hip dysplasia. Compendium of Cont Ed 13:643-654,1991.

RHODES WH, JENNY J. A canine acetabular index. JAVMA 137:97-100,1960.

RISER WH. Producing diagnostic pelvic radiographs for canine hip dysplasia. JAVMA 141: 600-603,1962.

RISER WH. Growth and development of the normal canine pelvis, hip joints and femurs from birth to maturity: A radiographic study. J Am Vet Rad Soc 14:25-34,1973a.

RISER WH. The dysplastic hip joint: Its radiographic and histologic development. J Am Vet Rad Soc 14:35-50,1973b.

RISER WH. Canine hip dysplasia: Cause and control. JAVMA 165:360-362,1974.

RISER WH. The dysplastic hip joint: radiologic and histologic development. Vet Pathol 12:279-305,1975.

RISER WH. A half century of canine hip dysplasia. Semin Vet Med Surg (Small Anim) 2:87-91,1987.

RISER WH, SHIRER JF. Hip dysplasia: coxofemoral abnormalities in neonatal German Shepherd Dogs. J small Anim Pract 7:7-12,1966.

RISER WH, SHIRER JF. Correlation between canine hip dysplasia and pelvic muscle mass: a study of 95 dogs. Am J Vet Res 28:769-777,1967.

RISER WH, RHODES WH. Producing diagnostic pelvic radiographs for canine hip dysplasia examination. An Hosp 2:167-171,1966.

RISER WH, COHEN D, LINDQUIST S, MÅNSSON CS, CHEN S. Influence of early rapid growth and weight gain on hip dysplasia in the German Shepherd Dog. JAVMA 145:661-668,1967.

RISER WH, LARSEN JS. Influence of breed somatotypes on prevalence of hip dysplasia in the dog. JAVMA 165:79-81,1974.

RUBIN LD. Tenotomy often helpful. Panel report, Hip dysplasia in dogs. Mod Vet Pract 60:255,1979.

SAMUELSON ML. Correlation of palpation with radiography in diagnosis and prognosis of canine hip dysplasia. Proc Canine Hip Dysplasia Symposium St. Louis, MO 110-116,1972.

SCARTAZZINI R. A radiologic study of normal and dysplastic hip joints in six breeds of large dogs. Acta Rad (Suppl) 319:183-185,1972.

SCHALES O. Genetic aspects of dysplasia of the hip joint. North Am Vet 37:476-478,1956.

SCHALES O. Hereditary pattern in dysplasia of the hip. North Am Vet 38:152-159,1957.

SCHNEIDER-HAISS M, LOEFFLER K. Die Bedeutung der Röntgenaufnahme mit gebeugten Hintergliedmassen bei der Untersuchung auf Hüftglenksdyspasie des Hundes. Kleintierpraxis 32:359-362,1987.

SCHNELLE GB. Some new diseases in the dog. Am Kennel Gazzette 52:25-26,1935.

SCHNELLE GB. Congenital dysplasia of the hip (canine) and sequelae. Scien Proceed AVMA meeting, pp253-258,1954.

SCHNELLE GB. Congenital dysplasia of the hip in dogs. JAVMA 135:234-235,1959.

SCHNELLE GB. The present status and outlook on canine hip dysplasia. Gaines Dog Research Progress Spring 1973.

SCHOENECKER PL, LESKER PA, OGATA K. A dynamic canine model of experimental hip dysplasia: Gross and histological pathology, and the effect of position of immobilization on capitol femoral epiphyseal blood flow. J Bone Joint Surg. 66A:1281-1288,1984.

SCHRADER SC. Triple osteotomy of the pelvis as a treatment for canine hip dysplasia. JAVMA 178:39-44,1981.

SCHRADER SC. Triple osteotomy of the pelvis and trochanteric osteotomy as a treatment for hip dysplasia in the immature dog The surgical technique and results of 77 consecutive operations. JAVMA 189:659-665,1986.

SEER G, HUROV L. Elbow dysplasia in dogs with hip dysplasia. 154:631-637,1969.

SLOCUM B, DEVINE TM. Pelvic osteotomy technique for axial rotation of the acetabular segment in dogs. JAAHA 22:331-338,1986.

SLOCUM B, DEVINE TM. Abstact. Dorsal acetabular rim radiograph for evaluation of the canine hip. Vet Surg 18:81,1989.

SLOCUM B, DEVINE TM. Dorsal acetabular rim radiographic view for evaluation of the canine hip. JAAHA 26:289-296,1990.

SLOCUM B, SLOCUM TD. Pelvic osteotomy for axial rotation of the acetabular segment in dogs with hip dysplasia. Vet Clinics of NA/SAP 22:645-682,1992.

SLOCUM TD, SLOCUM B. Intertrochanteric lateralization. AVORE meeting Sparks NV,1993.

SMITH GK. Distraction radiography for hip dysplasia diagnosis. Proceedings of the 1994 Annual Scientific Meeting of the Veterinary Orthopedic Society, Snowbird/Alta, Utah, pp 45-50,1994.

SMITH GK. Advances in diagnosing canine hip dysplasia. JAVMA 210:1451-1457,1997.

SMITH GK, BIERY DN, GREGOR TP. New concepts of coxofemoral joint stability and the development of a clinical stress-radiographic method for quantitating hip joint laxity in the dog. JAVMA 196:59-70,1990.

SMITH GK, GREGOR TP, RHODES WH, BIERY DN. Coxofemoral joint laxity from distraction radiography and its contemporaneous and prospective correlation with laxity, subjective score, and evidence of degenerative joint disease from conventional hip-extended radiography in dogs. Am J Vet Res 54:1021-1042,1993.

SMITH GK, HILL CM, GREGOR TP, OLSON K. Reliability of the hip distraction index in two-month-old German Shepherd Dogs. JAVMA 212:1560-1563,1998.

SMITH GK, POPOVITCH CA, GREGOR TP, SHOFER FS. Evaluation of risk factors for degenerative joint disease associated with hip dysplasia in dogs. JAVMA 206:642-647,1995.

SMITH RN. The normal and radiological anatomy of the hip joint of the dog. J small Anim Pract 4:1-9,1963.

SMITH RN. The pelvis of the young dog. Vet Rec 76:975-979,1964.

SMITH WS, IRETON RJ, COLEMAN CR. Sequelae of experimental dislocation of a weight-bearing ball and socket joints in a young growing animal. J Bone Jt Surg 40A: 1121-1127,1958.

SMITH WS, COLEMAN CR, OBIX ML, SLAGER RF. Etiology on congenital dislocation of the hip. An experimental approach to the problem using young dogs. J Bone Jt Surg 45A: 491-500,1963.

SNAVELY JG. The genetic aspects of hip dysplasia in dogs. JAVMA 135:201-207,1959.

STOLL S, BROWN SG, PEIRMATEI DL. Intertrochanteric lateralization. ACVS proceedings, San Francisco, CA 1995.

SPRINKLE TA, KROOK L. Hip dysplasia, elbow dysplasia and eosinophilic panosteitis. Cornell Vet 60:476-490,1970.

SPRUELL JSA. Excision arthroplasty as a method of treatment of hip joint disease in the dog. Vet Rec 73:533-536,1961.

STRANDE A. Undersøkelse over hyppigheten av hofteleddsdysplasi hos noen hunderaser. 9th Nordic Veterinary Congress, København 4-7 July 1962

STRANDE A. Excision of the femoral head for canine hip joint lesions. Nord Vet Med 20:75-82,1968.

STUNKARD JA, SCHWICHTENBERG AE, GRIFFIN TP. Evaluation of hip dysplasia in German Shepherd Dogs. Mod Vet Pract. 50:40-44,1969.

SWENSON L. What do we know about hip dypslasia today? Conference on "The Dog in Service of Humanity" Geilo Norway Can 7-9,1987.

SWENSON L. Personal Communication,1989.

SWENSON L, AUDELL L, HEDHAMMAR Å. Prevalence and inheritance of and selection for hip dysplasia in seven breeds of dogs in Sweden and a benefit: cost analysis of a screening and control program. JAVMA 210:207-214,1997.

TOMLINSON J, MCLAUGHLIN Jr R. Canine hip dysplasia: Developmental factors, clinical signs, and initial examination steps. Vet Med 26-33, January 1996a.

TOMLINSON J, MCLAUGHLIN Jr R. Canine hip dysplasia: Medically managing canine hip dysplasia. Vet Med 48-52, January 1996b.

TOWNSEND LR, GILLETTE EL, LEBEL JL. Progression of hip dysplasia in military working dogs. JAVMA 159:1129-1133,1971.

TOWNSEND LR. Hip dysplasia in military working dogs. Proc Canine Hip Dysplasia Symposium St. Louis, MO 127-130,1972.

TURNER TM. Total hip arthroplasty. Proc AAHA Annual Meeting pp305-306,1982.

TVEDTEN HW, CARRIG CB, FLO GL, ROMSOS DR. Incidence of hip dysplasia in beagle dogs fed different amounts of protein and carbohydrate. JAAHA 13,595-598,1977.

VAN DER VELDEN NA. Hip dysplasia in dogs. Vet Quart. 5:3-10,1983.

VAN DYKE JA, HOLLEY HC, ANDERSON SD. Review of iliopsoas anatomy and pathology. RadioGraphics 7:53-84,1987.

VASSEUR PB. Evaluation of carprofen. A nonsteroidal anti-inflammatory drug for osteoarthritis in dogs (Abst) Vet Surg 21:409,1992.

VASSEUR PB, JOHNSON AL, BUDSBERG SCD, LINCOLN JD, TOOMBS JP, WHITEHAIR JG, LENTZ EL. Randomized, controlled trial of the efficacy of carprofen, a non-steroidal anti-inflammatory drug, in the treatment of osteoarthritis in dogs. JAVMA 206:807-811,1995.

TODHUNTER RJ, ZACHOS TA, GILBERT RO, ERB HN, WILLIAMS AJ, BURTON-WURSTER N, LUST G. Onset of epiphyseal mineralization and growth plate closure in radiographically normal and dysplastic Labrador Retrievers. JAVMA 210:1458-1462,1997.

VAUGHAN LC, CLAYTON-JONES DG, LANE JG. Pectineus muscle resection as a treatment for hip dysplasia in dogs. Vet Rec 96:145-148,1975.

WALKER T, PRIEUR D. Intertrochanteric femoral osteotomy. Semin Vet Med Surg (Small Aniam) 2:117-130,1987.

WALLACE LJ, GUFFY MM, CARDINET III GH, FEDDE MR. Surgical rehabiliation of the dysplastic dog. Conference on Research to Expand the Usefullness of the Military Working Dog. 18-20 March 1970, p 79.

WALLACE LJ. Clinical investigations and surgery on pectineus muscle and its relationship to canine hip dysplasia. Scientific proceedings AAHA, 38th annual meeting, Las Vegas, pp 384-388,1971.

WALLACE LJ. Pectineus tendon surgery for the management of canine hip dysplasia. Vet Clin NA Small Anim Pract 22:607-621,1992.

WALLACE LJ, GUFFY MM, CARDINET III GH. Pectineus tendonectomy: A procedure for treating clinical canine hip dysplasia. Proc Canine Hip Dysplasia Symposium St. Louis, MO 133-137, 1972.

WHITTINGTON K, BANKS WC, CARLSON WD, HOERLEIN BF, HUSTED PW, LEONARD EF, MCCLAVE PL, RHODES WH, RISER WH, SCHNELLE GB. Report of panel on canine hip dysplasia JAVMA 139:791-806,1961.

WILLIS MB. The hip scoring scheme: A preliminary report. Vet Rec 115:661-663,1984.

WILLIS MB. Hip scoring: Review of 1985-86. Vet Rec 137:461-462,1986.

WILLIS MB. Progeny Tests for hip scores in Bernese Mountain Dogs. Personal communication 1990.

WILLIS MB. Personal communication,1997a.

WILLIS MB. A review of the progress in canine hip dysplasia control in Britain. JAVMA 210:1480-1482,1997b.

WRIGHT PJ, MASON TA. The usefulness of palpation of joint laxity in puppies as a predictor of hip dysplasia in a guide dog breeding programme. J small Anim Pract 18; 513-522,1977.

# Chapter 6

# Lumbosacral disease

## Introduction

A discussion of primary spinal stenosis, sacral osteochondrosis (OC), and transitional lumbosacral vertebral segments (TLSV) is included in this monograph because the diseases are familial and thought to be inherited. All three lesions tend to be present in disproportionately large numbers in the German Shepherd Dog. The lesions are congenital or developmental and can occur singularly or in concert with degenerative disc disease at the lumbosacral junction (LS) causing compression of the spinal nerve roots that course through the spinal canal at that level. The syndrome results in sensory and/or motor nervous dysfunction due to: (1) compression, (2) destruction, or (3) displacement of the nerve roots or their accompanying vasculature. It is possible for similar clinical signs to be associated with LS lesions that are secondary to traumatic, inflammatory, degenerative, or neoplastic disease. Many of these more common LS lesions, especially those affecting the interposed intervertebral disc can cause malalignment of vertebral segments with or without instability exacerbating the clinical signs.

The lesions present a confusing clinical picture when found in conjunction with hip dysplasia because it is difficult to determine which condition causes the clinical signs of pain, discomfort, and dysfunction seen in the hind limbs. In the absence of hip dysplasia, the clinical signs associated with an LS lesion mimic those seen with hip dysplasia and may mislead the clinician especially when examining a dog of a breed known to have a high incidence of HD. Thus, many differing LS lesions can cause what is described as a cauda equina syndrome (CES) in dogs creating clinical signs that may be confused with those of HD.

Congenital spinal stenosis is a primary narrowing of the spinal canal that may crowd the neural elements causing their compression (Morgan, et al 1987; Bailey and Morgan 1992). The stenosis is a cause of CES when it involves the last lumbar and/or first sacral segments (Bailey and Morgan 1983, Tarvin and Prata 1980, Indrieri 1988, Morgan and Bailey 1990) (Figure 6-1). Sacral "osteochondrosis" within the dorsal portion of the cranial cartilage end plate of the sacrum causes a weakness in the dorsal anulus fibrosus. This may result in an avulsion causing a bulge on the floor of the spinal canal that may cause compression of the spinal nerves (Hime and Drake 1965; Lang and Jaggy 1989; Lang, et al 1989) (Figure 6-2). A transitional lumbosacral vertebral segment is an anomalous vertebral segment at the lumbosacral junction that may cause a spinal instability that precipitates premature degeneration of the lumbosacral intervertebral disc with possible dorsal herniation (Morgan

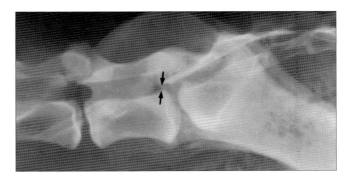

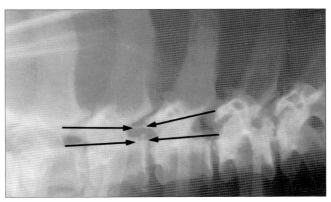

**Figure 6-1**
Lateral radiographs of a young male German Shepherd Dog with a primary spinal canal stenosis in the thoracic region and in the lumbosacral junction. Hind limb ataxia was present for 3 months and was progressive and the dog had pain on palpation of the lumbosacral region. The height of the canal decreases gradually in the mid-thoracic region (long arrows) while the narrowing is abrupt at the LS junction (small arrows). No evidence of LS instability was noted on stress radiographs. These lesions are thought to be congenital and familial.

**210** Lumbosacral disease

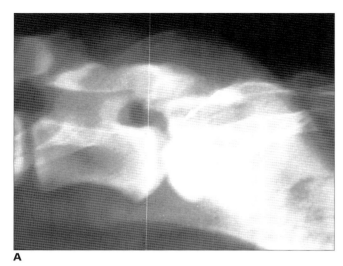

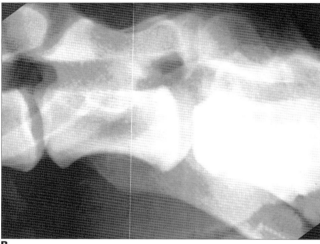

**Figure 6-2**
Lateral radiographs of the lumbosacral region of (A) a 1-year-old male and (B) a 7-year-old male German Shepherd Dog with "osteochondrosis" of the sacrum. In both dogs, a bony fragment has detached from the dorsocranial lip of the sacral endplate and is displaced dorsally into the spinal canal (arrows) causing compression of the spinal nerve roots within the spinal canal at that level. The fragment appears to be larger in A.

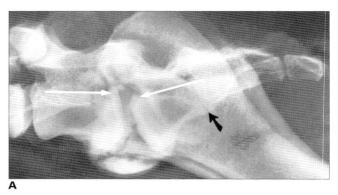

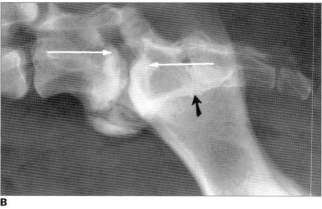

**Figure 6-3**
Lateral radiographs of a female mature Shepherd-cross with incoordination in the hind limbs. Comparison of the (A) neutral and (B) stressed positions illustrate instability at the lumbosacral junction characterized by disruption of the floor of the spinal canal (long white arrows) due to ventral shifting of the sacrum seen on the stressed views. The persistence of a disc space visible as a lucent line (black arrows) between the first and second sacral segments is diagnostic of a transitional vertebral segment. Because of the lumbosacral instability and disc degeneration, new bone, referred to as spondylosis deformans, has formed ventrally and laterally to the lumbosacral disc. In addition, the end plates adjacent to the lumbosacral disc are thickened indicative of chronic disc disease. The lumbosacral congenital anomaly when associated with disc disease is often a cause of cauda equina syndrome. The condition is familiar in certain breeds.

1968, 1972, Larsen 1977) (Figures 6-3, 6-4). It is important to understand that the cause of a cauda equine syndrome may be unrelated to any congenital or developmental lesion and be due only to lumbosacral disc degeneration (Figure 6-5).

## History

Various lumbosacral diseases cause a syndrome commonly noted in the older dog that is referred to as a cauda equina syndrome (CES). The name of the syndrome is derived from the anatomical structure, the cauda equina, which is defined anatomically as the sacral and caudal (coccygeal) segments of the spinal cord and associated nerve roots (Fletcher and Kitchell 1966, Hoerlein 1978, Evans and Christensen 1979). Some have included the last lumbar spinal cord segment and its nerve roots within the definition (de Lahunta 1977, Berzon and Dueland 1979, Lenehan 1983). The resulting clinical problem is a complex of neurological signs produced by pressure or injury to the caudal segments of the spinal cord, its associated nerve roots, or their blood supply (Walla 1986, Morgan and Bailey 1990). The three lesions discussed above can independently cause signs of a CES or can occur in combinations. However, these congenital/devel-

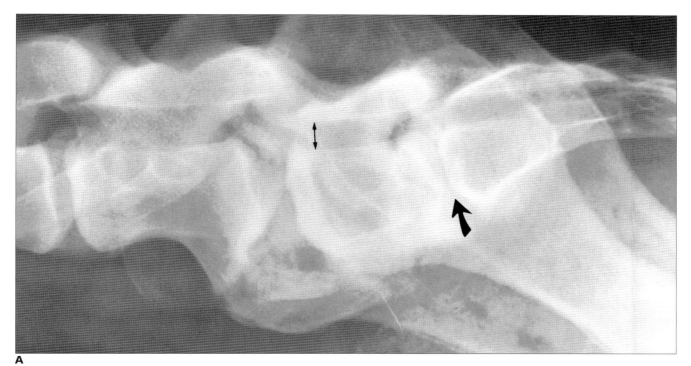

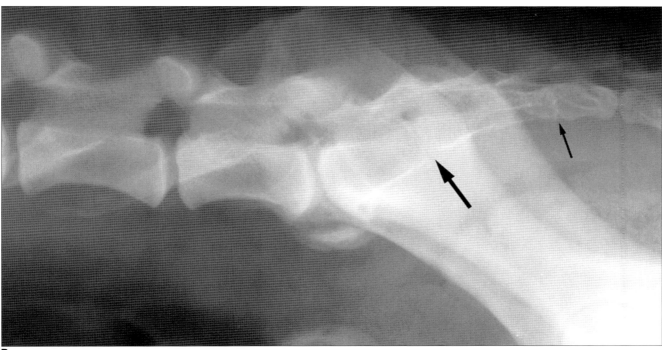

**Figure 6-4**
Lateral radiographs of the lumbosacral region of two dogs with a transitional vertebral segment. In both dogs, what should have been the LS disc shows signs of degeneration with spondylosis deformans. (A) The 9-year-old male German Shepherd Dog has a persistent disc between S1 and S2 (large arrow) and a spinal canal stenosis within the sacrum (small arrows). The widening of what was the LS disc space demonstrates instability. No clinical signs were present in this dog and these changes were noted incidentally on a radiographic study. (B) An 8-year-old male Australian Shepherd Dog has a transitional vertebral segment with incomplete fusion between S1 and S2 (large arrow). The disc between S3 and Cy1 is narrowed and almost fused (small arrow). Canal stenosis is not present. This dog was depressed and unwilling to move and had pain over the LS region probably associated with a protruding LS disc. Note how the extent of the secondary changes seen on the non-contrast radiographs is not directly related to the severity of the clinical signs.

opmental lesions are not the only causes of CES. Dorsally herniating intervertebral discs, fractures, inflammatory lesion, or tumors may create a space occupying mass within the spinal canal, while a fracture or subluxation, intervertebral disc degeneration, or other lesion can cause malalignment or instability at the LS junction any of which can cause a CES. The resulting clinical signs are similar regardless of the etiology and can be confused with signs caused by hip dysplasia and degenerative myelopathy. While any of these lesions alone can cause a CES, the presence of more than one lesion is additive and causes earlier appearance of more severe clinical signs. A more frequently occurring problem in diagnosis is the need to differentiate between the clinical signs of HD and those originating from an LS lesion. This is especially a problem in the German Shepherd Dog.

## Clinical signs

The most typical lesion causing a CES is an LS lesion characterized by a primary LS disc degeneration with dorsal protrusion of the disc. The typically affected dog in which this occurs is a member of a heavier breed and is presented for examination at an older age, usually 6 to 8 years. Thus, CES occurs in many dogs in the absence of any congenital or developmental lesion. It is often impossible to determine the etiology of the lesion by clinical or neurological examination and after the radiographic changes become more chronic; it may even be difficult to learn the specific etiology using this technique.

The degeneration of the LS disc is influenced in a number of ways. A transitional lumbosacral segment can cause an acceleration of the LS disc degeneration and clinical signs appear at an earlier age (Junghanns 1933). The dog with spinal canal stenosis is highly susceptible to compression of the nerve roots and even a small extradural mass or minimal vertebral instability can result in clinical signs of CES at a relatively young age. Sacral osteochondrosis results in a marked progression of LS disc degeneration with possible segmental malalignment and formation of a dorsally protruding mass into the spinal canal and can cause clinic signs at a young age.

The presence of LS instability in conjunction with other causes of CES exacerbates the clinical signs and these patients are presented earlier because of an accelerated LS disc degeneration. The clinical signs are complicated by the LS instability that causes a decrease in the height of the spinal canal and accentuates nerve root compression. Malalignment may result from LS instability and these lesions may be stable or unstable. When unstable, they may cause intermittent compression of the spinal nerves (Bailey and Morgan 1983; Jaggy, et al 1987; Morgan and Bailey 1990; Morgan, et al 1993).

The primary congenital and developmental lesions may be present alone and not produce clinical signs, but with a progressive LS disc degeneration, with or without malalignment and instability, clinical signs often result. Secondary soft tissue changes can be the primary cause of the canal stenosis or can exacerbate a previously existent primary canal stenosis.

Secondary changes around the diseased LS disc tend to stabilize the region. These include: (1) hypertrophy of the ligamentum flavum that extends between the vertebral arches making a roof for the spinal canal, (2) hypertrophy of the vertebral joint capsule laterally, and (3) protrusion of discal tissue from the floor of the canal. Since these are soft tissues, they are only seen on radiographs using contrast agents.

Specific clinical signs of cauda equina lesions include lower motor neuron signs in the hind limbs such as paresis or paralysis, hyporeflexia or areflexia, hypotonia or atonia, or denervation atrophy of striated muscle. Their presence assists in differentiation of a CES from hip dysplasia (Brecker and Pusey 1988; Bodner, et al 1990; Morgan and Bailey 1990). These lower motor neuron signs result in the following:

1. Deficits in placing reactions when walking, including proprioceptive placing,
2. Deficits in pelvic limb withdrawal reflexes,
3. Deficits in voluntary movement of the tail,
4. Loss of muscle tone causing weakness of the hind limbs and flaccidity of the tail,
5. Relaxation of the anal and urethral sphincters that are unresponsive to stimulation, and
6. Pain when exerting downward pressure over the lumbosacral area that forces extension of the lumbosacral joint.

Involuntary urination and defecation may develop in more severely affected dogs (Bodner, et al 1990; Morgan and Bailey 1990). If the LS junction is unstable, the acuteness and intensity of the pain is influenced by any physical action that increases the instability, such as arising, running or jumping or posturing to defecate. With LS stability, the compression of the spinal canal is more consistent and thus the clinical signs do not vary as markedly in intensity. Signs due to the secondary disc protrusion are chronic but are exacerbated by hyperextension of the pelvic limbs such as occurs with running or jumping. Any of these lesions may be asymmetrical and the clinical signs may be more severe on one side than the other.

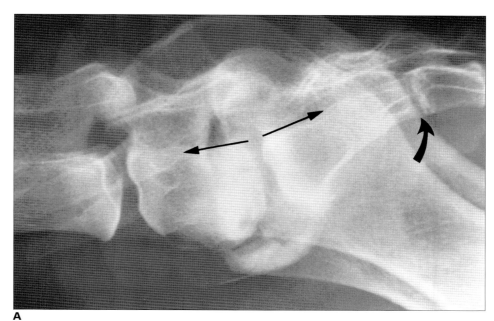

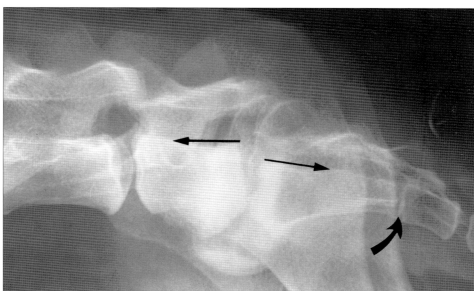

**Figure 6-5**
Lateral radiographs of a 7-year-old female Shepherd-cross with a history of weakness in the hind limbs and dribbling urine. Pain was evident over the sacral area on palpation. Extensive reactive bone (spondylosis deformans), sclerosis of the vertebral end plates, and disc space narrowing is evident on both neutral (A) and stressed (B) views. The stress view shows spinal canal stenosis resulting from LS instability (straight arrows). The only congenital lesion in this dog is the failure of complete closure of the disc space between S2 and S3 that has no clinical importance (curved arrows). The cauda equine syndrome in this dog is unrelated to any congenital or developmental lesion and is due only to lumbosacral disc degeneration.

The owner of a dog with CES often notices in particular that the dog cries out when it rises or that it has difficulty in standing or jumping. In addition, the dog has a tendency to stumble with the hind limbs, has increasing difficulty in jumping into the car, and may show signs of progressive hind limb lameness. The hind limb stride is shortened because hyperextension of the hind limbs is painful. The dog often appears to not know the location or position of the hind feet and has an increased sensitivity to grooming or petting of the pelvic area and may growl or attempt to bite. Because of the slow onset of the clinical signs and their lack of specificity, most owners delay in bringing the dog for examination and treatment until the clinical signs have been present for some time. By this time, the clinical signs have become more easily recognizable and determination of their cause can be easier. Unfortunately, this delay in presentation adversely influences the choice of treatment and its potential value.

Often the clinical signs can be confusing because they are similar in a dog with: (1) CES, (2) HD, or (3) a combination of the two. If the dog has hip dysplasia in association with the LS lesion, a particular problem exists in the interpretation of the clinical signs. The knowledge of a long-standing HD in a dog may cause the clinician to ignore the possibility of an LS lesion, thinking that all clinical signs are the result of the HD. It is possible that a dog with CES and normal hip joints is misdiagnosed because the patient belongs to a breed that commonly has HD and assumptions of HD are made without a thorough examination.

We suggested in the chapter on hip dysplasia (see Chapter 5) that pain in diseased hips causes a dog to try to limit movement of the hind limbs. One way to accomplish this is to use a "bunny hopping" gait which exaggerates motion at the lumbosacral joint as a means of increasing the range of stride in the hind limbs. This excessive motion at the site of a normally developed LS joint may cause a premature injury to the anulus fibrosus of the disc and eventual production of CES. However, the excessive motion at the site of a pre-existing LS lesion such as a transitional segment or sacral osteochondrosis causes the LS disc to degenerate more quickly.

It is helpful to recognize any sudden change in the nature of the clinical signs seen in a chronically dysplastic dog and should be a warning that an additional lesion may be responsible, such as a LS lesions or even a cruciate ligament lesion in the stifle joint.

## Physical examination

Pain can easily be elicited by applying downward pressure on the LS junction of the standing dog. Palpation of the LS region of the affected dog results in movement of the lumbosacral junction that causes wedging of the disc space and dorsal protrusion of the damaged disc. At this time, the dog may respond by trying to bite, by crying out, or by urinating. Unfortunately, a force directed downward on the lumbosacral junction in a standing dog also places an unusual force on the hip joints and the stifle joints, and the pain, or a part of the pain, evidenced might originate from either of those anatomical sites if affected. If the dog is positioned on its side during examination, pain that is elicited on palpation of the lumbosacral junction becomes more specific for that region.

Certain diagnostic rules can be followed in the differentiation of patients with a combination of lesions affecting the LS junction or the hip joints. In the dog with only a CES, the presence of HD is ruled out by radiographic evaluation of the hip joints. In the dog with suspected advanced HD, it is ruled in by radiographic examination of the pelvis while CES is ruled out by negative findings on physical and neurological examination. In the dog with the combination of CES and HD, the radiographic examination of the hip joints rules in HD while positive findings on the physical and neurological examination rules in the CES. It is also possible to differentiate between HD and CES through the use of physical examination of the hip joints and the use of specific radiographic techniques such as stress views and discography.

Diagnosis of dogs with cauda equina syndrome has been reviewed (Oliver, et al 1978; Denny, et al 1982; Lenehan 1983; Schulman and Lippincott 1988; Indriere 1988). A pattern of how separate factors influence development of CES has been developed (Figure 6-6).

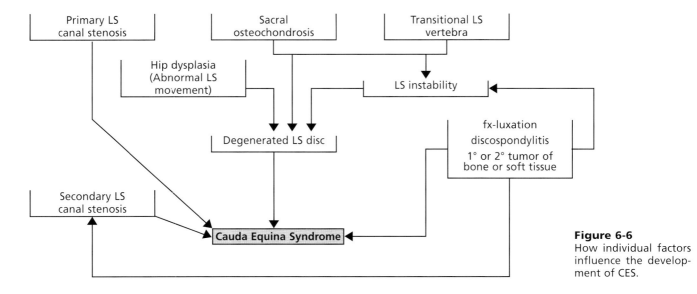

**Figure 6-6**
How individual factors influence the development of CES.

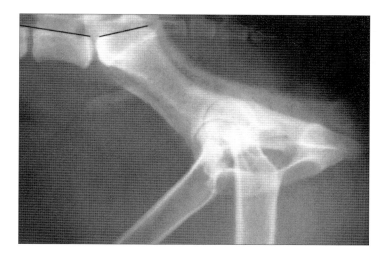
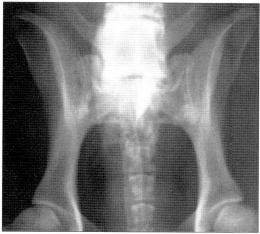

**Figure 6-7**
Normal lateral and ventrodorsal radiographs of the lumbosacral region of a mature dog. Note on the neutrally positioned lateral view that the line identifying the floor of the spinal canal continues with a 20° dorsal angulation. Note the difficulty in identification of the LS disc space on the VD view.

## Anatomy and development of the lumbosacral region

The vertebral body forms from a central ossification center and two secondary centers that develop into the vertebral end plates. The body of the vertebra has a uniform bone tissue density on the radiograph and has smooth end plates cranially and caudally which have a slightly increased bone density. The body of the last lumbar vertebra in the dog has a length that is two times as long as the height. Fusion of ossification centers has been described (Bailey and Morgan 1992). Interposed between the vertebral segments are intervertebral discs composed of the fibrous ring (anulus fibrosis) and a central nucleus (nucleus pulposus).

The arch forms from two centers of ossification that establish the limits of the spinal canal dorsally and laterally. The part of the arch that attaches to the vertebral body is the pedicle and the dorsolateral part of the arch is the lamina. Cranial and caudal vertebral notches from adjacent segments join to form the laterally facing intervertebral foramen through which pass the spinal nerves, arteries, and veins. Because of the thin bony plates that form the arch, the resulting shadows are only slightly denser than the surrounding soft tissues making identification of lesions in the arch difficult. The size of the enclosed spinal canal varies with members of the chondrodystrophoid breeds having a smaller canal (Morgan, et al 1987). The arch creates a spinal canal with a height one half the height of the body. This diminishes to less than one half at L7.

The various processes form from separate centers of ossification and include the spinous process protruding dorsally from the vertebral arch, cranial and caudal articular processes that originate between the pedicle and lamina, and transverse processes that project laterally and cranially. The thick spinous process on L7 is shorter than that seen on L6 and projects dorsocranially. The transverse process projects craniolateroventrally and is longest on L7. The caudal articular processes of the true vertebral joints of L7 projects caudally and have a laterally-facing articular surface that articulates with the medially-facing articular surface of the articular processes of the sacrum. The sacrum is formed by the fusion of three sacral segments. The height of the spinal canal within the sacrum becomes flattened as it narrows gradually with the diminishing size of the sacral bodies. The three spinous processes are fused in the dog. The cranial articular surface of the sacral body has a slight concavity and forms the base of the sacrum. The lateral aspects consist of laterally projecting wing-like structures that articulate with the ilia.

The lumbosacral articulation is such that on the lateral radiographic view of a normal dog, a line representing the floor of the spinal canal continues with an approximately 20° dorsal angle as measured in the neutrally positioned patient. With the hips in a flexed position, a line representing the floor of the spinal canal in a normal dog continues as a straight line. With the hips in an extended position, a line representing the floor of the spinal canal in a normal dog has a 30° to 45° angle. Thus, the normal range of LS movement seen on flexion and extension views of the hips ranges between 30° and 45° and is

# 216 Lumbosacral disease

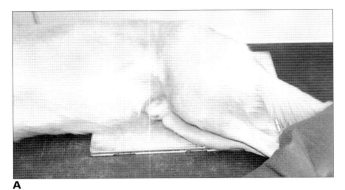

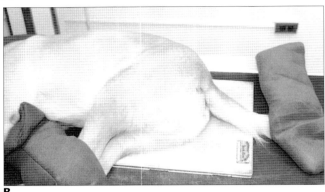

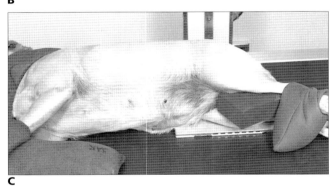

**Figure 6-8**
Photographs illustrate positioning of a dog on its side for making lateral views of the lumbosacral region in: (A) neutral, (B) flexed, and (C) extended positioning. The range of motion and alignment of the vertebral segments plus any instability at the lumbosacral junction are demonstrated on the resulting radiographs. Sandbags are used effectively to assist in positioning.

## Radiographic diagnosis

A routine radiographic study of the lumbosacral region includes ventrodorsal and lateral views (Figure 6-7). In addition, special radiographic techniques in the dog with suspect lumbosacral lesions include: (1) stress radiography, (2) discography, (3) subarachnoid myelography, and (4) epidural myelography. These studies assist in determining the specific cause of the cauda equina syndrome and the type of therapy indicated (Hathcock, et al 1988; Lang 1988; Morgan and Bailey 1990; Morgan 1993).

### Survey radiography

Lateral radiographs of the LS junction are made with the dog on its side with the hind limbs in a neutral position and permit evaluation of the: (1) width of the LS disc space, (2) character of the vertebral end plates, (3) height of the spinal canal, and (4) nature of lumbosacral alignment (Figure 6-8).
Usually the following combination of secondary changes is found in dogs affected with chronic LS disease: (1) collapse of the LS disc space, (2) vertebral end plate sclerosis, (3) vertebral osteophytes (spondylosis deformans), and (4) segmental malalignment with or without spinal canal stenosis. The unique changes associated with primary spinal canal stenosis, sacral OC lesion, or transitional vertebral segment may or may not be identified because of secondary bony changes. The presence of segmental malalignment is a reminder to use stress studies to determine the stability of the LS junction. The location or character of the cranial portion of the bony roof of the sacral canal on the midline is difficult to evaluate on the lateral view making detection of spinal canal stenosis often dependent on special radiographic procedures.

The VD radiograph is less informative than the lateral view in the evaluation of LS lesions. On the VD view, the LS disc can be studied more fully if the central x-ray beam is centered on the disc and angled caudocranially. The VD radiograph is of value in the detection of laterally located vertebral osteophytes that are secondary to disc degeneration that may compromise the size of the lateral intervertebral foramina.

### Stress radiography

A series of lateral radiographs of the LS region is made with the hips in a neutral, fully flexed, and fully extended position (Figure 6-8). This graphically illustrates the range and nature of motion at the LS space (Morgan, et al 1993). The motion is created by using the hind limbs

dependent on breed, physical condition, and age of the patient. In the presence of musculoskeletal disease affecting the hip or stifle joints or the LS intervertebral disc, this range of movement may be altered. In other patients, LS disease may result in segmental malalignment with or without instability, an increase in sacral movement dorsally or ventrally, as well as an increase in angulation of the floor of the spinal canal.

as a lever and the L7 vertebral body as the fulcrum. The range of motion permitted by the healthy LS disc is 30° to 45°. In a neutral position, the disc space with a healthy LS disc has minimal wedging with the apex dorsal. On full extension, the disc space with a healthy LS disc assumes a more prominent wedge shape with the apex dorsal. On full flexion, the disc space with a healthy LS disc assumes a wedge shape with the apex ventral. The range of motion with a diseased LS disc may be limited because of secondary fibrous and bony changes that stabilize the disc space (spondylosis deformans) or it may be increased because of destruction of the anulus fibrosus within the disc.

Lateral views permit evaluation of the relationship between the floor of the spinal canal at L7 and the sacrum. Normally, a continuous line drawn along the floor of the spinal canal has a slight dorsal 20° angulation at the LS disc. With stress the angle changes slightly but without formation of a "stair step" that indicates segmental malalignment with an abrupt dorsal or ventral displacement of the sacrum. This "break" in the line that indicates the floor of the spinal canal may be fixed, or its appearance may be influenced by movement of the hind limbs. The malalignment, whether stable or unstable, causes a fixed or variable narrowing of the spinal canal. More commonly, the sacrum is displaced ventrally on flexion of the hip joint; however, ventral sacral displacement may also be detected on extension of the hip joint. Evaluation of the clinical signs plus the degree of instability determines if surgical stabilization is required. It is possible to have marked malalignment between L7 and S1 but have no instability because of secondary bony changes.

## Epidurography

Epidurography is accomplished following the injection of a contrast medium between the bony wall of the spinal canal and the outer sheath of the spinal cord (dura) (Figure 6-9). It permits detection of a mass lesion within the epidural space. The injection is made through a 20-gauge spinal needle with the tip placed within the epidural space at the LS junction. Complete filling of the epidural space is difficult to maintain because it is poorly defined, contains fat, and has multiple openings through the laterally positioned intervertebral foramina permitting drainage of the contrast agent. However, the contrast agent generally outlines the dorsal and ventral surfaces of the spinal canal as seen on lateral radiographs. Additional lateral radiographs can be made with the needle remaining in position following repeated injections of additional contrast agent as are required to obtain maximum visu-

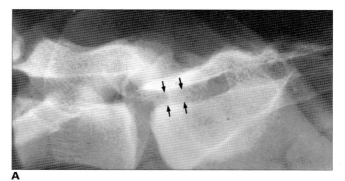

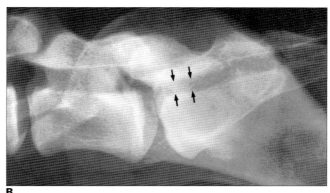

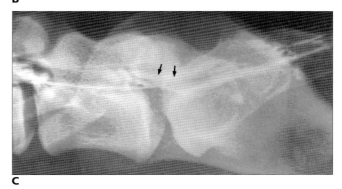

**Figure 6-9**
Non-contrast lateral lumbosacral radiographs were made in a 4-year-old male German Shepherd Dog with a hind limb lameness of 2 months duration at the time of examination. Slight atrophy of the muscles was noted in the left hind limb. Radiographs were made in a (A) neutral and (B) hyperextended position and illustrate a primary LS canal stenosis (arrows). On the (C) radiographs made following injection of a contrast agent into the epidural space, the LS canal stenosis (arrows) was clarified. The epidurogram was performed to rule out possible presence of dorsal disc protrusion as part of the cause of clinical signs. Because of only minimal protrusion of the lumbosacral disc, the dog was treated conservatively, but with little success. A dorsal laminectomy was performed 6 months after original entry with more satisfactory results.

## 218 Lumbosacral disease

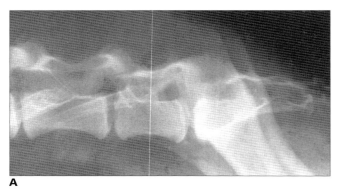

A

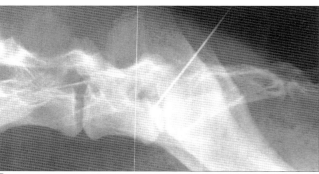

B

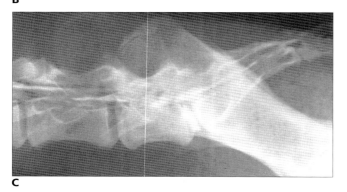

C

**Figure 6-10**
A mature German Shepherd Dog-cross had repeated signs of pain on jumping into a truck. (A) A non-contrast radiograph shows no evidence of lumbosacral disc disease. Stress studies showed no evidence of lumbosacral instability. (B) The discogram illustrates positioning of the needle tip and filling of a large cavity within the severely degenerated lumbosacral disc. Despite the abnormal discogram, (C) an epidurogram shows no evidence of dorsal disc protrusion. No evidence of canal stenosis, osteochondrosis, or transitional segment were noted. This study shows only the cavitation of the LS disc and tends to rule out a cauda equina syndrome as the cause of the clinical signs. Further clinical work-up is required to evaluate the cause of the hind limb pain. Since no cause for a cauda equina syndrome was found, the pain has to be most likely caused by a lesion associated with hind limb function such as orthopedic problem or possibly an infectious lesion. The dog was treated conservatively for early primary disc degeneration and ultimately lost to follow-up. This case illustrates a lumbosacral disc that is severely degenerated but without signs of LS instability or dorsal disc protrusion. Degeneration in a disc of this type could be expected to progress with collapse, secondary bony changes, and eventually a dorsal protrusion.

alization of a space-occupying lesion. Following removal of the needle, lateral radiographs can be made in stressed positions. The ventrodorsal view is of little value in epidurography. The epidurogram permits detection of spinal canal stenosis plus the influence of the thickened interarcuate ligament or dorsally protruded discal tissue. Epidurography combined with discography demonstrates the thickness of the intact dorsal anulus of the LS disc (Sisson, et al 1992; Barthez, et al 1994).

### Discography

Discography permits an understanding of the character of the intervertebral disc in the dog with a suspect CES. A 20-gauge spinal needle is positioned with the tip within the LS disc and a contrast agent is injected into the nuclear portion of the disc. The location of the needle tip can be determined radiographically prior to injection. Little or no contrast agent can be injected within a normal intervertebral disc or one with only early degeneration, whereas 2 to 3 cc or more of the contrast agent can be accommodated within a severely degenerated disc with cavitation (Figure 6-10). This technique shows the direction and extent of discal protrusion on both lateral and ventrodorsal views (Barthez, et al 1994). It is possible for the contrast agent to escape from the nucleus in a dorsal, ventral, or lateral direction through a partially torn anulus (Figures 6-11, 6-12). The discogram is often combined with an epidurogram since both studies can be performed following slight repositioning of the tip of a single needle.

### Myelography

Myelography is the filling of the subarachnoid space that lies between the inner two sheaths of the spinal cord with a positive contrast agent through a cisternal or lumbar tap using a 20- or 22-gauge spinal needle. This technique is usually not recommended as a technique for the evaluation of the LS canal because the subarachnoid space does not extend that far caudally and if it does, it usually does not fill with the contrast agent. Another problem with myelography in detection of an LS lesion is the normal elevation of the contrast-filled caudal subarachnoid space away from the floor of the spinal canal that prevents detection of a mass lying on the floor of the spinal canal. However, in the hands of some investigators, myelography is reported to be a valuable tool (Lord and Olsson 1976, Lang and Jaggy 1989).

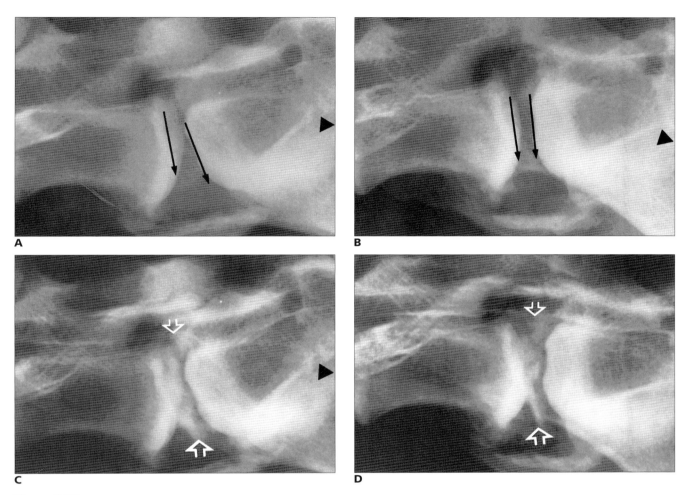

**Figure 6-11**
A 12-year-old male German Shepherd Dog had an acute onset of back pain with weakness in the hind limbs and an inability to arise. The hips were radiographically normal. On neurological examination, decreased muscle tone was noted in the hind limbs along with abnormal spinal reflexes. Non-contrast radiographs were made with the limbs in (A) extension and (B) flexion and demonstrated lumbosacral instability by noting the movement of the end plates (long arrows). (C, D) A discogram/epidurogram was performed and showed a diffusion of the contrast agent throughout a badly damaged disc with contrast medium extending to the ventral portion of the disc (large white arrows) and dorsally into the spinal canal (small white arrows). The dorsal disc protrusion was more prominent when the hind limbs were extended (C). The lucent zone between the first and second sacral segments indicated a failure of complete fusion of these segments (black arrow head) and a form of transitional segment. Because of the dog's advanced age, he was treated conservatively with little improvement in his signs expected.

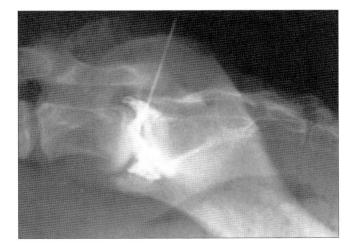

**Figure 6-12**
A lateral radiograph following discography of the lumbosacral disc with the needle remaining in position. The lumbosacral disc is badly degenerated and a large pool of the contrast agent fills the center of the disc, protrudes ventrally, and dorsally into the spinal canal where it creates a large epidural mass causing the cauda equina syndrome.

## Examination protocol

Not all of the special radiographic procedures achieve their maximum diagnostic level in each patient. Therefore, a protocol should be used that utilizes the procedures in a correct sequence to insure that the diagnosis can be made with the least technically demanding study and with the studies that are of least risk to the patient. The routine survey study and stress series can be performed safely and with absolute accuracy on a cooperative or sedated patient and should be performed first (Table 6-1). The discogram and epidurogram require experience to perform and are done on an anesthetized patient. However, they are of high diagnostic value and are the next examination(s) to be considered. Myelography requires anesthesia as well as a particular needle tip placement to perform the study satisfactorily and often does not demonstrate the LS region in larger non-chondrodystrophic dogs. For these reasons, this study is usually performed in search of other spinal lesions without anticipation of identification of an LS lesion.

**Table 6-1: Examination protocol for study of lumbosacral lesions**

1. Non-contrast neutral positioned lateral and ventrodorsal radiographs
2. Non-contrast lateral stress radiographs with full extension and full flexion of the hip joints
3. Discography with lateral radiographs made following injection of the contrast media into the disc
4. Epidurography with lateral radiographs made at several stages during injection of the positive contrast agent into the epidural space
5. Immediately after removal of the spinal needle, lateral stress radiographs are made with full extension and full flexion of the hip joints to enhance either the discogram or epidurogram
6. Immediately after removal of the spinal needle, dorsoventral contrast radiographs are made

## Differential radiographic diagnosis

Differential diagnosis of LS lesions is extensive since congenital, developmental, traumatic, inflammatory, neoplastic, and degenerative lesions can all affect this portion of the spine and cause clinical signs similar to those seen with CES. The degeneration of the LS disc occurs regularly but can be hastened by the presence of many of the above lesions. If a vertebral segment has a congenital or developmental lesion, the severity of canal stenosis can be influenced by an associated inflammatory lesion, trauma, or tumor. Once pronounced secondary bony changes have formed around a degenerative disc, the end plate sclerosis and vertebral osteophytosis can easily obscure the original disc disease or the canal stenosis (Morgan, et al 1993). Because of the slow progression of clinical signs associated with most lesions, secondary radiographic changes are usually present at the time of first examination and complicate diagnosis and determination of prognosis. All of this means that in the older dog, it is unlikely that the true cause of a cauda equina syndrome may be realized on non-contrast radiographs. Thus, the diagnosis of cauda equina syndrome is often made without knowing the initiating cause and treatment is based entirely on detection of a stenotic lesion using special radiographic studies. Even with diagnostic special radiographic studies, surgical exploration of the LS region may be the only method to determine the exact cause of the CES.

## Treatment

Treatment of primary spinal stenosis, sacral osteochondrosis (OC), and transitional lumbosacral vertebral segments (TLSV) are discussed together since the lesion to be corrected is one causing a CES. Any of these primary lesions can be associated with an epidural mass created by a degenerative disc or LS instability and influence the prognosis. Usually, the period of pain, the nature of the lameness, and the presence of other clinical and neurological signs determines the treatment to be attempted and the possibility of a return to normal activity.

### Medical treatment

Some affected dogs in which clinical signs are mild or in which apparent lumbosacral pain is the sole problem improve temporarily after strict confinement and restricted leash exercise for a period of 4 to 6 weeks. Use of analgesic drugs or corticosteroids has been recommended by some, however, they may result in a decrease in pain and the dog is inclined to increase its physical activity furthering progression of the compressive lesion. Therefore, their use must be accompanied by strict confinement. Conservative and medical therapy including rest, with or without drugs, only perpetuates the status quo of the CES, and clinical signs commonly recur in affected dogs treated in this manner.

## Chemonucleolysis

Chemonucleolysis is a unique treatment and follows the injection of the proteolytic enzyme chymopapain into the nucleus pulposus of the disc. Chymopapain is a proteolytic enzyme with selective digestive action on chondromucoprotein of the nucleus pulposus and with the least effect on the anulus fibrosus and has been used to reduce the size of the epidural mass caused by the protruding LS disc. Dissolution of the nucleus pulposus has been demonstrated histologically. The injection can be made through a spinal needle directed ventrally through the spinal canal into the disc. Narrowing of the affected disc space is seen radiographically within 24 hours following injection and indicates an acute LS instability that is created following injection of the enzyme. Activity of the dog must be strictly controlled for 3 to 4 days, to avoid physical activity that would result in further disc protrusion. Without this control, the dog may suffer greatly increased LS pain. In addition, restriction of movement decreases the chance that a stable LS junction will become unstable or that an already unstable LS junction will become increasingly unstable. It is understood that treatment of this type can do nothing for a primary canal stenosis caused by congenital bone disease or for a secondary canal stenosis caused by hypertrophy of the ligamentum flavum (interarcuate ligament) or hypertrophy of the periarticular tissue surrounding the true vertebral joints. The enzyme has a clinical effect only by its action on the protruding nucleus (Atilola, et al 1988 a, b).

## Surgical treatment

Dogs with recurrence of signs or dogs that are moderately to severely affected at the time of initial presentation (especially those with urinary/fecal incontinence) should be considered candidates for surgical therapy. Dorsal decompressive laminectomy of L7 and L1 segments is recommended (Figure 6-13). In a dog with a CES without instability in which the surgery can be limited to the midline, good success can be expected. Because the decompression is accomplished by removal of the arch of the vertebrae, it is not considered essential to explore the floor of the canal in an effort to remove a protruding dorsal anulus. In a patient with a lateral mass, compression may be combined with foraminotomy, the surgical increase of the size of the laterally located intervertebral foramina, or facetectomy, the surgical removal of the articular facets of the true vertebral joints. Either of these is considered in dogs in which compression of spinal nerves at the level of the intervertebral foramina is suspected. The surgery becomes more complicated because of the encroachment of compressive tissues on spinal nerves and because of the presence of laterally located spinal venous lakes. In animals with radiographically confirmed instability or significant retrolisthesis (a ventral slippage of the sacrum relative to the body of L7), fusion of the lumbosacral articulations may be necessary. It is important to evaluate the radiographic study prior to surgery, positively locating the LS junction and insuring that transitional segments do not affect the efficacy of the surgery. If a transitional segment results in movement between the anomalous segment and the sacrum, surgical stabilization at the level of the expected LS junction will not be effective. Instead, the surgery should be directed toward the site of instability.

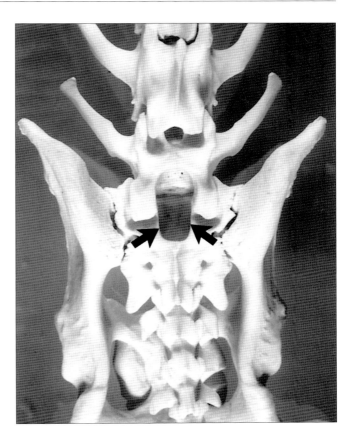

**Figure 6-13**
A photograph of a spinal specimen made from the dorsal side illustrating a decompressed laminectomy site at the LS junction (arrows). The surgery is shown to be limited to the midline. If neurological signs indicate, the procedure can be extended laterally so that it incorporates a foraminotomy or facetectomy.

Dogs should be confined for 2 to 4 weeks post-operatively. An early postoperative complication is seroma formation at the surgical site. Later problems include formation of a compressive laminectomy scar at the surgical site. Both may be avoided by use of appropriate surgical technique and postoperative patient management.

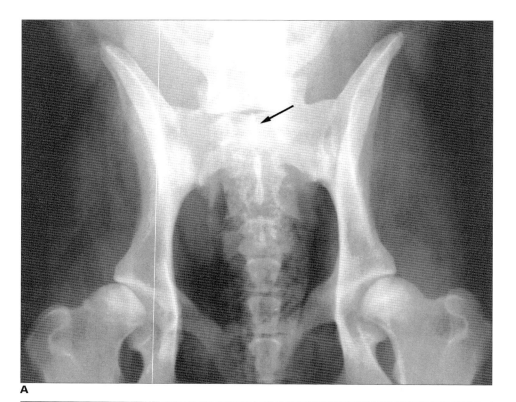

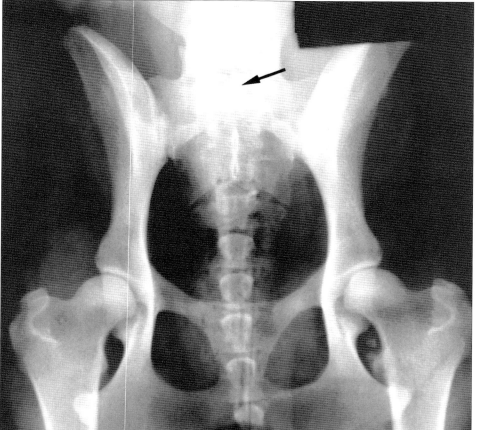

**Figure 6-14**
Ventrodorsal radiographs of the LS junction of two dogs with symmetrical transitional LS segments characterized by wing-like transverse processes. Both dogs were being examined to determine the status of the hip joints. (A) A 1-year-old female German Shepherd Dog has bilateral hip dysplasia with subluxation of both femoral heads and Morgan Lines bilaterally. The transitional LS segment is symmetrical, however, there is a slight obliquity of the pelvis and sacrum to the left. Note the separated spinous process of the anomalous segment (arrow). (B) A 2-year-old female Shepherd-cross has subluxation of the femoral heads. The transitional LS segment is symmetrical. Note the separated spinous process of the anomalous segment (arrow).

Attention to bladder emptying is necessary in dogs with bladder atony prior to surgery. The bladder should be manually expressed three times daily in such dogs. Urine should be submitted for culture and sensitivity testing prior to and 2 weeks after completion of surgery, and appropriate antibiotic therapy instituted as indicated by results.

## Prognosis

The prognosis is dependent on the severity of signs prior to surgery and the cause of the CES. Return to normal athletic function can be expected in dogs in which the nerve root compression is mild and the clinical signs are minimal. Dogs with more severe neurological signs such as bladder atony or a flaccid anal sphincter prior to surgery have the poorest diagnosis.

# Transitional lumbosacral vertebrae

## Definition

Transitional vertebral segments may occur throughout the spine and are located at junctions between two major sections of the spine and have been described earlier in dogs (Morgan 1968). The development of the last presacral vertebral segment in man has been described as "restless" (Junghans 1933) with frequent variations in the number of lumbar and sacral segments as well as morphological variations. These variations are of great interest in the dog, especially the separation of the first sacral segment that then appears as the last lumbar segment. This has been referred to as lumbarization of the first sacral segment.

Originally it was reported that the presence of the aberrantly formed vertebral segments was not painful, and transitional lumbosacral vertebral segments in the dog probably had little if any clinical significance in early life or perhaps throughout life (Morgan 1968, 1972; Bailey and Morgan 1983). Now it is known that lesions at the LS junction predispose to a weakness between these two sections of the spine and can cause instability leading to excessive motion around the aberrant disc with degeneration of the LS disc and creation of a CES.

The transitional segment can be bilaterally symmetrical or unilateral. In either situation, it is important to ascertain the affect of the anomalous segment on the strength of the sacroiliac joint (SI). If the joint(s) is weakened, a greater stress is placed on the aberrant LS disc due to the potential instability. It is presumed that this weakness is transmitted to the LS disc that undergoes an accelerated degeneration.

If the transitional segment is symmetrical, the last presacral disc is now located at what was the site of the bony junction between the first and second sacral segments (Figure 6-14). The SI joint is possibly strengthened by this type of anomaly if the transverse processes assume the form of the wings of the sacrum. Diagnosis on the ventrodorsal view is made by detection of the isolated spinous process of the anomalous segment along with the two wing-like processes. On the lateral view, diagnosis can be made by detection of the radiolucent disc space between what should have been S1 and S2, however, nothing can be learned about the nature of the attachment to the sacrum (Figures 6-3, 6-4).

The transitional segments with asymmetry typically have one transverse process that is wing-like and one that is typical of that seen with a lumbar segment. This type of sacral attachment is weakened and the LS disc typically is stressed abnormally as is characterized by the bony buildup around the discs and at the SI joint (Figure 6-15). The degree of pelvic obliquity varies somewhat dependent on the nature of the SI attachment (Figure 6-16).

With lumbarization of the first sacral segment, two of the original sacral segments remain. These may continue to present as a shortened sacrum or often a shifting of the first caudal segment occurs so that the number of sacral segments returns to three. This might be referred to as a sacralization of the first caudal (coccygeal) segment. However, determination of the exact number of lumbar and sacral segments is impossible without counting the total number of presacral segments. The number of segments is not critical; instead it is the nature of the spinal and sacral attachment to the pelvis that determines the character of the SI joint.

## Radiographic diagnosis

The basic radiographic changes describe the morphology of the vertebral segments and do not represent any error in the character of the bony tissue. Thus, determination of the shape, alignment, and method of segmental attachment is necessary for a description of the lumbosacral transitional segment (TLSV). The transitional segment can be recognized on both lateral and ventrodorsal views and its appearance is dependent on the symmetry of the SI articulations. If asymmetrical, an oblique attachment of the sacrum to the pelvis occurs that is best seen on the VD view. The resulting pelvic

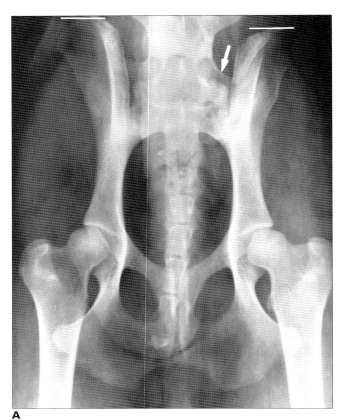 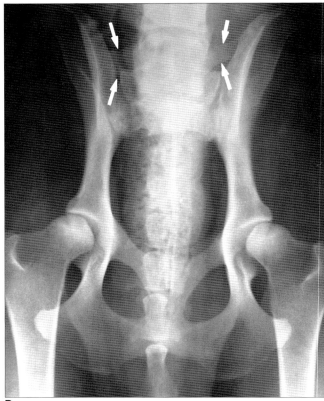

**Figure 6-15**
Ventrodorsal radiographs of the LS junction of two dogs with asymmetrical transitional LS segment characterized by the presence of transverse processes on the anomalous vertebral segment. It is thought that both SI joints are weakened. (A) In a 2-year-old male Australian Shepherd Dog the lateral processes are asymmetrical with the left being thicker and wing-like (arrow). However, it is difficult to determine if either process articulates with the ilium. Note the angulation of the pelvis to the sacrum with the right iliac crest further cranial than on the left (lines). Both femoral heads have minimal subluxation indicative of early hip dysplasia. The acetabular cups are not as deeply formed as in normal hips. (B) In a 2-year-old male Great Pyreenes both lateral processes remain separate (arrows) and seem to not articulate with the ilium. The pelvis is attached symmetrically. Both femoral heads subluxate indicating minimal dysplasia.

obliquity affects the placement of the acetabulum within the pelvis resulting is an acetabular roof that provides greater or lesser coverage of the femoral head.

Detection of the angulation of the floor of the spinal canal on the lateral radiograph marks the site of the old LS junction. Normally, a marked dorsal angulation of the floor within the sacrum is present at the site of its attachment to the last lumbar vertebra. With lumbarization of the first sacral segment, the angulation remains and the disc space shifts caudally so it is located between what were the first two sacral segments (Figures 6-3, 6-4). In the dog with a normal lumbosacral junction, the three spinous processes of the sacrum are fused with an undulation of the dorsal margin (Figure 6-7). With the anomalous segment, the spinous process of the transitional segment is separated. This is best identified on the VD radiograph (Figures 6-14, 6-15, 6-16). Also, the height of the spinal canal through the last lumbar segment, which really is the first sacral segment, is decreased (Figures 6-3, 6-4, 6-17). In addition, the effective height of the spinal canal may be further compromised due to malalignment following ventral slippage of the modified sacrum at the aberrant LS disc secondary to disc disease, and dorsal protrusion of the LS disc. Any or all of these can cause a compression of the cauda equina. Secondary bony changes are noted within the end plates adjacent to the old LS disc as it degenerates and spondylosis deformans often develops (Figures 6-3, 6-4) (Wright 1980).

On the ventrodorsal view, the altered method of attachment of the affected lumbar segment to the sacrum and to the pelvis can be seen, especially if the change is asymmetrical. With symmetrical shifting, the lesion may not be as easily recognized on this view (Figure 6-14).

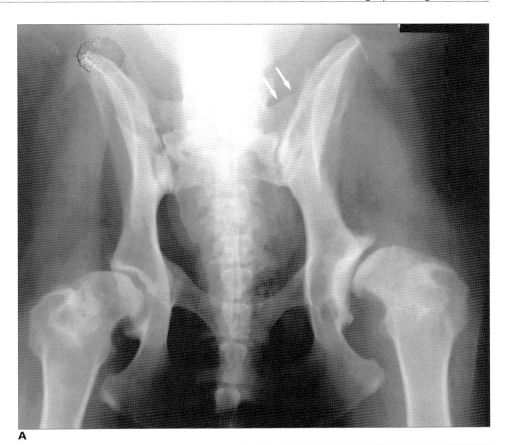

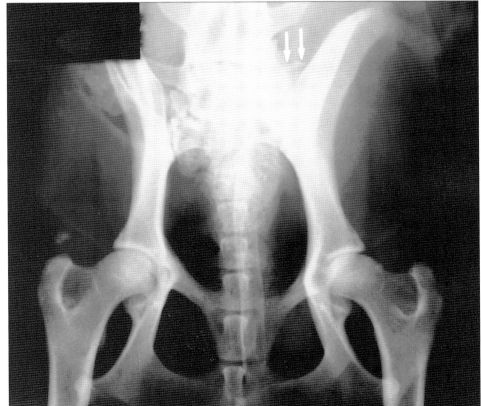

**Figure 6-16**
Ventrodorsal radiographs of the LS junction of two dogs with marked asymmetry in the transitional LS segment. It is thought that both SI joints are weakened. (A) In a 9-year-old male German Shepherd Dog, the lateral processes are asymmetrical with the left appearing as a thick lateral process (arrows) and the right a more normally appearing lateral lumbar process. Note the angulation of the pelvis to the left. The degree of hip dysplasia is severe, however there is more coverage of the femoral head on the right as a result of the pelvic obliquity. (B) In a 9-year-old male Brittany, the lateral processes are asymmetrical with the left appearing as a thick lateral process (arrows) and the right a more normal lateral lumbar process. The pelvis is attached asymmetrically with tilting of the pelvis to the left as a result of the badly malformed anomalous segment. The femoral heads seat deeply, however prominent osteophytes are seen on the caudal aspect of the femoral necks.

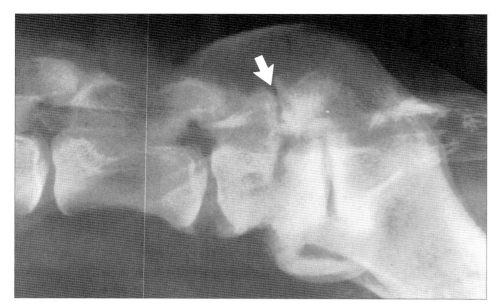

**Figure 6-17**
A lateral radiograph of a 12-year-old male German Shepherd Dog with marked secondary changes around the new disc space created by the anomalous segment. The secondary changes around L6 and L7 are limited to minimal spondylosis deformans. Excessive motion around the new disc space is assumed to be causing the secondary changes. Note the new bony changes dorsally that suggests that a part of the instability may be associated with the vertebral joints. This pattern is unusual.

However, with a transitional segment, the first process is separated and the remaining two are joined with the possibility of joining the spinous process of the first coccygeal segment (Figures 6-14, 6-15). The aberrant LS disc space is not as readily identified on the VD view because the space is angled to the x-ray beam. Secondary changes involving the sacroiliac joint can be identified.

The secondary radiographic changes noted in association with a transitional vertebral segment are progressive and dependent on the nature of the sacroiliac joints and the aberrant LS disc and as such are not usually recognized until later. The clinical signs are usually chronic and long standing prior to presentation, thus, the secondary radiographic changes are often prominent at the time of first clinical examination. These changes consist primarily of collapse of the original LS disc space with sclerosis of the end plates and ventral and lateral vertebral osteophytosis (spondylosis deformans). In some dogs, movement at the site of the new disc space permits development of secondary changes in the form of sclerotic end plates and spondylosis deformans (Figure 6-17). This is an unusual pattern of change.

## Heritability

In a group of German Shepherd Dogs evaluated for hip dysplasia, the frequency of transitional lumbosacral vertebrae (TLSV) was reported to be between 8 % and 11% (Morgan and Stephens 1985; Morgan, et al 1993). An earlier report of 4.3% was based only on ventrodorsal views of the pelvis and many symmetrically oriented anomalies were probably not detected (Larsen 1977). In similar studies, the frequency reported in Great Pyrenees was 1.5% (Larsen 1977) and 3% (Morgan and Stephens 1985); the frequency reported in Labrador Retrievers was 1.8% (Larsen 1977) and 3% (Morgan and Stephens 1985); and the frequency reported in Saint Bernards was 0.6% (Larsen 1977) and 0.0% (Morgan and Stephens 1985). Comparison between the breeds suggests a marked difference in frequency with the German Shepherd Dog involved to a much higher level than other breeds. It is assumed that these differences in frequency between the breeds have a genetic basis. In a study of Labrador Retrievers (see Chapter 9), TLSV was noted in the offspring of one sire breed with four different dams, in the offspring of two sires each breed with two different dams, and in two litter mates from another sire. This seems to offer proof that this anomaly is inherited.

The occurrence of degenerative disc disease in the aberrant LS disc is at least partially dependent on the morphology of the last presacral vertebrae and the relationship of its transverse processes to the pelvis (Morgan 1972). The degree of instability is dependent on the TLSV and is likely to precipitate degeneration of the anomalous disc. German Shepherd Dogs have a disproportionately high frequency of this anomaly (Morgan and Stephens 1985) and a statistically significant positive relationship was shown to exist between the presence of this congenital lesion and the development of the cauda equina syndrome (Morgan, et al 1993). The frequency of TLSV in a small group of German Shepherd Dogs with cauda equina syndrome was 38%. These studies suggest that the German Shepherd Dog with transitional LS segments is affected with a frequency of CES more than would be expected only by chance.

# Osteochondrosis of the sacrum

## Definition

"Osteochondrosis" of the sacrum is similar in appearance to "osteochondrosis" lesions found throughout the body except that this lesion is in a joint characterized by an intervertebral disc instead of a true joint. Radiographically it resembles an avulsion fracture, however, histologically, the resulting cartilaginous mass found on the floor of the spinal canal originates from disturbed endochondral ossification in the dorsal part of the growth cartilage of the sacral end plate (Figure 6-2). It is comparable to the irregular cartilage proliferation including degenerative changes and fissure formation noted in osteochondrosis in other sites (Olsson and Reiland 1978). Cartilage retention is followed by necrosis in the deepest layers of the lesion. The lesions vary from the common osteochondrosis in that the resulting displaced cartilage mass originating from the sacrum has a bony center. The resulting injury to the end plate leads to a faulty attachment of the dorsal anular fibers and increased mechanical stress on the LS intervertebral disc, which precipitates disc degeneration and can lead to a ventral slippage of the sacrum. Rupture of the disc in the area of the end plate defect leads to protrusion of disc material between the detached fragment and the sacrum. Thus, the "osteochondrosis" lesion predisposes LS disc degeneration and this, plus the resulting malalignment of the LS segments, becomes a common cause for cauda equina compression in certain dogs.

## Radiographic diagnosis

Radiographically, osteochondrosis of the cranial end plate of the sacrum is characterized principally on the lateral view by deformation of the dorsocranial corner with a resulting osseous fragment(s) lying free on the floor of the spinal canal. Usually the surrounding bone that forms the bed for the fragment has become sclerotic (Figure 6-2). The more chronic lesion is seen as a bony lip suggesting that the previously free chondral fragment has became reattached to the sacral lip. Radiographic and pathologic findings both suggest that the lipping and the free fragment are different degrees of "osteochondrosis" (Lang, et al 1992)

The radiographic diagnosis is based on the detection of the osteochondral fragment that originates from the dorsal lip of the sacrum on lateral and ventrodorsal survey radiographs. However, superimposition of the iliac wings and the sacroiliac joints can make it difficult to detect smaller "osteochondrosis" lesions on survey radiographs. Early disc space narrowing, end plate sclerosis, and spondylosis deformans at the LS disc may be seen secondary to the instability resulting from the OC lesion, perhaps suggesting this diagnosis when seen in a younger dog. In the older dog, disc space narrowing, end plate sclerosis, and spondylosis deformans is probably secondary to more classical disc degeneration unrelated to a sacral "osteochondrosis." Spondylosis deformans is minimal, when associated with the OCD lesion, as is secondary change involving the dorsal articular processes of the lumbosacral vertebral joints, suggesting that instability is not an important aspect of "osteochondrosis" of the sacrum.

Dorsal and lateral deviation and/or compression of the cauda equina caused by the osseous fragment or by the lip of bone may be seen on contrast radiographic studies. Either epidurography or discography may be of value in the identification of the injury and the dorsal protrusion of the disc. Hyperextension of the lumbosacral joint accentuates the spinal nerve compression. However, detection of a mass on the floor of the spinal canal at this site does not permit distinguishing between disc degeneration caused by an "osteochondrosis" lesion and an uncomplicated disc disease.

## Heritability

Sacral osteochondrosis has an obvious breed predisposition and is encountered within German Shepherd Dogs where it causes clinical signs in males at a ratio of 4.5:1. If dogs with cauda equina syndrome are examined, 30% of the German Shepherd Dogs are seen to be affected by a sacral osteochondrosis while less than 2% of other breed dogs with cauda equina syndrome are affected by a sacral osteochondrosis. Examination of 25 clinically normal German Shepherd Dogs detected slightly more than 6% to have sacral osteochondrosis (Lang, et al 1992) suggesting that the condition can be present without clinical signs. Genetic predisposition is suggested by the unusually high frequency within the German Shepherd Dog breed as well as finding affected littermates.

# Spinal canal stenosis

## Definition

Primary spinal canal stenosis is used by the authors to describe a form of congenital bony stenosis. It is thought to be familial, affects the vertebral segments of large breeds of dog, and if located at the LS junction, can be one of the causes of CES (Morgan and Bailey 1990). Spinal canal stenosis is noted in all parts of the spine, however, most frequently at the caudal cervical region, cranial thoracic region, and the lumbosacral region (Figures 6-1, 6-4, 6-9). The bone tissue is normal, however, the shape of the vertebra is affected with the length of the pedicles and lamina greatly shortened. While this shortening can cause pressure on the enclosed spinal cord and/or spinal nerves, it can also exist as a non-clinical lesion. Thus, in many dogs, a primary canal stenosis at the LS junction remains clinically silent until a secondary lesion compromises the height of the stenotic canal resulting in the onset of signs of a cauda equina syndrome.

Primary LS spinal canal stenosis in the dog has received attention in the past few years (Bailey and Morgan 1983; Oliver, et al 1978; Berzon and Dueland 1979; Lenehan 1983; Tarwin and Prata 1980; Denny, et al 1982). As in man, spinal canal stenosis is congenital and developmental in nature. Instability of the LS junction due to disc disease may be superimposed over a primary canal stenosis and thus create a clinically significant lesion (Lord and Olsson 1976). Spinal canal stenosis may occur with or without transitional vertebrae or osteochondrosis of the sacrum (Morgan and Bailey 1990). Any combination of lesions hastens and worsens the resulting clinical syndrome. While seen often in larger breeds, a primary spinal canal stenosis at the lumbosacral junction has been reported in smaller breeds as well (Tarvin and Prata 1980). The reports in the dog are generally limited to mid-thoracic lesion in Doberman Pinschers and LS lesions in German Shepherd Dogs.

Secondary canal stenosis due to a soft tissue lesion is much more common and is usually the result of dorsal bulging of the anulus fibrosus, hypertrophy and/or hyperplasia of the ligamentum flavum (interarcuate ligament), and thickening of the soft tissues around the articular facets. Any disease causing a mass that encroaches upon space within the spinal canal can be considered a cause of secondary canal stenosis.

## Radiographic diagnosis

Because primary canal stenosis is a congenital lesion of the bones forming the arch of the vertebral segment, bone tissue has normal density radiographically and only the size of the arch is affected. The width of the vertebral body is not affected so the width of the spinal canal remains normal. Only the height of the canal is diminished. The lesion of spinal canal stenosis is diagnosed on the lateral radiograph by noting the height of the spinal canal and comparing it with the height of the canal measured cranially and caudally. Spinal canal height normally decreases at the LS junction, however, with canal stenosis at this site, the change is abrupt with a magnitude of change such that the height is diminished to less than 50% of the canal height cranially. Disc spaces are not affected and thus degenerative changes are not seen in the younger dog. Primary canal stenosis is not seen regularly with TLSV or with sacral OCD lesions.

Myelography or epidurography are used to determine the effect of canal stenosis on the spinal nerves. The width and height of the subarachnoid space and the spinal cord can be evaluated on both lateral and VD views searching for a region of abrupt narrowing. The myelogram may not show subarachnoid filling to the effected level of the spinal canal. In this case, epidurography may be required to outline the area of canal stenosis. When canal stenosis is associated with other lesions, their effect on canal size may be noted as well.

## Heritability

Primary canal stenosis is commonly found in larger breed dogs and seems to affect males more frequently than females. Both Doberman Pinschers and German Shepherd Dogs appear to be affected more often than dogs of other breeds. Primary canal stenosis is assumed to be hereditary because of the strong familial pattern noted in affected dogs.

# References

ATILOLA MAO, BAILEY CS, MORGAN JP. Cervical chemonucleolysis in the dog: A surgical technique. Vet Surg 17:135-140, 1988a.

ATILOLA MAO, MORGAN JP, BAILEY CS, MIYABAYASHI T. Canine chemonucleolysis: An experimental radiographic study. Vet Rad 29:168-175, 1988b.

BAILEY CS, MORGAN JP. Diseases of the spinal cord. In: Ettinger SJ, ed. Textbook of veterinary internal medicine: diseases of the dog and cat, 2nd ed. Philadelphia: WB Saunders Co, p532-607, 1983.

BAILEY CS, MORGAN JP. Congenital spinal malformations In: Diseases of the Spine, Vet Clinics of NA:SAP 22:985-1015, 1992.

BARTHEZ PY, MORGAN JP, LIPSITZ D. Discography and epidurography for evaluation of the lumbosacral junction in dogs with cauda equina syndrome. Vet Rad & Ultrasound 35:152-157, 1994.

BERZON JL, DUELAND R. Cauda equina syndrome: pathophysiology and report of seven cases. J Am Anim Hosp Assoc 15: 635-643, 1979.

BODNER DR, DELAMARTER RB, BOHLMAN HH, WITCHER M, BIRO C, RESNICK MI. Urologic changes after cauda equina compression in dogs. J Urol 143:186-190, 1990.

BRECKER SJD, PUSEY CD. Spondylosis or cauda equina syndrome in farm animals and pets. J Neurol Neurosurg Psychiatry 2:309-311, 1988.

DE LAHUNTA A. Veterinary neuroanatomy and clinical neurology. Philadelphia: WB Saunders Co, 1977 p 61.

DENNY H, BIBBS C, HOLT PE. The diagnosis and treatment of cauda equina lesions in the dog. J Small Anim Pract 23:425-443, 1982.

EVANS HE, CHRISTENSEN GC. Miller's anatomy of the dog. 2nd ed. Philadelphia: WB Saunders Co, 1979 pp 974-998.

FLETCHER TF, KITCHELL R. Anatomical studies on the spinal cord segments of the dog. Am J Vet Res 27:1759-1767, 1966.

HATHCOCK JT, PECHMAN RD, DILLON AR, KNECHT CD, BRAUND KG. Comparison of three radiographic contrast procedures in the evaluation of the canine lumbosacral canal. Vet Rad 29:4-15, 1988.

HIME JM, DRAKE JC. Osteochondrosis of the spine of the foxhound. Vet Rec 77:445-450, 1965.

HOERLEIN BF. Canine neurology. 3rd ed. Philadelphia: WB Saunders Co, 1978.

INDRIERI RJ. Lumbosacral stenosis and injury of the cauda equina. Vet Clin North Amx3.

LANG J. Flexion-extension myelography of the canine cauda equina. Vet Radiol 29: 242-257, 1988.

LANG J, JAGGY A. Die Röntgenuntersuchung der Cauda equina des Hundes. Schweizer Archiv für Tierheilkunde 131:299-309, 1989.

LANG J, HÄNI H. SCHAWALDER P. A sacral lesion resembling osteochondrosis in the German Shepherd Dog. Vet Radiol 33:69-77, 1992.

LARSEN JS. Lumbosacral transitional vertebrae in the dog. J Am Vet Radiol Soc 18:76-79, 1977.

LENEHAN TM. Canine cauda equina syndrome. Compend Contin Educ Pract Vet 5:941-950, 1983.

LORD PF, OLSSON S-E. Myelography with metrizamide in the dog: A clinical study on its use for the demonstration of spinal cord lesions other than those caused by intervertebral disk protrusion. JAVRS 17:42-50, 1976.

MORGAN JP. Congenital anomalies of the vertebral column of the dog: a study of the incidence and significance based on a radiographic and morphologic study. J Am Vet Radiol Soc 9:21-29, 1968.

MORGAN JP. Radiology in veterinary orthopedics. Philadelphia: Lea & Febiger, 1972. pp 241-247.

MORGAN JP. Techniques of veterinary radiography 5th edition Iowa State University Press, Ames Iowa. 1993. pp239-254.

MORGAN JP, BAILEY CS. Cauda equina syndrome in the dog: Radiographic evaluation. J Small Anim Pract 31:69-77, 1990.

MORGAN JP, STEPHENS M. Radiographic diagnosis and control of canine hip dysplasia. Ames: Iowa State University Press, 1985. pp 104-117.

MORGAN JP, ATILOLA M, BAILEY CS. Vertebral canal and spinal cord mensuration: a comparative study of its effect on lumbosacral myelography in the Dachshund and German Shepherd Dog. J Am Vet Med Assoc 191:951-957, 1987.

MORGAN JP, BAHR A, FRANTI CE, BAILEY CS. Lumbosacral transitional vertebrae as a predisposing cause of cauda equina syndrome in German Shepherd Dogs: 161 cases (1987-1990). JAVMA 202:1877-1882, 1993.

OLIVER JE, SELCER RR, SIMPSON S. Cauda equina compression from lumbosacral malarticulation and malformation in the dog. J Am Vet Med Assoc 173:207-214, 1978.

OLSSON SE, REILAND S. The nature of osteochondrosis in animals. Summary and conclusions with comparative aspects on osteochondritis dessicans in man. Acta Radiol (Suppl) (Stockh) 358:299-306, 1978.

SCHULMAN AJ, LIPPINCOTT CL. Canine cauda equina syndrome. Compend Contin Educ Pract Vet 10:835-844, 1988.

SISSON AF, LECOUTEUR RA, INGRAM JT, PARK RD, CHILD G. Diagnosis of cauda equina abnormalities by using electromyography, discography, and epidurography in dogs. J Vet Int Med 6:253-263, 1992.

TARVIN G, PRATA RG. Lumbosacral stenosis in dogs. J Am Vet Med Assoc 177:154-159, 1980.

WALLA L. Die Kompression der Cauda equina beim Hund. Kleintierpraxis 31:315-322, 1986.

WRIGHT JA. Spondylosis deformans of the lumbo-sacral joint in dogs. J Small Anim Pract 1980. 21:45-58, 1980.

# Chapter 7

# Osteochondrosis of the femoral condyle

## Introduction

Osteochondrosis has been defined as a disturbance of cell differentiation in metaphyseal growth plates and joint cartilage. The cartilage cells fail to mature and vesiculate, and the matrix does not calcify leading to retention of cartilage. As a result, the cartilage of the epiphyses thickens and a delay or prevention of conversion to bone occurs. The resulting deficiency in blood supply causes the cartilage in its deepest portion to become necrotic. Following the death of the cartilage, a fissure may form, permitting synovial fluid to flow into this opening resulting in further injury to viable cartilage cells. Now the lesion becomes of clinical importance because material from the degenerating cartilage can now reach the joint cavity causing a sterile inflammatory reaction within the synovium and thus becomes painful. This osteochondritis dissecans lesion is usually shallow and creates a cartilage flap similar to that seen in the humeral head, however, the flap rarely calcifies in situ. Often the lesion appears deeper in the condyle and appears as a cyst-like cavity with an opening on the articular surface without a cartilaginous flap. This pattern suggests that the lesion took origin at an early stage of condylar development and possibly started in an area of faulty cartilage growth even prior to ossification. The majority of cases involve the weight-bearing aspect of the lateral femoral condyle (Arbesser 1974; Montgomery, et al 1989), however, lesions of the medial condyle have also been noted (Denny and Gibbs 1980, Harari 1998). An OCD-like lesion has been identified within the trochlea in an English Bulldog with an unstable lateral patellar luxation. This type of lesion is not commonly seen in dogs with a primary patellar luxation.

Lafeber, et al (1959), first reported osteochondrosis of the canine stifle of larger breeds and a description of the lesion was included in the text by Hickman (1964). Then, it seems to have been forgotten and not described again until the 1970's (Robins 1970; 1978; Morgan 1972; Olsson 1975; Knecht, et al 1977; Berzon 1979), with the majority of reported cases from continental Europe (Arbesser 1974; Punzet, et al 1975). The signalment, clinical history, and clinical signs of the patients were similar in all reports. It has consistently been reported that the male is more frequently affected than the female (Arbesser 1974, Denny and Gibbs 1980) and that the condition is usually bilateral (Arbesser 1974). Littermates were reported to be affected (Knecht, et al 1977; Woodard 1979). Many references were made of "osteochondrosis" affecting the stifle joint in addition to other joints in the same dog (Knecht, et al 1977; Alexander, et al 1981; Morgan, et al 1999). Several review articles are available (Montgomery, et al 1989).

Most affected dogs belong to large breeds including the Irish Wolfhound, German Shepherd Dog, and Great Dane. According to reports, the Labrador Retriever is not frequently reported to be affected (Denny and Gibbs 1980; Montgomery, et al 1989; Studdert, et al 1990; Morgan, et al 1999). In the giant breeds, such as the Irish Wolfhound and the Great Dane, the lesions tend to be large and the lameness is clearly a stifle lameness uncomplicated by an associated hip dysplasia, as is often seen in the German Shepherd Dog.

## Clinical signs

The primary clinical sign described in all published reports of young patients is lameness in the pelvic limbs more evident after exercise. The earliest age of onset of clinical signs is 3 to 4 months; 5 to 9 months for the majority of dogs, and more than 9 months in some dogs. The older cases are usually due to delayed recognition of signs by the owner, possibly because of bilateral involvement (Arbesser 1974; Punzet, et al 1975; Denny and Gibbs 1980; Montgomery, et al 1989). However, the lameness is usually gradual in onset and is persistent. The lameness is often observed for 2 to 4 months prior to presentation for treatment and may become intermittent in cases of longer duration.

In dogs bilaterally affected, "osteochondrosis" in the stifle joint may be somewhat difficult to diagnose clinically because rather than a lameness, there is an altered gait characterized by a decrease in the range of motion of the stifle joint resulting in a stiff gait. Because of the altered gait pattern, the dog may be suspected of having hip dys-

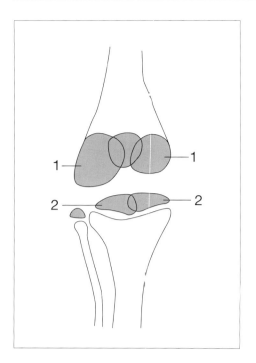
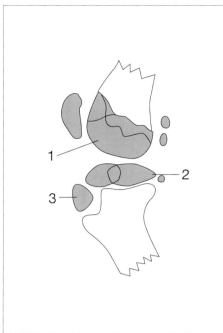

**Figure 7-1**
Drawings of the stifle joint showing ossification centers present during skeletal maturation. The femoral condyles (1) join with the trochlea to form the distal epiphysis of the femur. The tibial condyles (2) join with the tibial tuberosity (3) to form the proximal epiphysis of the tibia. The proximal fibular epiphysis, patella, and fabellae are seen as small separate centers of ossification.

plasia. Having ruled out hip dysplasia as a cause of the problem, attention should be directed to the stifle joint especially if some joint capsule thickening is noted along the medial aspect of the stifle joint. The ease in detection of the lesion is directly dependent on the lesion size. If the lesion is not large and the dog is not athletically active, a clinically silent lesion is possible. Because of this, many primary lesions may remain undiagnosed until later in life at which time they may be difficult to diagnosis because of the secondary changes of osteoarthrosis. The original lesion may also have partially healed and be no longer apparent radiographically.

In older dogs, lameness is observed only in those cases with large lesions, those with free intra-articular bony ossicles, and those with secondary osteoarthrosis (Arbesser 1974; Montgomery, et al 1989).

## Physical examination

Many of the giant breeds have a valgus deformity in the hind limbs centered on the stifle joint. This conformation may be associated with an osteochondrosis lesion of the lateral condyle. However it is arguable that the two conditions are associated. A varus deformity has also been described (Punzet, et al 1975) suggesting possible disease of the medial condyle, however, this association is also questionable. The frequency of stifle osteochondrosis is low enough to make it easy to suggest an association of that lesion with the much more common problem of valgus or varus deformity.

Patients affected bilaterally have difficulty in rising and when standing tend to adopt a crouched position with lateral rotation of the stifle joints as though trying to decrease weight bearing on the affected limbs (Denny and Gibbs 1980). Other dogs stand with the affected limb extended and abducted. These dogs may have shifting limb lameness.

In the authors' experience, the most classic presentation of osteochondrosis of the stifle joint is the finding on palpation of a thickening of the medial joint capsule without evidence of joint instability on palpation in a 6-month-old Great Dane. In the younger patient, passive motion of the joint produces discomfort.

In the dog with both hip dysplasia and "osteochondrosis" of the stifle joint, the clinical signs of hip dysplasia may overshadow those of the stifle and the stifle lesion is often overlooked, especially in those breeds in which hip dysplasia in common. Thus, this is another reason the condition is under reported.

## Anatomy and development of the femoral condyle

The developing stifle joint has a distal femoral epiphysis that forms from two separate centers of ossification representing the medial and lateral condyles and a center of ossification for the trochlea. These are visible at 2 to 3 weeks of age and the three centers join to form a separate distal femoral ossification center at 3 months. This center joins the distal femoral shaft at 8 to 11 months dependent on breed. The proximal tibia also has two separate centers of ossification that join to form the tibial plateau. They are also called condyles and are visible at 3 weeks of age and unite at 6 weeks of age. A third center of ossification is present in the proximal portion of the tibial tuberosity. It is first visible at the age of 3 months. The united centers forming the tibial plateau join with the center in the tibial tuberosity at the age of 7 months. The combined center of ossification joins the shaft of the tibia at 10 to 12 months of age dependent on breed. A small center of ossification represents the proximal epiphysis of the fibula and is present radiographically at 9 weeks and unites with the diaphysis by 8 to 12 months. The patella forms from a single center of ossification and is first visible at 9 weeks. It slowly increases in size until the time of skeletal maturation. Three small round ossification centers represent the fabella that are located on the caudal aspect of the stifle joint within the origin of the gastrocnemius muscle where they articulate with the distal femur and within the origin of the popliteus muscle. While usually having a smooth border, some are roughened and others may be formed from several separate centers of ossification and are referred to as bipartite or multipartite (Figure 7-1).

Until 3 months of age, the ossification of the femoral condyles precedes in a manner in which the margin of the bony ossification center appears roughened. This irregular outline should not be mistaken for osteochondrosis. However, by 4 months of age, this roughened border in the normal bone has become smooth. If a focal area of roughening remains after this age, the diagnosis of osteochondrosis must be entertained.

A second problem is associated with the difference in contour of the medial and lateral femoral condyles in the dog after reaching skeletal maturity. While the medial condyle is round, and full in appearance, the lateral condyle is smaller, doesn't have the full rounded appearance, and has a flattened surface. This can be mistaken for an osteochondrosis lesion.

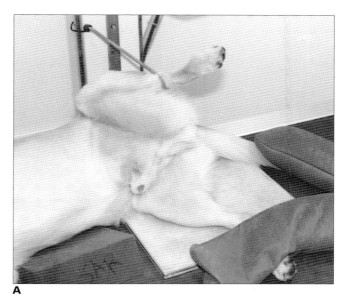

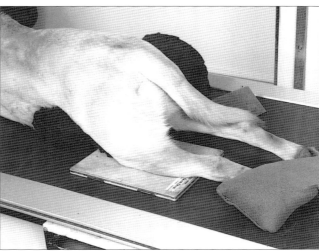

**Figure 7-2**
Photographs of a dog showing the positioning used in radiography of the stifle joint. The lateral view (A) is most easily made with the upper limb removed from the field of exposure while the foot on the affected limb is positioned using a sandbag or tie-down rope. Positioning for the caudocranial view (B) is more difficult. It is necessary to elevate the unaffected limb, tilting the pelvis, so that the sagittal plane through the stifle joint is perpendicular to the tabletop.

## Radiographic diagnosis

Two views are made of the stifle joint in the examination for osteochondrosis (Figure 7-2). Because of the small size of the joint, the views are made using "tabletop" technique. The lateral view is made with the patient laying on its side with the affected limb down and the unaffected limb removed from the field of view. Sandbags or tie-down ropes are used to position the limbs. This view

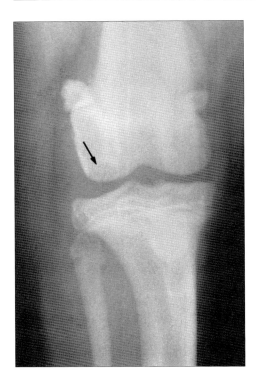 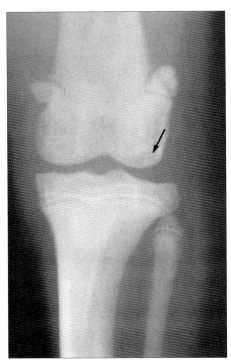

**Figure 7-3**
Radiographs of normal stifle joints with the limbs fully extended showing the smooth articular surfaces. Note the slight zone of lucency within the lateral condyle that represents the extensor fossa (arrows). This can be mistaken for an osteochondrosis lesion.

is made with slight obliquity to avoid perfect superimposition of the margins of the condyles that makes identification of a small lesion difficult.

The caudocranial view is made with the patient in sternal recumbency with the limb to be studied extended as far caudally as is possible (Figure 7-2). The unaffected limb is elevated by placement on sandbags resulting in elevation of that half of the pelvis. This creates a better position of the limb to be studied and avoids making oblique projections. This view is considered to be more diagnostic and is usually made with the femur at 30° to the tabletop and the x-ray beam angled 30° distoproximally. Thus, the caudodistal portions of the condylar margins are projected and a lesion, if present, causes an alteration in the contour of the condyle that is seen tangentially.

The normal femoral condyles have an intact, smooth articular surface (Figure 7-3). The manner in which the condyles are projected on the caudocranial view is dependent on the degree of extension of the limb and the angle of the central x-ray beam. There may be value in making more than one caudocranial view, although the lesion, if present, can be seen also on the lateral view. In the large dog, when full extension of the joint is more difficult to obtain, the intercondylar space is seen to be large and deep and the margin of the condyles appears rounded while the lateral condyle appears less full and somewhat flattened. The extensor fossa doesn't influence the margin of the lateral condyle with this positioning and any defect noted is "real" and indicates an "osteochondrosis" (Figure 7-4). In lighter breeds or heavy breeds that are anesthetized, the joint can be more completely extended for radiography and the intercondylar space is projected to be small and flattened. The margins of the condyles are smooth and complete; however, the extensor fossa creates a radiolucent area within the lateral condyle, which can be confused with an "osteochondrosis" lesion (Figure 7-3).

The same positional affect on the radiograph that can be obtained by positioning of the condyles can also be obtained through angulation of the x-ray beam within the midline of the limb. The most diagnostic view can be obtained by angling the x-ray beam so that the articular portions of the condyles are projected tangentially.

Bilateral involvement is noted in the majority of patients indicating the importance of radiography of both stifle joints regardless of the clinical signs. The principle lesion is a radiolucent area, appearing as a shallow or deep cavity, with or without sclerotic margins in the affected femoral condyle (Figure 7-4). The appearance of the lesion(s) is influenced by the radiographic view, the extension of the limb, the angle of the x-ray beam, and the extent of secondary modeling. On the lateral view, a flattening of a portion of the articular margin is often the principle abnormality. Often it is not possible to deter-

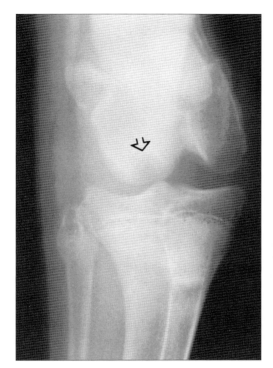 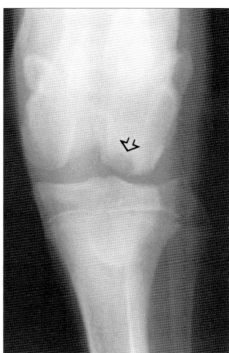

**Figure 7-4**
Caudocranial radiographs of both stifle joints of a young dog with large lesions of osteochondrosis in the lateral condyles (arrows). Note the valgus deformity. Often the bones are osteopenic from disuse.

mine which condyle is involved on this view. The lesion on this view may not be seen if there is perfect superimposition of the condylar margins.

In the caudocranial view, the appearance of the condylar defect depends on how the x-ray beam strikes the condylar articular surface plus limb position. It has been reported that lesions in the lateral condyle tend to be located caudally in the condyle, whereas, the lesions in the medial condyle tend to be located cranially (Denny and Gibbs 1980). Thus, the appearance of the lesions ranges from a flattened or irregular articular contour to a larger cystic appearing lesion with lysis extending deep into the underlying subchondral bone (Arbesser 1974, Denny and Gibbs 1980).

Wide variation in the description of the lesions may be the result of age at the onset of clinical signs, age at the time of radiography, size of the lesion, and degree of arthrosis. Also, lesions may present differently within the affected breeds, or even within affected families, thus influencing the descriptions within various reports (Denny and Gibbs 1980).

Separated joint bodies ranging up to 8 mm in size are noted frequently and are most easily identified on the lateral view (Denny and Gibbs 1980). It is possible that these free bodies represent either the original primary cartilage fragment(s) that have separated, gained a blood supply from the inflamed synovium and undergone endochondral ossification or may be due to osteochondroma formation secondary to the arthrosis. An uncommon complication of a lateral condyle "osteochondrosis" lesion is the development of a tenosynovitis of the tendon of the long digital extensor muscle with degenerative cartilage particles drifting into the tendon sheath.

With advancing age, the presence of secondary osteoarthrosis involves both the distal femur and the proximal tibia. The pattern of development is influenced by the size and location of the original lesion. Because of the wide separation between the femoral condyles and the tibial plateau, the original lesion usually remains visible on the radiograph even after the development of secondary bony changes.

Interestingly this lesion has been identified in larger members of the cat family (Figure 7-5). Generally, cats have few congenital or developmental lesions affecting the skeletal system. However, it is possible for all members of large cat families to have a genetic makeup predisposing them for "osteochondrosis." In the wild where they are under harsh conditions in which nutrition is limited, an expression of the lesions does not occur. However, in captivity where good nutrition is to be expected, the genetic defects may be expressed. This hypothesis applies to the larger breeds of cat and not the smaller breeds of domestic cats.

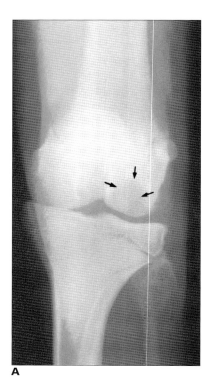 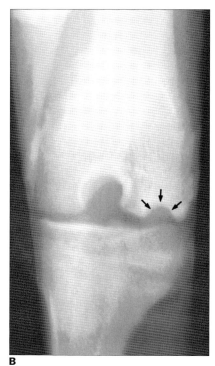 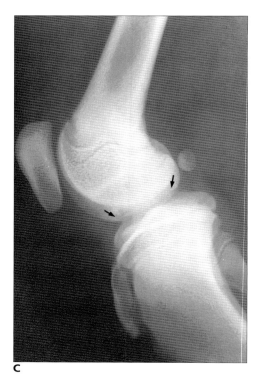

**Figure 7-5**
Caudocranial and lateral radiographs of the stifle joint of an 8 months old female Snow Leopard with lameness of 1 month. This is an excellent example of how positioning affects the projection of a large condylar lesion (arrows) on the caudocranial view. (A) If the limb is extended to a maximum and the central beam directed perpendicular to the tabletop, the more cranial, unaffected portion of the condyles is projected. (B) If the joint is flexed with a vertical x-ray beam or if the central beam is angled distoproximally, the more caudal portion of the condyle is projected. This results in better projection of the lesion in the more caudal portion of the condyles, with creation of a large intercondylar notch that results in the name, "tunnel view." The lesion can be identified on the lateral view (C) if careful attention is paid to the contour of each femoral condyle. A good appreciation is gained of the size of the lesion, the portion of the condyle affected, and the amount of affected articular surface on this view (arrows).

## Differential radiographic diagnosis

Differential radiographic diagnosis includes avulsion of the long digital extensor, which can create a radiolucent defect in the lateral femoral condyle as seen radiographically (Bardet and Piermattei 1983). However, that lesion is located further laterally on the caudocranial view and further proximal and cranial on the lateral view than a femoral condylar osteochondrosis. Because the avulsion is extra-articular, changes of secondary joint disease are not present. Aberrant origin of the cranial cruciate ligament (Dueland, et al 1982) may cause a secondary lucency that might be suggestive of osteochondrosis. Avulsion of the attachment of the popliteus muscle or head of the gastrocnemius muscle are uncommon causes of stifle joint lameness and might be confused with an "osteochondrosis" lesion radiographically.

While the radiographic changes of the conditions described above might be suggestive of an "osteochondrosis" lesion, the clinical picture varies markedly in the: (1) difference in age at time of presentation, (2) difference in the breeds that are involved, and (3) difference in the physical findings on palpation.

## Treatment

### Conservative treatment

Long term conservative treatment of lameness of the stifle joint is attempted frequently because the cause of the lameness remains unrecognized or because surgical treatment is not advised by the clinician or accepted by the owner. This conservative treatment consists of weight and exercise control and judicious use of analgesics. These patients often have the smaller lesions and this therapy may have a moderate degree of success. In the dogs with larger lesions, conservative therapy is not recommended and instead, surgical removal of the cartilage flap is probably of the most benefit, although a progressive osteoarthrosis is anticipated.

## Surgical treatment

Surgical treatment seems to be logical in the acutely lame dog hoping for a reduction in the duration of lameness with a healing of the primary lesion that might curtail the development of the secondary arthrosis. In the young dog, regardless of the size of the lesion, surgical removal of the cartilage flap if advisable for the following reasons: (1) to limit the synovitis reducing the production of degenerative cartilage products, (2) to encourage healing of the defect, and (3) to reduce the degree of osteoarthrosis. Following cartilage flap removal, the lesion is curetted to encourage invasion of the healing blood supply (Leighton 1981).

In the more chronic cases, where it is assumed that the cartilage flap has separated, the main purpose of the surgery is lavage of the joint in the hope that cartilage fragments can be flushed out and the chronic synovitis can be reduced.

The negative affect from the trauma of the arthrotomy when compared with the potential value of the lavage may balance out and leave the patient's clinical signs essentially unchanged. The advent of lavage through means of an arthroscopic technique may be thought of as the treatment of the future, when the required equipment becomes generally available.

## Prognosis

Prognosis for achieving a happy and comfortable pet seems to be indirectly correlated with the size of the lesion. For the dog with a small lesion, the prognosis is relatively good even with conservative therapy. In the dog with a medium size lesion, the prognosis is guarded, but it can be improved by surgical intervention. In the dog with a large lesion, even with surgery the prognosis is very poor and euthanasia may be a proper alternative. Because of the persistence of the injury to the articular surface, the prognosis for the dog to be an active athletic dog is always guarded.

## Heritability

Osteochondrosis of the femoral condyle seems to fall into the general pattern of heritability assigned to osteochondrosis in other sites and in other species. Because of the almost exclusive occurrence within large and giant breeds, a genetic tendency is suggested. However, the possible influence of rapid weight gain and heavy body weight on occurrence of the disease is suggested in case reports. These are influenced by heredity as well as by the nature of feeding the dog. Thus, osteochondrosis in the stifle joint must be considered in light of these facts with the apparent certainty that the disease does fit into a pattern seen in other inherited diseases.

Thus, the prudent breeder would be wise to avoid the use of affected dogs in their breeding program. However, remembering that use of a minimally affected dog with good traits coming from a background that appears to generally free of the disease may be a more acceptable practice than use of a dog that is free of the disease, but has numerous siblings or offspring that are affected. However, the breeder might choose to consider that the disease has such a low frequency that it is wise to completely exclude the phenotypically affected dog, along with all family members from all breeding programs.

# References

ALEXANDER JW, RICHARDSON DC, SELCER BA. Osteochondritis dissecans of the elbow, stifle, and hock: A review. JAAHA 17:51-56,1981.

ARBESSER E. Osteochondrosis dissecans der Femurkondylen beim Hund. Wien tierärztl Mschr 61:303-313,1974.

BARDET JF, PIERMATTEI DL. Long digital extensor and popliteal tendon avulsion associated with lateral patellar luxation in a dog. JAVMA 183:465-6,1983.

BERZON JL. Osteochondritis dissecans in the dog: diagnosis and therapy. JAVMA 175:796-799,1979.

DENNY HR, GIBBS C. Osteochondritis dissecans of the canine stifle joint. J Sm Anim Pract 21:317-322,1980.

DUELAND R, SISSON D, EVANS HE. Aberrant origin of the cranial cruciate ligament mimicking an osteochondral lesion radiographically. Vet Rad 23:175-177,1982.

HARARI J. Osteochondrosis of the femur. Vet Clinics of NA/SAP 28:87-94,1998.

HICKMAN J. Veterinary Orthopaedics. Oliver and Boyd, Edinburgh and London,1964.

KNECHT CD, VAN SICKLE DC, BLEVANS WE, AVOLT MD, HUGHES RB, CANTWELL HD. Osteochondrosis of the shoulder and stifle in 3 of 5 Border collie littermates. JAVMA 170:58-60,1977.

LAFEBER TJ, BECKWITH J, STROMBECK DR. What is your diagnosis? JAVMA 134:267-268,1959.

LEIGHTON RL. Surgical treatment of osteochondritis dissecans of the canine stifle. Vet Med SAC 74:1733-36,1981.

MORGAN JP, WIND A, DAVIDSON AP. Bone dysplasias in the Labrador Retriever: A radiographic study. JAAHA 35: 332-340, 1999

MONTGOMERY DD, MILTON JL, HENDERSON RA, HATHCOCK JT. Osteochondritis dissecans of the canine stifle. Cont Ed 11:1199-1205,1989.

MORGAN JP. Radiology in Veterinary Orthorpedics. Lea and Febiger, Philadelphia 1972, pp345-348.

OLSSON S-E. Lameness in the dog. A review of lesions causing osteoarthrosis of the shoulder, elbow, hip, stifle and hock. Proc 42nd Annu Mtg AAHA, 1975, pp364-370.

PUNZET G, WALDE I, ARBESSER E. Zur Osteochondrosis dissecans genu des Hundes. Kleintierpraxis 20:88-98,1975.

ROBINS GM. A case of osteochondritis dissecans of the stifle joints in a bitch. J Sm Anim Pract 11:813-817,1970.

ROBINS GM. Osteochondritis dissecans in the dog. Aust Vet J 54:272-279,1978.

STUDDERT VP, LAVELLE RB, BEILHARZ RB, MASON TA. Heritability of osteochondrosis in Labrador Retrievers. International Elbow Working Group, San Francisco CA,1990.

WOODARD DC. Osteochondritis dissecans in a family of bull terriers. Vet Med SAC 74:936,1979.

# Chapter 8

# Osteochondrosis of the talus

## Introduction

Osteochondrosis of the talus, the main weight-bearing bone in the hock joint, is similar in gross and histological appearance to osteochondrosis in other locations within the skeletal system (Alexander, et al 1981; Olsson 1981). The basic pathogenesis seen histologically is a failure of development of the immature joint cartilage. At the site of the lesion, the cartilage fails to undergo provisional calcification, and subsequently is not replaced by bone. This failure of endochondral ossification leads to retention or thickening of the cartilage followed by necrosis and dissecting fissures in the deep layers. Often in osteochondrosis of the talus, the cartilage flap is invaded by a capillary bed originating from the irritated synovium or from the joint capsule (Olsson 1975, 1976, 1984, 1987, 1993; Probst and Johnson 1993). Because of the re-establishment of a blood supply, the possibility of endochondral ossification exists even after separation of the cartilage flap from its bed. Because of the anatomy of the talus, the flap usually remains in situ and thus the ossification is noted in situ. In contrast, in osteochondrosis in the humeral head the flap, when in situ, lacks this soft tissue attachment and any secondary ossification cannot take place until the fragment falls free into the joint capsule.

The Rottweiler has frequently been reported to have osteochondrosis of the talus (Rosenblum, et al 1978; Mason and Lavelle 1979; Wisner, et al 1980) and in this breed, males have been reported to be affected more than females (Mason and Lavelle 1979) as is the case of osteochondrosis in other sites (Olsson 1987). In addition, the Labrador Retriever has been reported to be affected (Studdert, et al 1990). The age at the onset of clinical signs is 4 to 7 months. Many dogs are bilaterally affected (Rosemblum, et al 1978; Alexander 1980; Fitch and Beale 1998).

While early cases reported involvement of the medial ridge of the talus (Denny 1981; Koppel 1984; Breur, et al 1989; Brinker, et al 1990; Robins 1978), later reports described lesions in the lateral ridge as well (Johnson 1980; Aron, et al 1985; Robins, et al 1983; van Ee, et al 1988; Carlisle, et al 1990; Wisner, et al 1990). This delay in recognition of the lateral ridge lesions may have been due to the lesion in this location being more difficult to recognize radiographically.

## Clinical signs

The presenting clinical sign in a unilaterally affected dog is an obvious lameness characterized by a fixed position of the talocrural (tibiotarsal or hock) joint when the dog is standing or walking. Affected dogs tend to have a straight hind limb conformation and their entire movement is constrained. When running, the dog may have a tendency to carry the limb. As is usually the case, when a joint lesion is bilateral, the lameness may be less obvious because both limbs are painful and the gait is altered and characterized by reduced hind limb motion centered especially on the talocrural joint. In the bilaterally but unequally affected dog, the clinical signs in the form of lameness may be obvious in the most affected limb only. Eventually, in dogs so affected, a subtle lameness may be detected in the less affected opposite limb.

The reduced flexion of the hock joint, or the straighter than normal hock, is evident on standing and walking, although the length of stride may be reduced with signs of pain seen on movement. However, this may be difficult to evaluate because of an inability to compare the length of the stride with what should be considered normal. If affected bilaterally, the poor hind limb movement noticed by the owner often causes concern about hip dysplasia (Mason and Lavelle 1979).

## Physical examination

On physical examination of the patient with a medial lesion, thickening of the joint capsule over the medial malleolus is often detected. Pressure over this area causes pain and the dog responds by quick withdrawal of the limb. Because of the accessibility of the medial malleolus, even minor thickening of the joint capsule is detectable and the pain response is very prominent on slight pressure.

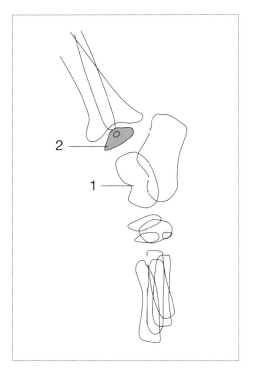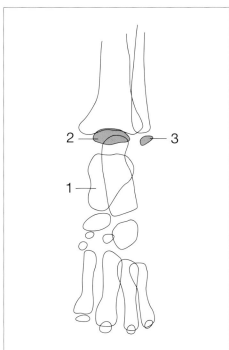

**Figure 8-1**
Drawings of a radiograph of the tarsal region in a puppy that show the single ossification center of the talus (1) and the adjacent ossification center of the distal tibial epiphysis (2). The small ossification center of the distal fibula is identified (3).

In the patient with a lateral lesion, the joint capsule thickness is less obvious, more difficult to detect, and slower to develop, probably because of the presence of the larger and more distally located lateral malleolus. Therefore, examination of this site is less rewarding. The diagnosis of a lateral lesion is therefore made by gait analysis and radiographic examination. Many assume the clinical signs and findings on palpation to be similar whether the lesion is medial or lateral, however, the secondary change in the form of joint capsule thickening is always more easily detected medially. Periarticular soft tissue thickening is dependent on chronicity of the lesion.

Capsular distention secondary to effusion is another finding that may appear in both acute and chronic cases and becomes more evident at the dog ages. This effusion is most often evident cranially and medially. On passive movement of the joint, the range of motion may be decreased and crepitation and pain may be evident. In particular, pain may be elicited upon forced flexion.

With advancement of osteoarthrosis secondary to osteochondritis dissecans of the talus, the condition generally becomes less painful with movement, but limb stiffness is obvious and gross thickening of the joint is evident. The signs associated with the osteoarthrosis are similar to those seen in any other joint so affected. In exceptional cases with a medial lesion, pieces of detached cartilage flap may lodge in the tendon sheath of the flexor hallucis longus muscle and cause a chronic tenosynovitis.

# Anatomy and development of the talus

All of the tarsal bones are visible radiographically by 4 weeks of age. Each tarsal bone forms from a single center of ossification that begins small and slowly increases in size until skeletal maturation at 8 to 12 months of age. Proximal to the talus, or tibial tarsal bone, is the distal tibial epiphysis. This appears ununited until 8 to 12 months of age. Adjacent to the talus on the lateral side is a separate center of ossification for the distal fibula. This closes later in skeletal maturation. In the younger patient, the trochlea of the talus is incompletely ossified and appears flattened. With further development, the rounded trochlear ridges form and the possibility of identification of an osteochondrosis increases (Figure 8-1).

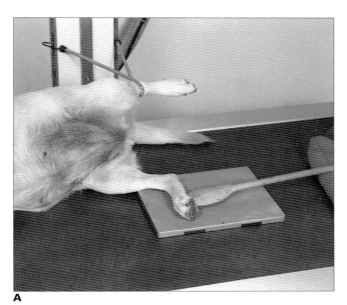 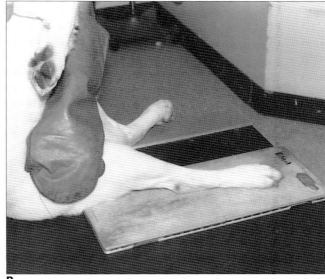

**Figure 8-2**
Photographs illustrate patient positioning for the lateral view (A) and the dorsoplantar view (B) of the tarsal region. It is recommended that the joint be positioned on the lateral view in a manner that removes the talus from superimposing the caudal malleolus.

## Radiographic diagnosis

Two views are usually made of the tarsus in the evaluation of osteochondrosis (Figure 8-2). The lateral view is made with the dog on its side with the affected side down with the uppermost limb removed from the region of the central beam. A comparison of two lateral views made with the foot positioned in a flexed position and a more extended position allows for more complete examination of the curvature of the trochlea.

The orthogonal view can be made with the dog in a sitting position with the limb extended and the beam directed in a dorsoplantar direction. This view can also be made with the dog on its sternum with the limb extended caudally and the beam directed in a plantarodorsal direction. The resulting radiographs are similar and influenced only by the degree of extended flexion (the straightness of the hock joint). An additional view of great value is the flexed dorsoplantar view made with the dog in dorsal recumbency with the limb flexed at the stifle and tarsal joint with the cassette elevated by placement on a stand or box. The tarsal joints are flexed at 15° and the central x-ray beam in directed vertically (Miyabayashi, et al 1991). Normal anatomy of this joint has been clearly described (Carlisle and Reynolds 1990).

The trochlear ridges must be carefully examined on the radiograph of a patient with suspected osteochondritis dissecans. On the lateral view in the normal dog, three curvilinear lines represent the articular margins of the trochlear ridges and the depressed center of the trochlea. These lines are seen to be concentric on the well-positioned lateral radiograph, with the larger lateral ridge positioned proximal to the medial ridge. The concentric ring representing a diseased ridge in an affected dog may appear to be "broken," have a portion "missing," or have a flattened margin (Figure 8-3). In the authors' experience, the lateral views of the affected young dog without secondary changes is more diagnostic than the oblique views in the detection of either cranial or caudal lesions on the medial or lateral ridges, but especially when the lesion is located more caudally. The lateral views are made more diagnostic by the use of different degrees of flexion. Any of the changes in contour of the articular surfaces should be considered diagnostic of "osteochondrosis" even though the lesion cannot be identified on the plantarodorsal view.

On the plantarodorsal or dorsoplantar views, the ridges and interposed depression are easily seen, however, the radiograph only projects a small portion of the contour of the trochlear ridges and, thus, may only identify a lesion if it is positioned so as to be "seen" tangentially by the central x-ray beam. The oblique views have been especially touted as helpful in identification of lesions on the lateral ridge. However, the caudal location of many lesions makes these views of little value. The use of the

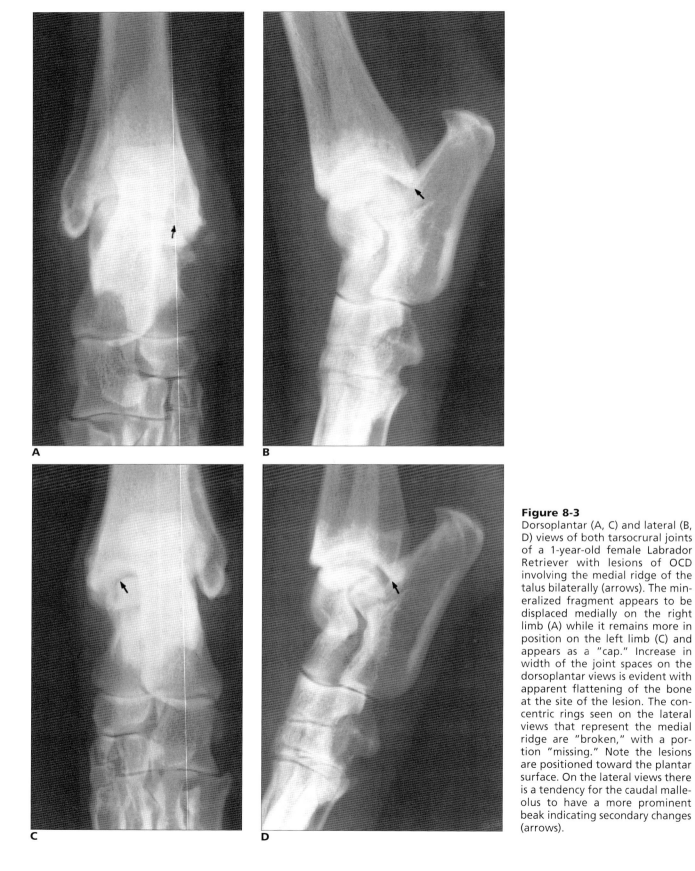

**Figure 8-3**
Dorsoplantar (A, C) and lateral (B, D) views of both tarsocrural joints of a 1-year-old female Labrador Retriever with lesions of OCD involving the medial ridge of the talus bilaterally (arrows). The mineralized fragment appears to be displaced medially on the right limb (A) while it remains more in position on the left limb (C) and appears as a "cap." Increase in width of the joint spaces on the dorsoplantar views is evident with apparent flattening of the bone at the site of the lesion. The concentric rings seen on the lateral views that represent the medial ridge are "broken," with a portion "missing." Note the lesions are positioned toward the plantar surface. On the lateral views there is a tendency for the caudal malleolus to have a more prominent beak indicating secondary changes (arrows).

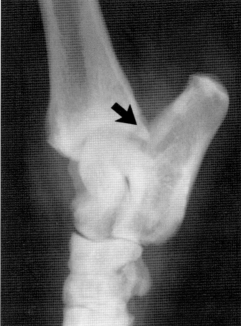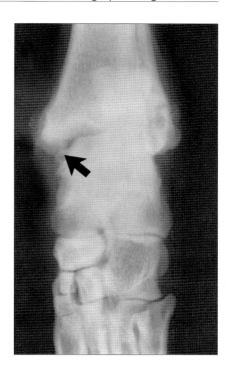

**Figure 8-4**
Dorsoplantar and lateral views of a talocrural joint of a 2-year-old male Rottweiler with bony changes typical of osteoarthrosis secondary to an osteochondrosis. In this dog, identification of the primary osteochondrosis of the medial ridge of the talus (arrow) is more difficult and the arthrosis might be thought to be secondary to trauma. On the lateral view, the joint is markedly modeled typical of that seen with an OCD lesion.

special dorsoplantar view is of value in correcting this problem.

With a lesion in the medial ridge of the trochlea of the talus, a prominent radiographic change noted on the dorsoplantar (plantarodorsal) view is an increase in width of the tibiotarsal joint space medially associated with flattening of the medial ridge of the affected bone (Figure 8-3). Later, this flattening becomes more rounded as bony modeling occurs. The increase in width of the joint space and flattened ridge result from the loss of bony tissue from the ridge of the trochlea. In some cases, a thin radiodense line is seen just proximal to the OCD lesion represents the presence of an undisplaced mineralized cartilage cap, indicating establishment of an intact blood supply to the cartilage flap. It may fragment at a later time and small pieces become displaced, seen on the radiograph as joint bodies, typically located cranially. If the cartilage flap remains intact, it can remain in situ and ossify. The subchondral bone within the distal tibia usually remains unchanged and does not appear to respond to the disruption of the opposing articular surface. This may change as the secondary arthrosis progresses.

If the lesion is within the lateral ridge, radiographic assessment is complicated by superimposition of the fibular tarsal bone in the dorsoplantar (plantarodorsal) view. The primary lesion in the lateral ridge appears similar to that seen in the medial ridge except that mineralization of the flap is less likely. The dorsolateral-medioplantar oblique view may be particularly useful in identification of these lesions (Wisner, et al 1990; Carlisle, et al 1990). Diagnosis of lesions in either ridge can be made using arthroscopy (Van Ryssen and van Bree H 1992, 1993). Secondary changes are similar to those expected in an osteoarthrosis, but tend to center adjacent to the lesion.

Enthesophytes form especially around the medial malleolus because of joint instability. Free ossified bodies, may be identified adjacent to the tip of the medial malleolus on the dorsoplantar (plantarodorsal) view and are thought to represent avulsion fractures (Rosenblum, et al 1978; Carlisle 1979; Johnson, et al 1980). However, free joint bodies adjacent to the articular surface of the medial malleolus are thought to originate from the OCD lesion. With chronicity, the degenerative joint disease progresses with enthesophytes seen cranially and caudally on the distal tibia and on the cranial, medial, and lateral aspect of body of the talus (Figure 8-4). A prominent secondary change is the pointing of the caudal malleolus of the tibia in an effort to increase the size of the articular surface in response to the joint laxity (Figures 8-3, 8-4).

## Differential radiographic diagnosis

The major differential diagnosis is found in the dog with post-traumatic changes in the talocrural joint in which the appearance of the secondary changes is similar to those that develop in the joint with an OCD lesion. If the arthrosis is extensive, visualization of the contour of the trochlea and identification of the OCD lesion is more difficult. This is not a problem in recommending treatment or determining prognosis for an affected dog, since the secondary osteoarthrosis is the cause of the clinical signs and is similar whether due to an osteochondrosis or trauma. However, in the potential breeding dog, the determination of the cause of the arthrosis has greater importance.

## Treatment

### Conservative treatment

Conservative treatment may play a role in management of OCD of the hock although many suggest that early diagnosis and surgical intervention are essential to the prevention of chronic lameness (Olsson 1975; Leighton 1979; Mason and Lavelle 1979; Johnson, et al 1980). However, the author's experience is that in most cases, regardless of the type of treatment, progressive arthrosis can be expected (Smith, et al 1985).

### Surgical treatment

Surgical treatment may be compromised by the limited access to the joint via the joint capsule (in contrast to an approach via the osteotomy of the medial malleolus). A wider approach is not considered because of the possibility of interfering with the integrity of the medial collateral ligament and thus, with the stability of the joint. An osteotomy of the medial malleolus in a young dog provides a better access to the joint, but the softness of the malleolus in a dog of this age results in failure of stabilization of the osteotomy site. These problems in surgical approach may prevent the detection of lesions in less accessible parts of the joint either cranial or caudal and may lead to overlooking the presence of free fragments. The smallness of the joint space often makes lavage ineffective further compromising the results of the surgery.

Notwithstanding all of these problems, the effectiveness of the surgery is increased if it is performed early, with the removal of the loose cartilaginous flap and curettage of the underlying cartilage defect. The immediate result is that the dog is more comfortable. However, the articular surface remains incongruent and the secondary arthrosis will progress rapidly, especially if a major portion of the weight-bearing surface is involved. Still, it is hoped that by early removal of the fragment, a part of the cause for development of the arthrosis is removed. One report suggested that surgical treatment had little affect on limiting the progression of osteoarthrosis and did not reduce the level of lameness later in life or increase the dog's use of the limb (Smith, et al 1985). However, these dogs underwent surgery after prominent bony changes were present indicating marked osteoarthrosis was already present. Despite all of these warnings, the clinician may be rewarded by seeing a patient with extreme pain and lameness change into a playful happy puppy following surgery. This suggests that the pain from the synovitis due to the cartilage fragment and cartilage products may be much more severe than the pain from the chronic osteoarthrosis.

## Prognosis

Generally, the prognosis for use of the limb is poor because of late detection of the lesion and the rather extensive development of secondary osteoarthrosis at the time of diagnosis. If the best results are to be obtained, diagnosis and treatment should be done early. The frequent bilateral involvement further affects the prognosis. Because of the guarded prognosis for this disease, any affected dog should be considered a poor candidate for any type of work or athletic activity regardless of the type of treatment or the age of the dog at the time of treatment.

## Heritability

The frequency of occurrence of OCD of the talus in Rottweilers and Labrador Retrievers suggests a breed predisposition. Littermates have been reported to be affected as well as a sire producing several affected dogs, thus, pointing to the likelihood of osteochondrosis of the talus being an inherited disease (Olsson 1976; Johnson, et al 1980; Olson, et al 1980). Thus, the prudent breeder would be wise to avoid the use of affected dogs in their breeding program. Since the disease has a low frequency, the complete exclusion of the phenotypically affected dog, along with all family members, from all breeding programs might be considered.

# References

ALEXANDER JW. Osteochondritis dissecans of the hock in the dog. Cal Vet 2,9-11,1980.

ALEXANDER JW, RICHARDSON DC, SELCER BA. Osteochondritis dissecans of the elbow, stifle and hock - a review. JAAHA 17:51-56,1981.

ARON DN, MAHAFFEY MB, ROWLAND GN. Free chondral fragment involving the lateral trochlear ridge of the talus in a dog. JAVMA 186:1095-1096,1985.

BREUR GJ, SPAULDING KA, BRADEN TD. Osteochondritis dissecans of the medial trochlear ridge of the talus in the dog. Vet Comp Orthop Trauma 4:168-176,1989.

BRINKER WO PIERMATTEI DL FLO GL. Osteochondritis dissecans of the talus. In: Handbook of small animal orthopedics and fracture treatment. 2nd ed. Philadelphia: WB Saunders Co. 1990 pp.441-443.

CARLISLE CH. Osteochondritis dissecans of the canine tarsus: a radiographic study. Abstract. 1st Scientic meeting, Radiology Chapter, Australian College of Veterinary Scientists May 14, 1978. J Am Vet Radiol Soc 20:79,1979.

CARLISLE CH REYNOLDS KM. Radiographic anatomy of the tarsocrurial joint of the dog. J Sm Anim Pract 31:273-279,1990.

CARLISLE CH ROBINS GM REYNOLDS KM. Radiographic signs of osteochondrosis dissecans of the lateral ridge of the trochlea tali in the dog. J Sm Anim Pract 31:280-286,1990.

DENNY HR. Osteochondritis dissecans of the hock joint in the dog. Veterinary Annual 21:224-228,1981.

FITCH RB BEALE BS. Osteochondrosis of the canine tibiotarsal joint. Vet Clinics of NA/SAP 28:95-113,1998.

JOHNSON KA. Osteochondritis dissecans of the lateral ridge of the tibial tarsal bone in a dog. Aust Vet J 56:615-616.1980.

JOHNSON KA, HOWLETT CR, PETTIT GD. Osteochondrosis in the hock joints in dogs. JAAHA 16:103-113, 1980,

KOPPEL E. Osteochondrosis disseccans im Sprunggelenk des Hundes. Kleintierpraxis 29:291-300,1984.

LEIGHTON RL. Osteochondritis dissecans of the hock in a dog. Vm/SAC 85:325-329,1979.

MASON TA, LAVELLE RB. Ostseochondritis dissecans of the tibial tarsal bone in dogs. J Sm Anim Pract 20:423-432,1979.

MIYABAYASHI T, BILLER DS, MANLEY PA, et al. Use of a flexed dorsoplantar radiographic view of the talocrural joint to evaluate lameness in two dogs. J Am Vet Med Assoc 199:598-600,1991.

OLSON NC, MOSTOSKY UV, FLO GL, TVEDTEN HW. Osteochondritis dissecans of the tarsocrural joint in three canine siblings. JAVMA 176:635-637.1980.

OLSSON S-E. Lameness in the dog. A review of lesions causing osteoarthrosis of the shoulder, elbow, hip, stifle, and hock joint. Proceedings 42nd Annu Mtg AAHA 1975, pp 364-370.

OLSSON S-E. Osteochondrosis - A growing problem to dog breeders. Progress. Gaines Dog Research Center. Summer Edition, 1:4-11,1976.

OLSSON S-E. Pathophysiology, morphology, and clinical signs of osteochondrosis in the dog. In: Bojrab MJ,ed. Pathophysiology in Small Animal Surgery, Philadelphia Lea & Febiger 1981 pp 604-617.

OLSSON S-E. Pathogenesis and pathology of osteochondritis dissecans of the hock joint in the dog. Proceed ALCOV, 2nd Int Meeting of dog articular surg, Morzine-Avoriaz Jan 17-19, 35, 1984.

OLSSON S-E. General and local aetiologic factors in canine osteochondrosis. Vet Quart 9:268-278,1987.

OLSSON S-E. Pathophysiology, morphology, and clinical signs of osteochondrosis in the dog. In: Disease mechanisms in small animal surgery. 2nd ed. Philadelphia: Lea & Febiger, 1993; 793-795.

PROBST CW, JOHNSTON SA. Osteochondrosis. In: Textbook of small animal surgery. Vol 2. Philadelphia: WB Saunders Co, 1993 pp 1962-1965.

ROBINS GH. Osteochondritis dissecans in the dog. Aust V J 54:272-279,1978.

ROBINS GM, READ RA, CARLISLE CH, WEBB SM. Osteochondritis dissecans of the lateral ridge of the trochlea of the tibial tarsal bone in the dog. J Sm Anim Pract 24:675-685,1983.

ROSENBLUM GP, ROBINS GM, CARLISLE CH. Osteochondritis dissecans of the tibio-tarsal joint in the dog. J Sm Anim Pract 19:759-767,1978.

SMITH MM, VASSEUR PB, MORGAN JP. Clinical evaluation of dogs after surgical and nonsurgical management of osteochondritis dissecans of the talus. JAVMA 187:31-35,1985.

STUDDERT VP, LAVELLE RB, BEILHARZ RB, MASON TA. Heritability of osteochondrosis in Labrador Retrievers. Presentation 1990 International Elbow Working Group, San Francisco CA.

VAN EE RT, GIBSON K, ROBERTS ED. Osteochondritis dissecans of the lateral ridge of the talus in a dog. JAVMA 193:1284-1286,1988.

VAN RYSSEN B, VAN BREE H. Arthroscopic evaluation of osteochondrosis lessions in the canine hock joint: A review of two cases. JAAHA 28:295-299,1992.

VAN RYSEN B, VAN BREE H. Arthroscopy of the canine hock joint. JAAHA 29:107-115,1993.

WISNER ER, BERRY CR, MORGAN JP, POOL RR, WIND AP, VASSEUR PB. Osteochondrosis of the lateral trochlar ridge of the talus in seven Rottweiler dogs. Vet Surg 19:435-439,1990.

# Chapter 9

# Bone dysplasias in the Labrador Retriever: A radiographic study (Morgan, et al 1999)

## Introduction

Breeders of Labrador Retrievers have been aware for many years of the problem of heritable hip dysplasia in the Labrador Retriever. Heritable bone or joint diseases have been reported during the last 15 years to exist commonly in the shoulder joint (osteochondrosis) (Vaughan 1968, Smith and Stowater 1975), elbow joint (joint incongruity, ununited anconeal process, medial coronoid process disease, or osteochondrosis of the humeral condyle) (Grøndalen 1979, Olsson 1983), and tarsocrural joint (osteochondrosis) (Olson, et al 1980; Smith, et al 1985) of the Labrador Retriever.

The presence of these diseases is not always obvious to an owner because the lameness may be subtle. If the disease is present bilaterally, an abnormal gait without an obvious lameness is produced. Initial studies have found these diseases to be present even in bench (conformation) champions in which clinical signs were overlooked during competition involving gait evaluation. One reason these diseases have become so common in the Labrador Retriever may be that affected dogs without obvious lameness have been used inadvertently for breeding. The increased popularity of the dog may also have contributed to the incidence of the diseases through indiscriminate breeding.

Recently, transitional lumbosacral vertebral segments (TLVS) have been suggested as a cause of cauda equina syndrome (Morgan, et al 1993). Because clinical signs of cauda equina syndrome may be confused with hip dysplasia, examination of the lumbosacral junction was included in the study. Since the stifle joints were routinely included in the radiographic examination of hip dysplasia, the incidence of osteochondrosis of the stifle joint was also documented. The results from 1018 dogs are included.

## Materials and methods

The presence of osteochondrosis of the humeral head, distal femoral condyle, and talar trochlea, in addition to elbow dysplasia, hip dysplasia, and lumbosacral vertebral transitional disease were recorded. No distinction was made between osteochondrosis and osteochondritis dissecans. Only dogs 12 months of age or older were included.

## Radiographic studies

Radiographic studies were made using the following protocol: (1) a single mediolateral view of each shoulder joint with the forelimb extended cranially; (2) two mediolateral views of each elbow joint, one tightly flexed (<90), and one extended (120); (3) one ventrodorsal (VD) view of the pelvis and hind limbs using conventional positioning with the hind limbs extended caudally that permitted evaluation of the hip joints, stifle joints, and the lumbosacral region, (Rendano and Ryan 1985); and (4) plantarodorsal and mediolateral views of each tarsus. Mild tranquilization was used in preparation of the dogs for study when required.

Shoulder joints were judged normal if the humeral head was of uniform bony density and presented with a smooth contour of the bony epiphysis. Shoulder joints were judged affected if a defect in the caudomedial contour of the bony epiphysis of the humeral head was noted. A shoulder in which a small smooth periarticular bony lip on the caudal aspect of the humeral head was the only abnormal finding was evaluated to be within normal limits.

Elbow joints were judged normal if the bones fit tightly and no evidence of osteoarthrosis was noted. Elbow joints were judged affected if osteoarthrosis was present as indicated by reactive new bone (periarticular osteophytes or enthesophytes) involving the (1) anconeal process, (2) area adjacent to the ulnar trochlear notch, and (3) lateral epicondylar ridge. Features of osteoarthrosis were seen in conjunction with any of the following: (1) joint incongruity, (2) medial coronoid process disease, (3) a radiolucent zone within the anconeal process diagnostic of an ununited anconeal process, or a (4) defect within the bony contour of the medial aspect of the humeral condyle diagnostic of an osteochondrosis. Elbow joints with only minimal incongruity or minimal new bone formation were evaluated to be within normal limits.

Hip joints were judged normal if the bones forming the hip joint fit tightly and there was no evidence of new bone formation on the femoral head, neck, or acetabulum. Hip joints were judged affected if any of the following were noted: (1) joint laxity, (2) incongruity between femoral head and acetabulum, or (3) secondary bony changes, in particular, on the caudal aspect of the femoral neck (Morgan and Stephens 1985). Hip joints with minimal joint laxity and no signs of new bone formation or signs of minimal new bone formation and no joint laxity were evaluated to be within normal limits. Distraction techniques were not used.

The stifle joints were judged normal if the contour of the condyles was smooth and intact. Stifle joints were judged affected if a defect was noted within the bony contour of either condyle on the craniocaudal projection (Montgomery, et al 1989).

The tarsocrural joints were judged normal if the contours of the trochlea were smooth and intact and no evidence of osteoarthrosis was present. The tarsocrural joints were judged affected if any of the following were seen: (1) a defect in the bony contour of either trochlear ridge or either view, (2) free intra-articular bony fragments, or (3) spurring of the caudal tibia on the lateral view with modeling of the articular surface (Smith, et al 1985). A site was evaluated as affected whether the lesion was detected unilaterally or bilaterally.

The lumbosacral region was judged affected if any of the following were noted: (1) a radiolucent disc space between the normally fused first and second sacral segments, (2) laterally-positioned wing-like sacral processes from the anomalous segment, (3) sacral asymmetry characterized by a lumbar transverse process opposed by a sacral wing on the anomalous segment, or (4) separation of the spinous processes of the sacrum (Morgan 1998). A dog was evaluated as affected if one or more sites were judged positive for disease.

## Results

The total of 1018 dogs (370 male, 648 female) was divided by ages (Table 9-1). The frequency of normal dogs and dogs affected in at least one site, was calculated (Table 9-2). Of the six sites studied, one affected site was found in 250 dogs (24.6%), two affected sites in 68 dogs (6.7%), three affected sites in 12 dogs (1.2%), with no dogs having four,

**Table 9-1: Age in months of a Labrador Retriever population in a radiographic study of inherited bone and joint disease.**

| | |
|---|---|
| 12 to 24 | 585 |
| 24 to 36 | 273 |
| 36 to 48 | 55 |
| 48 to 120 | 105 |
| Totals | 1018 |
| Average age | 24.4 |
| Median age | 18.01 |

**Table 9-2: Status of dogs as determined radiographically in 1018 Labrador Retrievers, by sex.**

| | Normal | | Affected |
|---|---|---|---|
| Total | 688 (67.6%) | Total | 330 (32.4%) |
| Male | 230 (62.2%) | Male | 140 (37.8%) |
| Female | 458 (70.7%) | Female | 190 (29.3%) |

five, or six sites affected. The majority of lesions were present bilaterally.

Shoulders were affected in 38 dogs (3.7%) (Table 9-3) in which humeral head osteochondrosis was the only positive finding in 26 (2.6%). Elbows were affected in 180 dogs (17.7%) (Table 9-4) in which elbow dysplasia was the only positive finding in 111 (10.9%). Hips were affected in 128 dogs (12.6%) (Table 9-5) in which hip dysplasia was the only positive finding in 65 (6.4%). The femoral condyle was affected in seven dogs (0.7%) (Table 9-6) in which osteochondrosis of the femoral condyle was the only positive finding in 4 (0.4%). Tarsocrural joints were affected in 32 dogs (3.1%) (Table 9-7) in which osteochondrosis of the trochlea was the only positive finding in 14 (1.4%). In dogs having more than one site affected, the most frequent combination of elbow and hip dysplasia was noted in 43 dogs (4.2%).

An anomalous vertebral segment was noted at the lumbosacral junction in 37 dogs (3.6%) (Table 9-8). It was possible to examine the offspring from the sire or dam of 14 dogs with LS lesions. TLSV was noted in the offspring of one sire breed with four different dams, in the offspring of two sires each breed with two different dams, and in two littermates from another sire. The occurrence of each disease by sex is summarized (Table 9-9).

**Table 9-3:** The occurrence of osteochondrosis of the shoulder either singly or in combination with other lesions as determined radiographically in 1018 Labrador Retrievers, by sex.

| Sex | Shoulders | Shoulders – alone | In combination with |||||
|---|---|---|---|---|---|---|---|
| | | | Elbows | Hips | Elbows, Hips | Elbows, Tarsus | Hips, Tarsus |
| Both sexes | 38 (3.7%) | 26 (2.6%) | 4 | 3 | 2 | 2 | 1 |
| Male | 18 (4.9%) | 11 (3.0%) | 2 | 2 | 0 | 2 | 1 |
| Female | 20 (3.1%) | 15 (2.3%) | 2 | 1 | 2 | 0 | 0 |

**Table 9-4:** The occurrence of elbow dysplasia singly or in combination with other lesions as determined radiographically in 1018 Labrador Retrievers, by sex.

| Sex | Elbow | Elbows – alone | In combination with |||||||| 
|---|---|---|---|---|---|---|---|---|---|---|
| | | | Shoulders | Hips | Stifles | Tarsus | LS anomaly | Shoulders, Hips | Shoulders, Tarsus | Hips, Tarsus |
| Both sexes | 180 (17.8%) | 111 (10.9%) | 4 | 43 (4.2%) | 2 | 5 | 4 | 2 | 2 | 7 |
| Male | 87 (23.5%) | 56 (15.1%) | 2 | 16 (4.3%) | 1 | 4 | 2 | 0 | 2 | 4 |
| Female | 93 (14.4%) | 55 (8.5%) | 2 | 2 (4.2%) | 1 | 1 | 2 | 2 | 0 | 3 |

**Table 9-5:** The occurrence of hip dysplasia singly or in combination with other lesions as determined radiographically in 1018 Labrador Retrievers, by sex

| Sex | Hips | Hips – alone | In combination with |||||||| 
|---|---|---|---|---|---|---|---|---|---|---|
| | | | Elbows | Shoulders | Stifles | Tarsus | LS anomaly | Shoulders, Elbows | Elbows, Tarsus | Shoulders, Tarsus |
| Both sexes | 128 (12.6%) | 65 (6.4%) | 43 (4.2%) | 3 | 1 | 3 | 3 | 2 | 7 | 1 |
| Male | 50 (13.5%) | 23 (6.2%) | 16 (4.3%) | 2 | 1 | 1 | 2 | 0 | 4 | 1 |
| Female | 78 (12.0%) | 42 (6.5%) | 27 (4.2%) | 1 | 0 | 2 | 1 | 2 | 3 | 0 |

**Table 9-6:** The occurrence of osteochondrosis of the stifle singly or in combination with other lesions as determined radiographically in 1018 Labrador Retrievers, by sex.

| Sex | Stifle | Stifle – alone | In combination with ||
|---|---|---|---|---|
| | | | Elbows | Hips |
| Both sexes | 7 (0.7%) | 4 (0.4%) | 2 | 1 |
| Male | 3 (0.8%) | 1 (0.3%) | 11 | 1 |
| Female | 4 (0.6%) | 3 (0.5%) | 1 | 0 |

Table 9-7: The occurrence of osteochondrosis of the tarsus singly or in combination with other lesions as determined radiographically in 1018 Labrador Retrievers, by sex.

| Sex | Tarsus | Tarsus – alone | In combination with | | | | |
| --- | --- | --- | --- | --- | --- | --- | --- |
| | | | Elbows | Hips | Elbows, Hips | Shoulders, Elbows | Shoulders, Hips |
| Both sexes | 32 (3.1%) | 14 (1.4%) | 5 | 3 | 7 | 2 | 1 |
| Male | 17 (4.6%) | 5 (1.4%) | 4 | 1 | 4 | 2 | 1 |
| Female | 15 (2.3%) | 9 (1.4%) | 1 | 2 | 3 | 0 | 0 |

Table 9-8: The occurrence of transitional lumbosacral vertebral anomalies singly or in combination with other lesions as determined radiographically in 1018 Labrador Retrievers, by sex.

| Sex | LS anomaly | LS anomaly – alone | In combination with | |
| --- | --- | --- | --- | --- |
| | | | Elbows | Hips |
| Both sexes | 37 (3.6%) | 30 (2.9%) | 4 | 3 |
| Male | 10 (1.0%) | 6 (0.6%) | 2 | 2 |
| Female | 27 (4.2%) | 24 (3.7%) | 2 | 1 |

Table 9-9: The occurrence of osteochondrosis of the shoulder, stifle, and tarsus and elbow and hip dysplasia as determined radiographically in 1018 Labrador Retrievers divided by sex.

| Sex | Shoulder | Elbow | Hips | Stifle | Tarsus | LS anomaly |
| --- | --- | --- | --- | --- | --- | --- |
| Both sexes | 38 (3.7%) | 180 (17.8%) | 128 (12.6%) | 7 (0.7%) | 32 (3.1%) | 37 (3.6%) |
| Male | 18 (4.9%) | 87 (23.5%) | 50 (13.5%) | 3 (0.8%) | 17 (4.6%) | 10 (1.0%) |
| Female | 20 (3.1%) | 78 (14.4%) | 78 (12.0%) | 4 (0.6%) | 15 (2.3%) | 27 (4.2%) |

## Discussion

The Labrador has been the most common breed used by Guide Dogs For The Blind, and has found enthusiastic acceptance in other service oriented groups as well (Canine Companions For Independence, search and rescue, and contraband detection). Basic to this popularity is the breed's benevolent personality and athletic ability. Knowledge of the frequency of potentially crippling orthopedic disorders in the breed is therefore of great importance to its fanciers. The heritable nature of certain of the osteochondroses, joint dysplasias, and transitional vertebral segments has been established (Swenson 1987; Morgan, et al 1993; Padgett, et al 1995; Swenson, et al 1997 a, b).

This report draws attention to the multiplicity of inherited bone and joint abnormalities in the Labrador Retriever. This is a very large case series and as such it is a detailed accounting of many lesions observed among individuals of this breed. It is important to understand any bias possibly present in these selected individuals. If the radiographic studies were evaluated as normal, owners were rewarded with a statement to this affect. The cost of the survey study performed at the specially scheduled radiographic clinic was less than that charged for a similar series made in a private practice. These two factors stimulated interest in the study, but tended to cause owners to present dogs assumed to be normal. Thus, the findings in the study are probably not representative of the entire breed and the frequency of affected dogs is thought to be greater than the 1/3 reported.

The affect of sex on the frequency of disease was noted. Shoulder osteochondrosis, elbow dysplasia, and tarsal osteochondrosis were noted more frequently in male dogs. The LS anomaly was noted more frequently in the female dog. Because the lesions are developmental and can be detected early in life, the age of dogs played no role in the results.

Combinations of disease were noted and elbows and hips were often affected in the same dog. This means that if a dog has one of these diseases there is a greater likelihood of its having the other disease. This strongly supports the concept that the dysplasias and osteochondroses are both influenced by a genetic composition that includes a predisposition for a rapid growth rate or a heavier body weight which may be further influenced by environmental factors such as a high energy diet (Hedhammer, et al 1974; Kasström 1975; Olsson 1976, 1987).

The value of stud dogs and brood bitches is based on their ability to produce offspring with desirable traits, lacking undesirable traits such as bone and joint dysplasias. Evaluation of breeding stock can be based on phenotypic assessment of the individual but evaluation is stronger when it includes the status of progeny and siblings. Limited preliminary data not included in this chapter suggests further support for the belief that affected individuals, those with positive phenotypes, are more likely to produce affected offspring. However, affected offspring were found subsequent to the matings of normal phenotype individuals and, thus, the value of progeny and sibling evaluation becomes apparent.

Periarticular osteophytosis was a prominent radiographic finding surrounding the humeral heads in many 1-year-old dogs and was often found bilaterally. This was a solitary radiographic finding without any detectable alteration to the normal contour of the humeral head and without any osteophytosis involving the caudal aspect of the glenoid cavity. Because of failure to identify the primary lesion of osteochondrosis of the humeral head or extensive secondary arthrosis, the dogs were evaluated as normal. The finding of a minimal "Morgan Line" as a solitary finding in a dog over 2 years of age in conjunction with a well formed femoral head seating within a deep acetabulum was treated in a similar manner (Klimt, et al 1992).

## Conclusions

A report of the incidence of joint dysplasias, osteochondroses, and transitional lumbosacral segments in over 1000 Labrador Retrievers is based on radiographic studies. Of the 1018 dogs evaluated, 688 (67.6%) dogs were judged to be radiographically normal and 330 (32.4%) dogs were evaluated as affected in at least one site. Elbow and hip dysplasia were noted to occur together more frequently than expected if random. Elbow dysplasia and shoulder and tarsal OCD were found more frequently in the male. A survey of the sires and dams of dogs affected with LS anomaly suggested the condition to be inherited.

# References

GRØNDALEN J. Arthrosis with special reference to the elbow joint of young rapidly growing dogs. 11 Occurrence, clinical and radiographical findings. Nord. Vet.-Med. 31; 69-75, 1979.

HEDHAMMER, WU F-M, KROOK L, SCHRYVER HR, DE LAHUNTA A, WHALEN JP, KALLFELZ FA, NUNEZ EA, HINTZ HF, SHEFFY BE, RYAN GD. Overnutrition and skeletal disease. An experimental study in growing Great Dane Dogs. Cornell Vet 64:(Suppl) 5,1-160, 1974.

KASSTRÖM H. Nutrition, weight gain and development of hip dysplasia. An experimental investigation in growing dogs with special reference to the effect of feeding intensity. Acta Radiol (Suppl) (Stockh) 344:136-178, 1975.

KLIMT U, TELLHELM B, FRITSCH R. Die Bedeutung der "Morgan-Linie" für die Untersuchung auf HD beim Hund. Kleintierpraxis 37:211-217, 1992.

MORGAN JP. Transitional lumbosacral vertebral anomaly in the dog: A radiographic study. Submitted for publication 1998.

MORGAN JP, BAHR A, FRANTI CE, BAILEY CS. Lumbosacral transitional vertebrae as a predisposing cause of cauda equina syndrome in German Shepherd Dogs: 161 cases (1987-1990). JAVMA 202:1877-1882, 1993.

MORGAN JP, STEPHENS M. Radiographic diagnosis and control of canine hip dysplasia. ISU Press, Ames Iowa 1985.

MORGAN JP, WIND A, DAVIDSON AP. Bone dysplasias in the Labrador Retriever: A radiographic study. JAAHA.

MONTGOMERY DD, MILTON JL, HENDERSON RA, HATHCOCK JT. Osteochondrosis of the canine stifle. Cont Ed 11:1199-1205, 1989.

OLSON NC, MOSTOSKY UV, FLO GL, TVEDTEN HW. Osteochondrosis of the tarsocrural joint in three canine siblings. JAVMA 176:635-637, 1980.

OLSSON S-E. Osteochondrosis- A growing problem to dog breeders. Gaines Progress, Summer 1976, p1-11.

OLSSON S-E. The early diagnosis of fragmented coronoid process and osteochondrosis of the canine elbow joint. JAAHA 19:616-626, 1983.

OLSSON S-E. General and local aetiologic factors in canine osteochondrosis. Vet Quart 9:268-278, 1987.

PADGETT GA, MOSTOSKY UV, Probst CW, Thomas MW, Krecke CF. The inheritance of osteochondrosis and fragmented coronoid process of the elbow joint in Labrador Retrievers. JAAHA 31:327-330, 1995.

RENDANO VT, RYAN G. A positioning and labeling guide for radiographs to be submitted to the Orthopedic Foundation for Animals. Vet Rad 26: 170-186, 1985.

SMITH CW, STOWATER JL. Osteochondrosis of the canine shoulder joint: A review of 35 cases. JAAHA 11:658-662, 1975.

SMITH MM, VASSEUR PB, MORGAN JP. Clinical evaluation of dogs after surgical and nonsurgical management of osteochondrosis of the talus. JAVMA 187:31-35, 1985.

SWENSON L. What do we know about hip dysplasia today? Presented at "The Dog in Service of Humanity", Geilo, Norway May 7-9, 1987.

SWENSON L, AUDELL L, HEDHAMMAR Å. Prevalence and inheritance of and selection for hipdysplasia in seven breeds of dogs in Sweden and a benefit: cost analysis of a screening and control program. JAVMA 210:207-214, 1997a.

SWENSON L, AUDELL L, HEDHAMMAR Å. Prevalence and inheritance of and selection for elbow arthrosis in Bernese Mountain Dogs and Rottweilers in Sweden and benefit: cost analysis of a screening and control program. JAVMA 210:215-221, 1997b.

VAUGHAN LC. Osteochondrosis of the head of the humerus in dogs. J Sm Anim Pract 9:283-94, 1968.

# Chapter 10

# Schemes for control of disease

## Introduction to control of dysplasia through use of registries

Registries are based on the assumption that the diseases described in this monograph, plus many other diseases, are inherited traits, with the mode of inheritance usually being polygenic. That means that the traits will not be expressed if the appropriate genes are not present. Heritability estimates vary depending on the disease, the particular study reported, and the effect of various environmental factors that are involved in the calculations. Attempts to limit the occurrence of these diseases should concentrate on selection of the breeding stock. Dogs afflicted with the diseases should not be used in breeding programs. Dogs producing offspring with any of the diseases should not used for breeding in the future. Phenotypically normal, first-degree relatives of affected dogs should not be used for breeding. There is a value for breeders to cooperate in the collection of appropriate data for progeny-testing breeding stock, especially males.

First attempts at control of HD were undertaken by the Swedish Kennel Club (Svenska Kennel Klubben or SKK). Their attempts gave us our first indication that there was no value in establishing a plan unless the breeders agreed to follow it. Also, it was necessary that the plan be such that as many dogs as possible could be evaluated. Level of transmissibility from early studies was suggested to be around 0.4 to 0.6 indicating the percentage of genetic influence. With numbers this high, a decrease in the prevalence of HD should be expected if selective breeding were conducted. Having undergone many changes, the current program of the SKK is now a model to be considered and has developed to the point that they will have examined 1 million radiographs by the turn of the century. Most results are now recorded and knowledge of progeny and littermates can be ascertained. This information includes the dog's name and the findings are in an open registry and are made available to the breed clubs for their distribution. This is referred to as an official information or open information.

The Orthopedic Foundation for Animals (OFA) was established in the United States over 25 years ago and currently has evaluated over 500,000 radiographs and has served effectively as a method of standardizing radiography of the hips and film evaluation in that country. It was established at a time radiographs were evaluated by many "experts" and evaluations varied widely. The OFA clearly established rules to be followed in making the radiographic examination of the hip joints and in the evaluation of the status of the hips. However, because of the method of organization, no incentive existed for the owner or veterinarian to submit radiographs of dogs thought to be dysplastic since no information on dysplastic studies can be distributed by the organization. The scheme is therefore of value only to identify dogs certified to have normal hips. No information on progeny is available and information concerning percentages of involvement in breeds is certainly suspect because of a great bias in selection of radiographs submitted. Some breeds in the USA have been reported by this group to have a decreased frequency of dysplasia. However, these determinations are made only from radiographs submitted. Frequently dogs with obvious signs of dysplasia are screened by the submitting clinican and not sent to the OFA. Also, only dogs used for breeding or competition are evaluated since there is no incentive for companion dogs to be evaluated. Thus, any decrease in frequency of dysplasia detected by the OFA must be evaluated with caution (Corley and Hogan 1985). This bias has been described recently when it was reported that only 56% of clients at a university hospital who requested and paid for the making of OFA hip radiographs submitted them to the OFA. Dogs whose radiographs were not submitted had a 10-fold higher incidence of HD than dogs whose films were submitted for official OFA interpretation. This bias varies widely depending on breed with 74% of Rottweiler and 21% of Golden Retriever radiographs being submitted to OFA for evaluation (Smith 1997).

It appears that there are only minimal changes in prevalence of HD noted in the past years in the United States. It is possible that some of the reasons are that dog breeders are a constantly changing group. It is also possible that dysplastic dogs are being bred regularly. Certainly the lack of any restriction by a national breed club to only register puppies from radiographically free sire and dam permits a free selection of dogs used for breeding. A final consideration is the question as to why there is no statement from the American Veterinary Medical Association (AVMA) about methods of controlling HD other than that pertaining to techniques of positioning the patient for radiographic examination (Feldmann 1974).

It would be most desirable that a registry should be able to accumulate data on progeny and littermates and all information should be available to a person seeking information in the selection of a sire or dam to use for breeding. Only in this way can positive results be expected in the control of an inherited disease. With the use of progeny information, the interpretation of a single radiograph becomes less important and dogs thought to be questionable can be eliminated from breeding because of the evaluation of siblings.

In practice you deal with one owner and one dog. The advice given an owner concerning breeding of this individual dog is made difficult since you are forced to extract as much information from a single examination that produced one radiograph. This difficulty is especially true because of the practice of destroying other siblings thought to be dysplastic before they are examined often thinking that this is the "right" thing to do. This effectively hides information concerning the presence of dysplasia in the family. This practice leads to production of litters with dysplasia from normal sire and dam and grandsire and grandam that are certified to have normal hips radiographically.

The efforts of other schemes or evaluation systems are discussed in the following pages. It is hoped that by a review of the history of schemes used in the control of heritable disease in the past that information can be available that will permit greater progress to be made in the future.

It is hoped that this history of attempts to control both hip and elbow dysplasia will be of interest to the reader both because of the nature of the schemes put in operation but also because of the interesting individuals who played roles in the establishment of these schemes. If this book were to be dedicated, it should be to the authors of the reports contained within this chapter since they represent some of the leaders in veterinary medicine who have devoted a great part of their lives in an effort to limit the pain and suffering of both affected dog and the owners.

## References

CORLEY EA, HOGAN PM. Trends in hip dysplasia control: analysis of radiographs submitted to the orthopedic foundation for animals, 1974 to 1984. JAVMA 187:805-809, 1985.

FELDMANN BM. Letter to the editor. JAVMA 165:876-877, 1974.

SMITH GK. Canine Hip Dysplasia: Advances in Diagnosis. submitted to JAVMA 1997.

# Control of hip dysplasia in Sweden

Joe P. Morgan, DVM, Vet. med. dr
Department of Surgical and Radiological Sciences
School of Veterinary Medicine
University of California
Davis, California 95616

Lars Audell, DVM
Radiology Consultant
Gudby Gard
194 92 Upplands Vasby
Sweden

One of the earliest programs established for control of inherited bone and joint disease was the program in Sweden to control HD that was centered at the Royal Veterinary College in Stockholm under the direction of Professor Sten-Erik Olsson, and was instituted in 1958. A study of HD in a large kennel at the Swedish Army Dog Training Center had revealed that the condition was genetically influenced and a later study on a larger material from the same kennel gave further support to the concept that it was hereditary in nature with heritability between 0.4 and 0.6. With this information, a HD control program for the German Shepherd Dog breed was started in cooperation with the Swedish Kennel Club (SKK) on January 1, 1959. Sweden thereby became the first country in which active measures were taken to control canine HD.

The early study was based on the concept that potentially well-recognized dogs required a certificate of having normal hips. The Kennel Club requested a certificate of normal hip joints for German Shepherd Dogs which were to: (1) be awarded a show or working championship, (2) compete in a stud class, (3) be awarded a special breeding prize for working dogs, and (4) be imported into Sweden and registered in the SKK. Dogs were examined if they were over 6 months of age. It was possible for the program to begin in Sweden because of the unique population of dogs. Most dogs (70%) are purebred and many of these dogs (90%) are registered in the SKK. The number of stray dogs is minimal permitting a close account of breeding activity.

Early on, mixed feelings were expressed about the program, however, most breeders were interested and cooperative and there was general acceptance of the program. Consequently, an increased demand for radiography was noted throughout the country by clinicians and clinics. Through 1970 the radiographs were evaluated at the Department of Clinical Radiology of the Royal Veterinary College in Stockholm.

From the introduction of the program, a list of German Shepherd Dogs with normal radiographic studies was published monthly in the Journal of the Swedish Kennel Club. A stamp was placed into the registration books of these dogs that had normal hip joints. Only dogs with normal hip joints were registered by the Kennel Club and received a notation in the registration book. Hips were classified as normal or, if dysplastic, were graded using grades 1 to 4. Borderline cases were recommended to return for repeated examination.

After about 6 years of this program, serious criticism about its effectiveness was raised. The program was said to cause owners of German Shepherd Dogs to be overly concerned with the status of the hip joints of their dogs and the position of normal hip joints achieved such great importance that other characteristics in the animal were ignored and not given adequate attention. Breeders told that actually, the evaluation of normal hip joints was given little attention when dogs were selected for breeding, despite the importance that was suggested. In addition, most German Shepherd Dogs used for breeding were never entered in dog shows and were thus not evaluated. Since the problem of HD was not limited to the German Shepherd Dog, it was argued that other breeds should be included in a new program.

Evaluation of the frequency of HD in the German Shepherd Dog showed that HD was more of a problem in Sweden after the first 10 years of selective breeding than before this breeding program was started. A suggestion was made that dogs with certain desirable traits that were possible linked to HD, were being selected for breeding (Henricson, et al 1972).

Because of these reasons, the program was discontinued and all restrictions placed on the German Shepherd Dogs were abandoned on January 1, 1967. Instead, the SKK decided to support a voluntary program for all breeds by offering public recognition of dogs that were radiographed and were found to have normal hip joints. Owners and breeders were advised to use only dogs with normal hip joints for breeding, however, dogs judged to have grade I HD were also considered useful as breeding stock if they were mentally and physically sound. The data at that time indicated that dogs with grade I dysplasia had a similar frequency of dysplasia in their offspring as dogs with normal hip joints (a slight difference was not demonstrated until later studies). The monthly list of radiographed dogs in which the hip joints were normal was eventually discontinued and the result of the radiographic examination, whether positive or negative, was included in the registration book of each dog which was radiographed. This function and the special registry for radiographic studies were transferred to the SKK on January 1, 1971. The program was placed under the control of Dr. Lars Audell from August 1972.

In 1973, the age of dogs examined was increased from 6 months to 9 months and from 6 months to 12 months for the giant breeds.

Still, little progress was noted in eradication of HD despite the length of time the program had been in effect. It appeared that the measures taken had little effect on breeding results. At that time, it was considered suitable to analyze the progress to determine the reason for the apparent lack of progress. The analyses revealed that for several affected breeds one half of all puppies were from parents either suffering from dysplasia or those in which the status of the hips was unknown. This indicated that even with the widespread publicity given to the program, many were breeding without giving attention to the presence of HD. Thus, it could hardly be expected that any dramatic improvement in the incidence of the disease could be made.

Since 1973, the owners were required to sign a statement that all results are to be registered by the SKK and that the information was to be within the public domain. In 1977, all dogs had to have their identification number tattooed in the left ear or on the inner aspect of the thigh at the time of radiography. In 1979, results of all radiographic evaluations of hip joint conformation registered by the SKK became easily available to the public. As a service to breeders, it has been possible since 1983 to obtain information on the status of hip joints of any individual dog for which radiographs have been evaluated. It was also possible to obtain information concerning: (1) all the progeny of any individual dog, (2) all dogs within a breed in relation to year of birth, and (3) all breeding dogs in relation to year of birth and litters born. Consequently, it has been possible since 1983 for a breeder to obtain information on hip joint status of parents, grandparents, and littermates of these dogs as well as the status of the dog to be bred. In response to requests from the national clubs for several breeds, it has been mandatory since 1984 that the status of the hip joints is known for the sire and dam if progeny are to be registered by the SKK.

**Table 10-1: Historical factors that may have played a role in the willingness of owners to have dogs radiographed and their willingness to submit radiographs for evaluation and the possible influence of these factors on the frequency of HD recorded in a given year.**

|  |  |
|---|---|
| 1971 | A change takes place in the method of evaluation of radiographs. One radiologist (PeO Gustaffson) becomes responsible for the evaluation replacing a panel of radiologists from the Veterinary School. The membership of the panel had varied in the past and could consist of a single person. In retrospect, the high differences in frequency of HD often seen with similar differences simultaneously in many breeds probably show inter-reader differences rather than changes in the dog population. |
| 1972 | A second important change reflects the assumption of managing of the film evaluation by the SKK which results in better cooperation with and service to the owners and breeders. |
| 1973 | From the end of 1972, another change occurs in film evaluation with the assignment of a single radiologist (Lars Audell) who continues to be responsible for evaluation today. Three grades of arthrosis are noted separately from the determination of dysplasia. A new grading of excellent is introduced in breeds with high prevalence of HD. The evaluation of borderline is excluded. All dogs with normal hips receive an indication of "h" in their registration book. The age of examination is changed to 9 months (and 12 months for the giant breeds). Owners are required to sign that the results are open to obtain an officially scrutinized evaluation. |
| 1974 | Massive information is distributed throughout the country in meetings and in articles in Hundsport (SKK sponsored journal for dog owners and breeders) to encourage the evaluation of as many dogs as possible. In order to get as many of the affected dogs as possible into the program, all dogs with moderate or severe dysplasia are evaluated free of charge. |
| 1975 | Progeny results are published in Hundsport |
| 1976 | All new results from film evaluation are centrally computerized in an open registry at SKK. |
| 1977 | SKK employs a specialist in genetic diseases in dogs (Åke Hedhammar). Tattooing becomes a requirement to have the results recognized officially by the SKK. |
| 1978 | A large increase in the evaluation of Retrievers born in 1977 is noted. |
| 1979 | Tattooing becomes mandatory for identification. The SKK introduces a program for eradication of some genetic diseases. |
| 1980 | The minimum age for evaluation of radiographs of the hips becomes one year for all breeds. Parvovirus infection causes a marked decrease in the number of dogs radiographed in Sweden because of the fear of taking a healthy dog to a clinic or hospital. |
| 1984 | The insurance companies refuse to pay for treatment or life insurance of dysplastic dogs unless both parents have normal hips. Information about hips and elbows was discussed at a conference regarding genetic diseases arranged by the veterinary profession and the Swedish Kennel Club. |
| 1986 | It becomes mandatory to have official HD results of both parents in order to register puppies in many breeds. |
| 1990 | Some breeds demand that parents must be free of HD in order to register puppies. |
| 1993 | The result of a HD radiographic examination is no longer noted in the registration book, unless requested by the owner. |
| 1996 | A separate certificate indicating the results of a HD radiographic examination becomes mandatory instead of the stamp in the registration book. |

Another important action by the medical insurance companies in Sweden occurred in 1984 that assisted in calling attention to the problem of breeding dysplastic dogs. Approximately 40% of the dog population in Sweden are covered by a form of medical insurance. In that year, the companies determined that they would not pay for the cost of treating an insured dog with HD unless both parents were radiographically free of dysplasia at the time of breeding. Also, at this time, some breed clubs began the practice of not registering puppies unless the parents were radiographed and the status of the hips was known (normal or dysplastic). This number has grown to include over 70 breeds at this time.

The effect of these measures has been widespread (Figure 10-1) and has had marked influence on the attitude of the breeders toward the problem of HD (Table 10-1). The lead by the SKK and the insurance companies has resulted in a dramatic shift toward use of dogs as breeding stock that have been evaluated and found not to have HD, which has been accompanied by a decreased prevalence of HD in most breeds.

On January 1, 1980, it was determined that all dogs must be 12 months of age or older to be radiographed and officially registered.

At this time, early 1980s, a study was begun that would explain to breeders the positive consequences of selection of breeding stock and show that the results of the Swedish State Dog Training Center are applicable and transferable to other breeding stock. Certain points should be considered in the choice of a "normal" dog such as the status of the parents, littermates, and progeny and this information was made known to interested parties. If these animals are known to be free of dysplasia, the risk to the offspring is reduced considerably. In 1983, data concerning radiographic evaluation was offered to breed clubs for distribution as they felt was appropriate.

The number of dogs of all breeds radiographed increased considerably. In the early 1960s, about 1000 dogs were examined each year. This increased to approximately 5,000 dogs by the 1970s, 10,000 by the 1980s, and 18,000 by the 1990s (Figure 10-2).

As a result of this long history, there is pressure on the breeders making it difficult to breed a dysplastic dog. For example, among registered breedings throughout the country in 1988, only 282 used affected dogs. Dogs with the following grades of dysplasia were used: grade I, 200; grade II, 70; grade III, 10; and grade IV, 2. The number of breedings in which both dogs were judged radiographically normal increased from only 10% in 1970 to a level of 61% in 1980, while the number of un-screened dogs used for breeding decreased from 60% in 1970 to 10% in 1980 (Hedhammer 1989)

However, while certain breeds have over 75% of the registered puppies radiographed (Rottweiler and Bernese Mountain dog), other breeds have only 50% of the registered puppies radiographed (German Shepherd Dog and Golden Retriever). The total for all breeds is only 1/3 (of all puppies registered are radiographed).

The frequency of dysplasia was studied in breeds randomly selected and the improvement in hip conformation in response to normal to normal matings was determined. The breeds selected were the German Shepherd Dog (Figure 10-3), Rottweiler, Bernese Mountain Dogs, Saint Bernard, Irish Setter, English Setter, Gordon Setter, and Labrador Retriever. In seven of the eight breeds, the percentage of normal offspring increased and the average improvement was almost 2% per year over a 9-year period. This was possible because of an increase in the percentage of normal to normal matings over the same time period that ranged between 25% and 48%. An average of almost 40% of the offspring of these seven breeds was evaluated annually radiographically. Simply stated, the status of dysplasia within breeds of dogs was seen to improve markedly as a result of mass selection based on a phenotype determined radiographically. No attempt was made to control various environmental factors that have been reported to influence the trait. Thus, as has been predicted by heritability estimates, the phenotypic expression of dysplasia in dogs can be controlled based on genetic principles only (selection of breeding stock).

At the present time over 300,000 patients have been radio-graphed with the results recorded by the SKK. The program now includes studies for elbow arthrosis indicative of elbow dysplasia. Over 200 clinics send around 20,000 hip radiographs and 8,000 radiographs of the elbows to Dr. Lars Audell for evaluation each year. One additional feature that helps to make the study successful is that dogs with hips judged dysplastic at grade II or higher and dogs with elbows judged with moderate arthrosis or higher are recorded at no expense to the owner. The charge for making the radiographs is 800:- Swedish Kronor (approximately $100 US) and includes the cost of tattooing.

A major part of the success of this program is that, since 1973, all radiographs are reviewed by a single radiologist, with the conformation of the hip joints classified as normal or dysplastic using grades of dysplasia of 1, 2, 3, and 4. The grading system is a modification of that originally suggested by Schnelle in 1954 using joint laxity and con-

**258** Schemes for control of disease

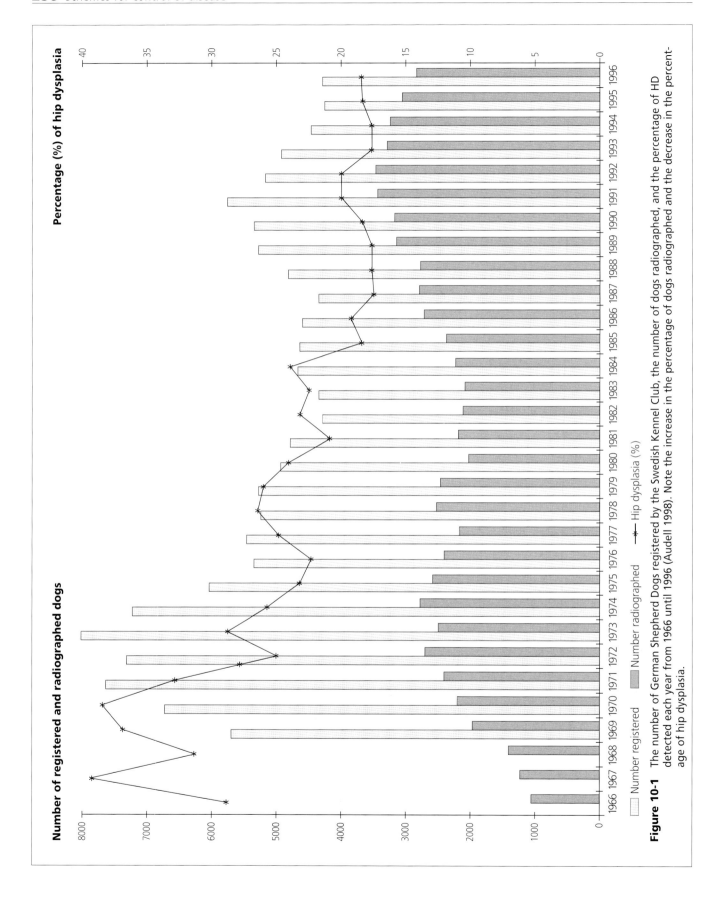

**Figure 10-1** The number of German Shepherd Dogs registered by the Swedish Kennel Club, the number of dogs radiographed, and the percentage of HD detected each year from 1966 until 1996 (Audell 1998). Note the increase in the percentage of dogs radiographed and the decrease in the percentage of hip dysplasia.

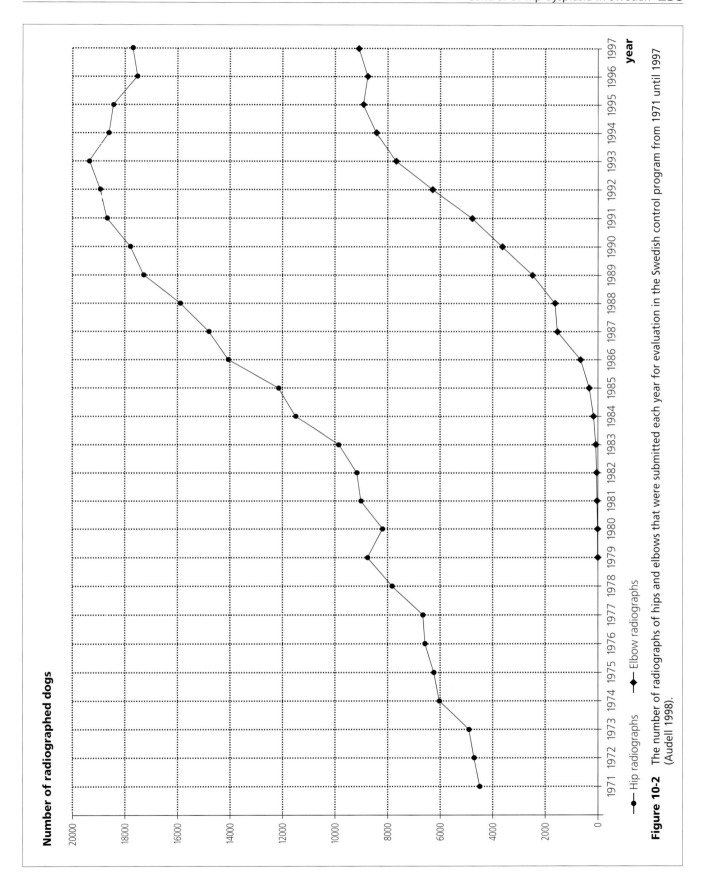

**Figure 10-2** The number of radiographs of hips and elbows that were submitted each year for evaluation in the Swedish control program from 1971 until 1997 (Audell 1998).

**260** Schemes for control of disease

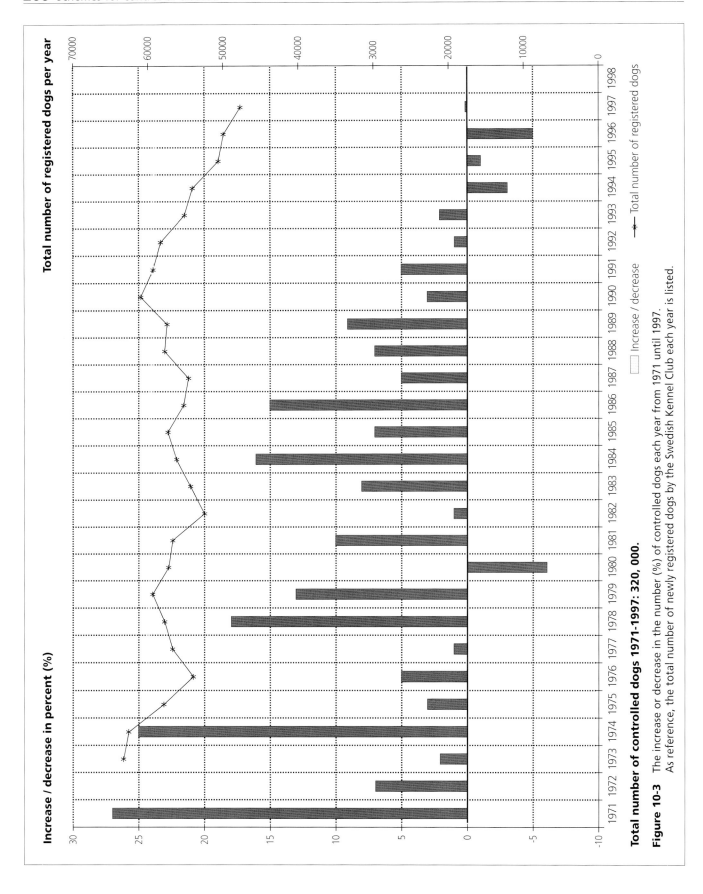

**Figure 10-3** The increase or decrease in the number (%) of controlled dogs each year from 1971 until 1997. As reference, the total number of newly registered dogs by the Swedish Kennel Club each year is listed.

**Total number of controlled dogs 1971-1997: 320, 000.**

formation of the acetabulum. An important modification is that the severity of osteophyte formation and osteoarthritic deformation secondary to HD is graded separately so as to not influence the evaluation of joint conformation. Also, because of the special problem with dogs with deep acetabula but obvious signs of laxity, re-examination at an older age is recommended before a final evaluation is given.

The results from a recent study (1997) provide the reader the latest data from the long-standing Swedish program. A total of 83,229 dogs born between 1976 and 1989 were included in the report and represent seven breeds (German Shepherd Dogs, Golden Retrievers, Labrador Retrievers, Newfoundlands, Rottweilers, Bernese Mountain Dogs, and Saint Bernards). Most dogs were examined when they were between 12 and 18 months of age. These breeds were selected for analysis because they represent those with high and medium-high prevalence of HD.

During the period studied, the prevalence of HD of any grade, as well as that of individual grades 2, 3, and 4, decreased in all breeds. The decrease in prevalence was most prominent in Rottweilers where prevalence of grade 1 HD decreased from 20% to 7% and the prevalence of HD grades 2, 3, and 4 decreased from 16% to 6%. Smaller decreases have been reported for other nationwide screening programs and decreases of this magnitude have been documented earlier, but only in small populations of dogs in which the breeding was well controlled. It is assumed that differences in the decrease of HD among the breeds can be attributed to variations in the intensity of selection of breeding stock that were applied over the time of the study as well as differences in prevalence at the beginning of the study.

It is important to understand the breadth and depth of the Swedish program. By 1976, more than 70% of the male and 60% of the female German Shepherd Dogs, Golden Retrievers, Labrador Retrievers, Rottweilers, and Bernese Mountain Dogs that were being used for breeding were already screened for HD. These percentages were even higher in 1988. Almost all litters born during 1988 were offspring of dams that had been screened for HD. In comparison, in 1976 only 30% of the male and 50% of the female Newfoundlands had been screened while only 20% of the male and 50% of the female Saint Bernards had been screened. By 1983 to 1985, the percentages in these breeds increased and were similar to the percentages for the other breeds.

The study reported in 1997 explored the effect of sex on the prevalence of HD and the disease was found to be significantly higher in females than in males for German Shepherd Dogs, Golden Retrievers and Saint Bernards. This is in accordance with findings of previous surveys from Sweden and other countries, however, it has not been noted in many other studies. A sex-related difference in prevalence of HD could be explained by the effect of secondary sex characteristics coded by genes on the sex chromosomes such as difference in growth rate.

In all breeds, age at the time of examination had a significant effect on percentage of dogs determined to have HD. This was evident even when offspring from dysplastic parents were not included. To minimize age bias in a screening program, it is, therefore, important to evaluate as many individuals as possible at the same age or in a narrow age interval. This was done in this report. The study reported that all heritability estimates were moderate to high and range generally between 0.40 and 0.60 supporting earlier reported figures that were similar.

Examination of progeny was of special importance in the recent report and again the prevalence of HD found in progeny was lowest when both parents had normal hip joints and was highest when both parents were dysplastic. Importantly, the prevalence of HD found in progeny was also high when the status of the hips was not known. (This suggests that the status might have been known to be dysplastic and was ignored by the breeder). This type of positive relation existed between the prevalence of HD of any grade and matings of dysplastic parents resulted not only in more dysplastic progeny but also in progeny with more severe grades of HD.

Benefit vs cost analysis of a large-scale program of this type is important because the breeder is asked to participate and pay a large amount of the cost of administration of such a program. This important aspect of a control scheme is seldom evaluated. One method of evaluation of the economic benefit of the program is to calculate the benefit through consideration of the increased number of puppies that were normal compared to the number expected to be dysplastic if change in breeding practices had not occurred. When the estimated number of dogs saved from only moderate, severe, and very severe HD within the entire populations of dogs in Sweden is multiplied by the cost of purchasing a dog of these breeds (equal to $700) the value of these dogs is estimated to be almost $6 million. The total cost of the Swedish HD screening program from 1976 through 1988 was estimated to be nearly $4 million. The economic benefit of the program showed that the benefit/cost ratio was greater than 1 in all breeds but the Newfoundlands and Saint Bernards. The benefit of the decreased prevalence of grade 1 HD was not included, and this represents an additional bonus (Swenson, et al 1997).

Another method of evaluation of the cost benefit associated with the success of the program is to examine the expected costs of medical and surgical treatment that would have been required to care for the dysplastic dogs. This was estimated within the German Shepherd Dog breed. The decrease in dysplasia frequency within the approximately 32,000 German Shepherd Dogs occurred with a drop of affected dogs from 35% to a level of 22% dysplasia. Considering that this decrease did not occur within one year but was spread across the 12 years of the study, approximately 3,500 GSDs were born with normal hips that would have otherwise been dysplastic. If the cost of examination and treatment of each of these dysplastic dogs were $1000 during their life, this cost would have been $3,500,000. If this is added to the $2,500,000 cost of procuring the puppies, the total benefit is approximately $6,000,000. It is impossible to predict the cost to breeder and/or buyer in negotiating a financial settlement in the event that a dysplastic puppy is sold. Nor, can the cost of a damaged reputation of a breeder be estimated. Finally, the cost in having to change plans to breed an animal because of the unexpected detection of HD cannot be estimated but is very real to a breeder. The results from this ongoing study which provides data from the largest single material available clearly shows that screening programs such as operated by the SKK with information linked to ancestral background in a stud book in an open registry will soon pay for itself.

The progress attainable in the eradication of HD depends on how consistently the breeding plan is followed and on the degree of precision with which breeding values of the breeding stock can be estimated. In traits such as HD, which have high heritabilities (>0.3) and a high frequency, there is a lot to gain, owing to the threshold character of HD by using family records to predict the breeding values of proposed breeding animals. These include records of full- and half-siblings and parents, and perhaps even grandparents. This will be the most effective way to further improve a breeding program. Progeny testing of sires will also improve a breeding program. Progeny testing of dams will also improve a breeding program, but bitches have often made their major contribution of puppies before the status of the hip joints can be sufficiently evaluated. The report clearly states that the status of dysplasia within breeds of dogs can improve markedly as a result of mass selection based on a phenotype determined radiographically.

## References

HENRICSON B, OLSSON S-E. Some practical problems involved in control of hereditary defects in dogs. 18th World Veterinary Congress 1964.

SWENSON L, AUDELL L, HEDHAMMAR Å. Prevalence and inheritance of and selection for hip dysplasia in seven breeds of dogs in Sweden and a benefit/cost analysis of a screening and control program. JAVMA; 210,207-214,1997.

HEDHAMMER Å. Kennelklubbens bekämpningsprogram. Hip dysplasia. Past, present and future, Falkenberg Sweden 19 March 1989.

SWENSON L. What do we know about hip dysplasia today? Conference on "The dog in service of humanity", Geilo, Norway 7-9 May 1987.

# Fédération Cynologique Internationale (FCI)

PROFESSOR EM. SAKI PAATSAMA (deceased)
Department of Surgery
College of Veterinary Medicine
Helsinki, Finland

## Utrecht 1974

The Scientific Committee of the Fédération Cynologique Internationale (FCI) held their first workshop in Utrecht in 1974 to deal with the problem of HD. They assigned one or more experts in the different countries to evaluate radiographs and sign certificates concerning HD. From the breeders' point of view, it was desirable to arrange contact between these HD-panels in order to compare the various national methods. The meeting created a committee to standardize the terminology and classification of HD as well as to plan a uniform, internationally valid certificate.

The following were elected to the committee: W. Brass (Hannover), U. Freudiger (Bern), L.F. Müller (Berlin), S. Paatsama (Helsinki), C.C. van de Watering (Utrecht), and as secretary and the representative of the FCI, N.A. van der Velden (The Netherlands). This committee met many times in the following years and was assisted by S-E Olsson (Stockholm) and Chr. Saar (Berlin). A report of the committee was published in the Journal "Kleintierpraxis" 23:169-180, 1978.

## Barcelona 1980

S. Paatsama, as the President of The World Small Animal Veterinary Association, reported that the Scientific Committee of the FCI introduced in 1979 an International Certificate to reduce to a minimum the problems surrounding the increased movements of dogs across international frontiers. The certificate incorporated the suggested classification standards of the FCI Scientific Committee covering canine HD and included five different national classifications. It was recognized that Great Britain and the United States of America had their own classification standards.

The President suggested at the World Congress in Barcelona (Spain) in 1980, that in the next World Congress in Las Vegas (USA) in 1982, a discussion should be undertaken that would lead to the approval of an international HD-certificate to achieve uniformity also between the countries not belonging to the FCI. It was felt that the WSAVA was the correct body to deal with the realization of an international certificate.

In his report to the general assembly of the FCI in Dortmund 1981, J. Bouw (The Netherlands), Chairman of the Scientific Committee of the FCI, stated the importance of the acceptance of such an international HD certificate. He announced that the meeting on HD for the countries belonging to the FCI would be held in Hannover (Germany).

## Hannover 1981

The invitation for this meeting in Hannover on December 12 and 13, 1981 was sent to all members' countries by the General Secretariat of the FCI. Representatives of the following countries took part: Austria, Belgium, Denmark, Finland, Germany, Italy, The Netherlands, Norway, Sweden, Switzerland, and Yugoslavia. Based on the principles of the report of the HD Committee of the FCI, radiographs were presented, discussed, and evaluated. A wide conformity was achieved in the evaluation and classification.

However, it was not possible to agree on an internationally uniform classification for HD. Therefore, the traditional classification scheme used in each country would be printed on the back of the international certificate (Table 10-2). At this time, the international classification A1 to E2 is in use in three FCI countries. No international HD certificate is in use.

## Dortmund 1991

At a meeting in Dortmund on June 14, 1991, with 15 member countries of FCI represented, changes were made as follows with the following new rules being recommended:

a) The minimum age for the diagnosis is 1 year, for giant breeds 1 1/2 years.
b) The dogs are to be identified by some recognized system, eg, legible tattooing or microchip. The same identification number has to be on the pedigree and on the x-ray film.
c) The minimal identification of the x-ray films needs the identification number (tattoo/microchip/registration), the date of x-ray examination, and marks of the right or left hip.
d) The owner must sign to confirm that the dog being x-rayed is the one stated on the request. The owner should also give authority for the radiograph to be retained by the diagnostic body. (It is recommended that a clause be inserted giving the diagnostic body authority to utilize the results in such manner as considered desirable). The veterinarian has to confirm that he/she has checked and confirmed the identification of the dog. He/she should indicate whether anesthe-

sia or sedation was used and that the dog was sufficiently relaxed.
e) The radiograph should be stored centrally.
f) The final diagnosis is to be based at least on one radiograph in position I (with extended hind legs). A second x-ray in position II (with flexed hindlegs) may be used.
g) The minimum size of the x-ray film in position I must be such as to include both hips and patellae.
h) The technical quality of the radiographs has to be such as to allow accurate diagnosis of the hip status.
i) If the above listed rules are not fulfilled the radiograph has to be rejected.
j) Radiographs should be read by the persons/panel approved by the club in which the dog is registered.
k) Each national panel should have a possibility of appeal. Issues of principles, eg, involving a breed can be submitted to the HD panel of the Scientific Committee of FCI.

Examples of the large and giant breeds that must be at the minimum age of 1 ½ years for the evaluation of hip status:
- Bull mastiff
- Doggue de Bordeaux
- Great Dane
- Leonberger
- Maremma
- Mastiff
- Mastiff Neapolitan
- Newfoundland and Landseer
- Pyrenean Mountain Dog
- St. Bernard

Also, at the meeting in Dortmund in 1991, changes were made as follows relative to the description of classes, applicable to dogs, aged between 1 and 2 years, provided there is correct positioning using position I. This classification scheme may be adopted for older dogs, but secondary arthritic changes have then to be evaluated according to the age of the dog. (This resulted in new rules and classification instead of using A1 to E2, A to E.)

## A: No signs of HD

The femoral head and the acetabulum are congruent. The craniolateral rim appears sharp and slightly rounded. The joint space is narrow and even. The acetabular angle according to Norberg (adapted for position I) is about 105°. In excellent hip joints the craniolateral rim encircles the femoral head somewhat more in laterocaudal direction.

## B: Near normal hip joints

The femoral head and the acetabulum are slightly incongruent and the acetabular angle according to Norberg (adapted for position I) is about 105° or the center of the femoral head lies medial to the dorsal rim of the acetabulum and the femoral head and the acetabulum are congruent.

## C: Mild HD

The femoral head and the acetabulum are incongruent, the acetabular angle according to Norberg is about 100¡ and/or there is a slightly flattened craniolateral rim. Irregularities of no more than slight signs of osteoarthritic changes of the margo acetabularis cranialis, caudalis, or dorsalis or on the femoral head and neck may be present.

## D: Moderate HD

Obvious incongruence between the femoral head and the acetabulum with subluxation. Acetabular angle according to Norberg more than 90° (only as a reference). Flattening of the craniolateral rim and/or osteoarthrotic signs.

## E: Severe HD

Marked dysplastic changes of the hip joints, such as luxation or distinct subluxation, acetabular angle according to Norberg less than 90°, obvious flattening of the margo acetabularis cranialis, deformation of the femoral head (mushroom shaped, flattening) or other signs of osteoarthrosis.

This classification has been made based on the radiological features only. It is as objective as possible.

**Puerto Rico 1997**

The Hip Dysplasia Committee of the FCI met in Puerto Rico in June 1997 and discussed the points of importance which arose in the HD meeting organized by WSAVA at the World Conference in Birmingham earlier in the year. It was noted that before it is possible to agree concerning the development of an International Certificate, the differences in the evaluation systems between different countries must be solved. It is necessary that methods of evaluation must be consistent. Unfortunately, in many countries, the quality of the radiographic examination and the radiographic evaluation do not reach a satisfactory level that will be required to obtain this agreement. Difficulties appear to center around the failure of all countries to use the positioning as described in the Dortmund Protocol. Failure to find an agreement concerning radiographic evaluation remains one reason why the percentage of HD is so variable between different countries and especially in breeds, many of which have the same origin. The big challenge will be how to organize an education program and a method of certification examination that will be accepted by all. It is obvious that a first concern is to accomplish this within the countries that are members of the FCI.

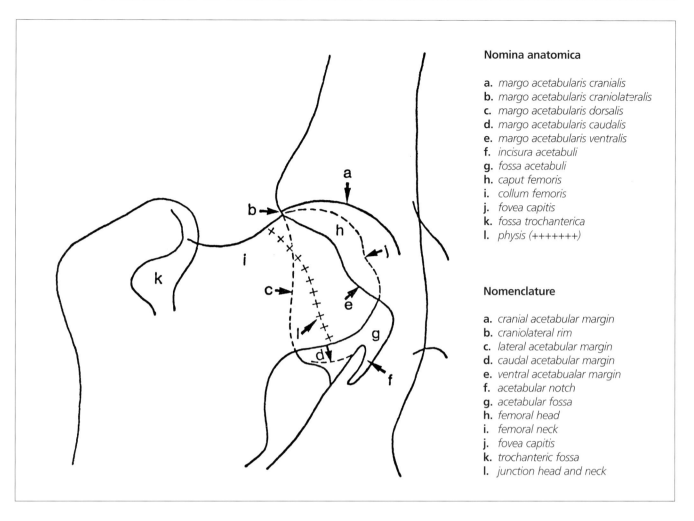

**Figure 10-4**
Nomenclature used in describing the radiograph of the hip joint.

**Table 10-2: International certificate**

| Classification, Einstufung | Classification, Klassifizierung | Country – Land | | | | | Classification, Einstufung |
|---|---|---|---|---|---|---|---|
| | | SF Finland Finnland | NL The Netherlands Niederlande | D Germany Deutschland | S Sweden Schweden | CH Switzerland Schweiz | |
| 1 | No signs of hip dysplasia Kein Hinweis für HD | Ei-dysplasia "hyvät" | Negatief geheel gaaf (1) | Kein Hinweis für HD | Utmärkt | Frei | 1 |
| A | | | | | | | A |
| 2 | | Ei-Dysplasiaa | Negatief niet geheel gaaf (2) | | U.A. | | 2 |
| 1 | Transitional Case Übergangsform (verdächtig für HD) | Rajatapaus | Transitional case (Tc) | Übergangsform (verdächtig für HD) | | | 1 |
| B | | | | | | | B |
| 2 | | | | | | | 2 |
| 1 | Mild Leichte HD | I | Licht positief (3) | Leichte HD | I | I | 1 |
| C | | | | | | | C |
| 2 | | | | | | | 2 |
| 1 | Moderate Mittlere HD | II | Positief (3½) | Mittlere HD | II | II | 1 |
| D | | | | | | | D |
| 2 | | | Positief (4) | | | | 2 |
| 1 | Severe Schwere HD | III | | Schwere HD | III | III | 1 |
| E | | | | | | | E |
| 2 | | IV | Positief optima forma (5) | | IV | IV | 2 |

# Hip dysplasia and its control in Great Britain

PROFESSOR DONALD D. LAWSON
Department of Surgery
Glasgow University Veterinary School
Glasgow, Scotland

In the period after the Second World War, dog breeding in Britain increased substantially and this increase, coupled with a lack of appreciation of the risks of introducing genetic defects, resulted in both dog owners and breeders being confronted by a "new" spontaneous hind limb lameness. This was a real problem, especially in the larger breeds of dog. The cause of the problem soon became established as canine hip dysplasia (CHD), which, after some time, became accepted as an inherited defect.

The breed society that was most concerned initially in the UK was the German Shepherd Dog League (GSDL) which had expanded considerably and had imported a large number of dogs from various European countries to help improve the breed in the UK. The majority of the membership of the society was located in the south of England and it is of some interest that the earliest recognition of the presence of the lameness associated with CHD occurred in that part of the country and that it progressed northwards only after a period of time. Presumably this feature was due to the movement of dogs that had won show certificates and had then been acquired by breeders in different parts of the country.

By the 1950s, the GSDL had become sufficiently concerned about the incidence of CHD associated lameness that they approached the British Veterinary Association (BVA) to request assistance in establishing a scheme to help control CHD. By this date evidence had been produced in various countries, that CHD was an inherited defect, although this opinion was not universally accepted, especially by those who wished to ascribe blame to other factors. One part of the argument rested upon the observation that the dogs were not noted to show lameness until they were some months old and it was suggested that this supported the concept that CHD was not inherited. Perhaps the most notable exception to the acceptance of CHD as an inherited disease was related to establishment of a "trials testing" program in West Germany, which was based on the concept that if animals were able to complete a major obstacle course without showing any form of lameness they were to be considered satisfactory for breeding selection. The "trials testing" program was finally abandoned when it was clearly established that many clinically sound dogs could be shown radiographically to have evidence of the structural changes of the hip joints that were ascribable to CHD.

In Sweden, a scheme had been established in which animals had their hips radiographed and "graded" according to the observable hip abnormalities. This discriminated between dogs that were considered to be normal and those with minor, moderate, or gross abnormalities. A similar system had been developed in the US, which also employed "grading," and as with the Swedish scheme, the x-ray interpretation was based on an "overall impression" of the observed changes. In neither instance was reporting on the individual aspects of the joints attempted.

The grading terminology that was employed in both Sweden and the US was very similar: normal = 0, minor dysplasia = 1, moderate dysplasia = 2, marked dysplasia = 3, and gross dysplasia = 4. This scale varied somewhat over a period of time as the more minor abnormalities seen in CHD became more appreciated.

In the discussions that took place in the UK, it was felt that the "grading systems" that had been established did not employ a sufficiently detailed radiographic assessment of the identifiable structural changes that occurred and that it would be helpful to report on each part of the hip joints separately since it had been noted that the changes occurred in a somewhat "random" manner. It was also felt that the "grading schemes" were open to misuse by breeders who believed that there was little or no difference between dogs that were in adjacent grades, possibly because the grades were recorded numerically and the difference between grades 1 and 2 could appear to be small. As a result, breeders were liable to make assumptions that were not justified in relation to the elimination or control of CHD. It was hoped that the proposed UK scheme would overcome these difficulties.

By the time the GSOL approached the BVA, it had been generally accepted that CHD had a genetic basis, but the mode of inheritance was not established. The reason for the progression of the clinical condition during growth had also not been fully explained. Attempts to identify a "simple mode of inheritance" had been made in various countries but were unacceptable because the very marked variations found in CHD did not conform to any pattern that could be accounted for by a single genetic factor.

A study in the UK set out the hypothesis that only a "polygenic mode of inheritance" fitted the observable findings that occurred in CHD. Studies on the development of the structural abnormalities that developed in cases of CHD indicted that they were liable to be progressive, especially during the growth period, and this gave rise to the claim that CHD was both polygenic and multifactorial. The environmental factors affecting "the final degree of expression" (ie, the degree to which the abnormalities develop) were not directly responsible for producing the hip changes, but produced their effects only when the hips were unstable. This gave rise to the observation that CHD was "that abnormality of the development of the hip joint that results in its instability," and this implies that the structural changes of the hips that develop in CHD are all secondary to the instability present.

The two environmental factors that were specifically incriminated as being responsible for these secondary structural abnormalities were: (1) over feeding to produce rapid growth in young pups which resulted in excessive weight gain and so abnormally high weight loading on the hip joints, and (2) excessive exercise and "freedom" in immature animals which promoted the damaging effects of the abnormal weight bearing on the immature hip joints. It was emphasized, however, that these factors were effective only if the hip joints were unstable.

The variation of phenotype abnormalities that occur in hips affected by CHD shows a very wide range; from normal, at one end, to extremely abnormal at the other, with every degree of affection between being identifiable. This, when coupled with the fact that the structural changes do not occur in a regular manner, but in different degrees in the various parts of the hip joint, indicated that it was necessary to have a system of reporting that was capable of recording each part of the hip joint separately while still providing an overall assessment of the hip status.

A report was produced which set out an analytical approach to the reporting of x-rays for the assessment of CHD. This was the basis of the development of the BVA/Kennel Club HD Scheme. In the paper, each of nine features of each hip joint was reported upon separately and given a letter to signify whether it was normal (A) or abnormal (B), and for two "features" greater degrees of abnormality were identified. This approach was adopted to ensure that changes present in each part of the joint were reported upon separately because of the way in which the changes were observed to occur. It was also designed to meet the claims of many dog breeders that there was a lack of uniformity in the x-ray interpretation employed in many of the established schemes.

The age at which breeding selection could satisfactorily be made was also the subject of concern. Many breeders, quite naturally, wished to make decisions at an early age and so limit the costs of keeping affected litters. It could be shown that severely affected animals could be detected as young as 12 to 16 weeks of age and rejected but, unfortunately, evaluation at this young age proved to be impractical in making positive breeding selection since many animals would show evidence of CHD only after they had reached skeletal maturity at about 12 months of age. Minor structural changes in the hips could readily pass undetected at a young age and, for this reason, it was decided that certificates stating that an animal had no evidence of CHD should not be issued before it was 12 months of age. In the US some time later, it was proposed that certification should be deferred until the animals were 2 or even 3 years of age because cases had occurred where structural changes of the hips had been positively identified for the first time only when they had reached that age. The experience gained with the BVA/KC HD Scheme, however, substantiated the use of 12 months as the minimum age for examination where a detailed analytical interpretation was employed.

When the BVA/KC HD Scheme was first established, it utilized a series of plus marks, rather than the letters cited in the article, to indicate the degree of abnormality detected in each of the nine features of the hips. The certification produced reported only one of three results: (1) "Within the agreed standards of normality" - which meant that no abnormality of any of the nine features had been detected, (2) "Breeders letter" - which was issued when only very minor abnormality was detected and indicated that breeding from such an animal was preferable to breeding from another which was either more severely affected or where the CHD status was unknown, and (3) "Fail" - which indicated that the extent of the abnormalities detected was liable to be associated with the probability of the animal involved transmitting CHD to its offspring and that this was a greater risk than was acceptable if control of CHD was a genuine consideration.

The background of this form of reporting was that it had been well established that dogs and bitches that were clinically sound could frequently be demonstrated to have evidence of CHD on x-ray and that the polygenic mode of inheritance indicated that any attempt to control CHD required to employ the "first principles of breeding," that is, "like breeds to like." As a result it was indicated to breeders that only animals certified to be within the first two categories should be selected for breeding.

The original BVA/KC HD Scheme was employed by dog breeders in a somewhat variable manner, possibly because many of them were not fully convinced of the necessity for control of CHD and because they could readily identify that many of the animals that were classed as "failures" were clinically sound. The "failure" group necessarily embraced a very wide range of degrees of hip abnormalities. The classification used had the effect of potentially severely restricting the breeding stock and as a result was not universally popular. Breeders were under increasing pressure to produce greater numbers of pups and they also were required to keep in mind other inherited conditions that had to be controlled.

The BVA/KC HD Scheme was an advisory one and no specific pressure was placed upon breeders, other than by breed societies that wished to control CHD. The Scheme existed essentially for the benefit of breeders and consequently the dog owners. Whatever the reasons, the overall uptake of the HD Scheme was less than the situation warranted and varied both between breeds and between groups in the larger breeds.

At this time, an exhibition displaying material from CHD schemes from Sweden, the US, Germany, and the UK was mounted at an annual congress of the BSAVA and this made it possible to compare the evaluation in each scheme. The BVA/KC HD Scheme was the only one that employed the detailed analytical approach and it could be seen that this form of assessment was more precise.

Additional schemes that were attempted:

1. With a view to assisting breeders whose kennels had many affected dogs, the BVA set up a "Kennel Scheme" that was designed to assess all the animals in a breeding kennel, employing the BVA/KC HD Scheme assessment, so that a comparison could be made between the potential breeding stock and the best kept for breeding. This process was carried out for a small number of breeding kennels that were in serious trouble and it was known to be effective. Breeders did not adopt it, however, and it was discontinued after a short period.

2. Manual assessment of the degree of joint laxity, carried out on 6 to 12 week old pups. This is an adaptation of the Ortolani Sign, as used in the human for the detection of congenital dislocation of the hip. It involved the use of general anesthesia and "measured" the joint laxity digitally. A real difficulty arose from the fact that congenital dislocation of the hip occurs only very rarely in dogs and so the abnormal mobility looked for in the dog is not the return of the femoral head into the acetabulum, but the very slight increase in lateral displacement of the great trochanter that can occur when the femur is pushed laterally while the pelvis is being held in position. The abnormal movement range is in the range of 1 to 2 mm and is difficult to detect by hand with any accuracy especially in young, small pups. The procedure proved to be both dangerous and of such limited value that it continued for only a short period.

3. The use of the "fulcrum position" in which a cylinder is positioned between the thighs and the stifles pressed forcibly medially prior to x-ray. Even before this procedure was described in literature, a trial involving Greyhounds had been carried out in the UK in which it was shown that it was possible to cause the femoral heads to be displaced laterally by forcibly pressing the heavily muscled thighs together. After the fulcrum position paper was published, a trial carried out in Glasgow demonstrated that in animals that had gross dysplastic changes, it was not uncommon for "fulcrum" effects to be absent due to the degree of reaction that had developed around the joints, while in dogs with little or no evidence of CHD the lateral displacement of the femoral heads could be produced fairly readily and these observations cast real doubt on the significance of the procedure.

4. Radiographic assessment of dogs at the age of 16 to 20 weeks also proved unattractive although it was possible to identify animals with gross CHD, it was not able to obtain the positive breeding selection which still required assessment at 12 months or over.

### The BVA/KC HD Scoring Scheme

An approach was made on behalf of the German Shepherd Dog Improvement Foundation by Dr. M. B. Willis to the BVA to alter the original scheme to a "grading scheme." However, when it was pointed out that it was only the BVA/KC HD Scheme that employed an analytical interpretation, he agreed with the suggestion that it would be preferable to modify the existing scheme so that it could produce a score for the animals examined. The modification involved devising specific criteria for each of the degrees of abnormality that could be discerned for each of the nine "features" of the hips. Criteria were designed to cover the full range of abnormalities that occur in CHD so as to provide a clear indication of the extent of the phenotype abnormality present in each instance.

The criteria for each feature were devised separately, since it was known that the structural changes that occurred did not follow a regular pattern but were sometimes more evident in one part of the joint than in another. As a result, it was implicit that the score recorded for any given feature would apply to it alone and it was not to be expected that the same level of score would be recorded uniformly for all features in any given case. Indeed, in some instances, the main finding would be subluxation, with only very minor evidence of exostoses or bone loss, while in others, extensive structural changes could be present with lesser degrees of subluxation recorded.

The score values for all of the features, except one, ranged from 0 to 6 and were derived by examining a series of radiographs together with their prepared bone specimens. Each score point had its own description which could be discriminated from its neighboring points and was, necessarily, intended to embrace a range of changes. No attempt was made to correlate the score values for any given feature with those of other features because of the variation in their occurrence mentioned earlier. For the caudal acetabular edge (Ca.A.E.) only 5 points could be described because of its relatively small size and its projection as seen on the film. The scoring criteria are listed in Table 10-3.

The total score is the sum of the scores recorded for the two hips and gives a good representation of the "hip status" of the animal under investigation. It serves as a basis for comparison with other animals of the same breed.

Since the environmental factors that affect the final degree of expression cannot be quantified by radiographic assessment, it is necessary to accept that they promote the effects of instability on joints and that their effects can be considered as "markers" revealing the effects produced by joint instability, even when it exists in quite small degree.

There are important limitations that are inherent in any HD scheme but the use of set criteria materially assists in having uniformity in reporting. Examiners are required to discriminate as to which side of a score "boundary" they are to record the score and this requires both care and frequent reference to the criteria.

Since the scheme produces a numerical score, there is a temptation to view the results in a simple numerical manner rather than to accept that the scores are necessarily devised for a condition that shows considerable variability and they should be accepted as a "guide," rather than as "absolute."

It is possible to collate the scoring obtained for any given breed of dog, where a sufficient number of individuals have been scored, and to set out the range of scores recorded and the calculated breed mean score (BMS). This activity has been undertaken by geneticists on behalf of the breed societies, with Dr. M. B. Willis, who is an agricultural geneticist with a strong interest in dogs, especially German Shepherd Dogs, playing the major role. The BMS provides a figure that indicates the overall hip status of the breed to that date, provided a sufficient number of animals have been scored. Since it employs all the scores recorded since the beginning of the scoring scheme, it is increasingly conditioned by the scores that have been recorded from the start and does not provide a "current" value statement. The number of dogs evaluated, the range of scores, and the BMS are shown in Table 10-4.

In making these calculations, it is important to acknowledge that the scoring process contains inherent limitations and that it is not possible to utilize the score points as if they all are of identical numerical value. The BMS represents the degree of the problem, Hip Status, that exists within a breed, but it does not provide a score value that can be safely employed as a basis for breeding selection. Indeed, if it is used in this way, the best possible result that could be predicted is the maintenance of the status quo. If improvement in CHD status is the objective, it is essential to select for breeding only animals that show either no demonstrable abnormality or, only very minor defects with scores that are well below BMS. (This is, in essence, exactly the same advice that was provided under the original BVA/KC HD Scheme.)

Unfortunately, some breeders have mistakenly come to accept the BMS as a basis for breeding selection and this has been largely responsible for the slow progress made in the control of CHD within certain sections of some breeds. The fact that some breeders regard the BMS as the specific value for breeding selection is shown when they become very concerned if the score that their dog obtains is even one point over BMS.

Table 10-3: British Veterinary Association/Kennel Club Hip Dysplasia Scheme criteria for scoring with a listing of the nine features to be evaluated and the six score points that could be assigned to each feature.

| Score Point | Norberg Angle | Subluxation | Cranial acetabular edge (CrAE) | Dorsal acetabular edge (DAE) | Cranial effective acetabular rim (CrEAR) | Acetabular fossa (AF) | Caudal acetabular edge (CaAE) | Femoral head & neck exostosis | Femoral head recontouring |
|---|---|---|---|---|---|---|---|---|---|
| 0 | +15% and over | Femoral head well centred in acetabulum | Even curve, parallel to femoral head throughout | DAE has slight curve | Sharp, clean cut junction of DAE and CrAE | A fine bone line curves medial and caudal from caudal end of CrAE | Clean line | Smooth rounded profile | – |
| 1 | +10% to +14% | Femoral head centre lies medial to DAE. Lateral or medial joint space increases | Lateral 1/4 CrAE flat and lateral or medial joint space diverges slightly | Loss of S curve only in the presence of other dysplastic change | Very small exostosis or very small facet at CrAE | Slight increase in bone density medial to AF. "Fine line" hazy or lost | Small exostosis at lateral CrAE | Slight exostosis in "ring formation" | Femoral head does not fit in circle due to exostosis or bone loss |
| 2 | +5% to +9% | Femoral head centre super-imposed on DAE. Medial joint space | CrAE flat throughout most of its length | Very small exostosis on cranial DAE | Very small exostosis or very small facet and/or minor bilabiation | Fine line lost AF and ventral AE hazy due to new bone. Notch at CaAE clear | Small exostosis at lateral and medial CaAE | Slight exostosis visible on skyline and/or density on medial femoral head | Some bone loss and/or femoral head/neck ring of exostosis |
| 3 | 0% to +4% | Femoral head centre just lateral to DAE. 1/2 femoral head within acetabulum | CrAE flat and slight bilabiation | Obvious exostosis on DAE especially cranially and/or minor "loss of edge" | Facet and/or small exostosis and/or bilabiation | Incomplete remodelling of acetabulum with medial face lateral to AF. Ventral AE lost. AF hazy. Notch irregular | Large exostosis and narrow notch at CaAE | Distinct exostosis in "ring formation" | Obvious bone loss and exostosis giving slight conical appearance |
| 4 | -1% to -5% | Femoral head centre clearly lateral to DAE. 1/4 femoral head within acetabulum | CrAE flat and moderate bilabiation | Exostosis well lateral to DAE and/or moderate "loss of edge" | Obvious facet and/or obvious exostosis and/or marked bilabiation | Marked remodelling. Medial face of acetabulum clearly lateral to AF. Ventral AE lost. Notch partly closed. | Marked exostosis and "hooking" of lateral end of CaAE | Obvious complete collar of exostosis | Gross remodelling. Obvious bone loss and exostosis gives mushroom appearance. |
| 5 | -6% to -10% | Femoral head centre well lateral to DAE. Femoral head just touches DAE | CrAE flat and gross bilabiation | Marked exostosis all along DAE and/or gross "loss of edge" | Gross exostosis and/or facet and/or gross bilabiation | Gross remodelling. Dense new bone throughout acetabulum. CaAE notch lost and AF obscured | Gross distortion due to mass of new bone in acetabulum. Notch lost completely | Massive exostosis giving mushroom appearance | Very gross remodelling with marked bone loss and much new bone |
| 6 | -11% and over | Complete pathological dislocation | Entire CrAE slopes cranially | Massive exostosis from cranial to caudal DAE | Complete remodelling of CrEAR. Massive exostosis and/or gross facet | Complete remodelling and new articular surface, well literal to AF. Notch lost | – | Massive exostosis and infill of trochanteric fossa and below femoral head | Femoral head is improperly shaped due to mal-development of temporal head centre |

### Table 10-4: Hip scores by breed
Data current to March 10, 1997 (Data on the BVA/KC scores are produced by kind permission of Dr. M. B. Willis, geneticist.)

| Name of breed | Number of dogs assessed | Best score obtained | Worst score obtained[1] | Mean score of breed | Rank[2] |
| --- | --- | --- | --- | --- | --- |
| Clumber spaniel | 418 | 0 | 102 | 43.09 | 1 |
| Otterhound | 101 | 4 | 102 | 42.16 | 2 |
| Sussex spaniel | 88 | 7 | 101 | 38.48 | 3 |
| Newfoundland | 2032 | 0 | 106 | 30.56 | 4 |
| Bullmastiff | 494 | 0 | 104 | 29.75 | 5 |
| Gordon setter | 1364 | 0 | 104 | 25.51 | 6 |
| Briard | 451 | 0 | 99 | 22.72 | 7 |
| St Bernard | 180 | 0 | 70 | 21.56 | 8 |
| Old English sheepdog | 1035 | 0 | 100 | 21.14 | 9 |
| English setter | 1516 | 0 | 95 | 19.94 | 10 |
| Golden retriever | 18556 | 0 | 106 | 19.52 | 11 |
| German shepherd dog | 26142 | 0 | 106 | 18.73 | 12 |
| Brittany | 175 | 0 | 74 | 18.53 | 13 |
| Welsh springer spaniel | 788 | 0 | 104 | 18.45 | 14 |
| Bouvier des Flandres | 124 | 4 | 76 | 18.21 | 15 |
| Shetland sheepdog | 81 | 2 | 100 | 18.12 | 16 |
| Hungarian puli | 301 | 1 | 102 | 17.81 | 17 |
| Irish water spaniel | 455 | 0 | 102 | 17.8 | 18 |
| Mastiff | 149 | 0 | 81 | 17.62 | 19 |
| Airedale terrier | 709 | 0 | 91 | 17.1 | 20 |
| Polish lowland sheepdog | 236 | 5 | 59 | 16.97 | 21 |
| Cavalier King Charles spaniel | 229 | 2 | 92 | 16.79 | 22 |
| Tibetan terrier | 561 | 0 | 90 | 16.63 | 23 |
| Cocker spaniel | 223 | 5 | 89 | 16.49 | 24 |
| Boxer | 249 | 0 | 64 | 16.29 | 25 |
| Bernese mountain dog | 2490 | 0 | 102 | 16.2 | 26 |
| Labrador retriever | 25708 | 0 | 104 | 16.14 | 27 |
| Italian spinone | 427 | 0 | 89 | 15.9 | 28 |
| Irish setter | 513 | 0 | 100 | 15.89 | 29 |
| Field spaniel | 58 | 0 | 51 | 15.89 | 30 |
| Large Munsterlander | 249 | 0 | 88 | 15.86 | 31 |
| Kerry blue terrier | 46 | 4 | 53 | 15.5 | 32 |
| Standard poodle | 260 | 4 | 74 | 15.48 | 33 |
| Nova Scotia duck tolling r. | 88 | 0 | 63 | 15.2 | 34 |
| Chow Chow | 557 | 0 | 102 | 14.4 | 35 |
| Anatolian shepherd dog | 123 | 0 | 68 | 14.34 | 36 |
| Giant schnauzer | 119 | 0 | 66 | 14 | 37 |
| Alaskan malamute | 144 | 2 | 66 | 13.97 | 38 |
| Maremma | 105 | 2 | 83 | 13.86 | 39 |
| Rottweiler | 7115 | 0 | 99 | 13.6 | 40 |
| English springer spaniel | 392 | 0 | 102 | 13.58 | 41 |
| Border collie (working sd) | 3220 | 0 | 89 | 13.4 | 42 |
| Tibetan mastiff | 73 | 3 | 45 | 13.39 | 43 |
| Elkhound | 286 | 0 | 61 | 13.38 | 44 |
| Weimaraner | 896 | 0 | 89 | 13.34 | 45 |
| Soft coated wheaten terrier | 191 | 2 | 62 | 13.08 | 46 |
| Samoyed | 866 | 0 | 94 | 12.95 | 47 |
| Rough collie | 524 | 0 | 89 | 12.81 | 48 |

**Table 10-4 (continued)**

| Name of breed | Number of dogs assessed | Best score obtained | Worst score obtained[1] | Mean score of breed | Rank[2] |
|---|---|---|---|---|---|
| Swedish vallhund | 73 | 2 | 29 | 12.76 | 49 |
| Hungarian vizsla | 294 | 2 | 59 | 12.74 | 50 |
| Pyrenean mountain dog | 260 | 0 | 94 | 12.7 | 51 |
| Keeshond | 41 | 3 | 63 | 12.51 | 52 |
| Great Dane | 173 | 0 | 59 | 12.37 | 53 |
| Rhodesian Ridgeback | 667 | 0 | 88 | 12.04 | 54 |
| Leonberger | 328 | 0 | 74 | 11.99 | 55 |
| Chesapeake Bay retriever | 226 | 0 | 52 | 11.95 | 56 |
| Curly coated retriever | 156 | 1 | 59 | 11.25 | 57 |
| Bearded collie | 1629 | 0 | 78 | 11.18 | 58 |
| Belgian shepherd dog | 784 | 0 | 104 | 11.11 | 59 |
| Japanese akita | 1154 | 0 | 92 | 10.94 | 60 |
| German wirehaired pointer | 162 | 0 | 77 | 10.78 | 61 |
| Hovawart | 109 | 0 | 79 | 10.53 | 62 |
| Australian shepherd dog | 169 | 2 | 71 | 10.51 | 63 |
| Irish red/white setter | 153 | 0 | 52 | 10.32 | 64 |
| Dobermann | 680 | 0 | 70 | 10.14 | 65 |
| Dalmatian | 63 | 0 | 39 | 9.79 | 66 |
| German shorthaired pointer | 220 | 0 | 57 | 9.74 | 67 |
| Flat coated retriever | 2691 | 0 | 85 | 9.14 | 68 |
| Siberian husky | 1231 | 0 | 43 | 6.43 | 69 |
| Irish wolfhound | 61 | 0 | 86 | 6 | 70 |
| Smooth collie | 39 | 0 | 17 | 5.24 | |
| Shar Pei | 37 | 5 | 81 | 18.46 | |
| Saluki | 37 | 0 | 14 | 4.8 | |
| Afghan hound | 34 | 0 | 54 | 9.04 | |
| Japanese shiba inu | 33 | 0 | 35 | 9.88 | |
| Norwegian buhund | 30 | 2 | 42 | 12.56 | |
| Tibetan spaniel | 30 | 2 | 31 | 11.24 | |
| Pointer | 28 | 0 | 60 | 11.54 | |
| Affenpinscher | 27 | 7 | 52 | 15.22 | |
| Malinois | 27 | 0 | 60 | 10.97 | |
| Hungarian Komondor | 26 | 4 | 72 | 16.64 | |
| Pyrenean sheepdog | 25 | 3 | 77 | 16.41 | |
| Finnish lapphund | 25 | 9 | 21 | 13.79 | |
| Schnauzer | 23 | 6 | 70 | 23.17 | |
| Bloodhound | 23 | 8 | 62 | 22.08 | |
| Welsh corgi (Pembroke) | 20 | 9 | 50 | 24.2 | |
| Staffordshire bull terrier | 19 | 7 | 23 | 13.1 | |
| Miniatur poodle | 18 | 6 | 58 | 16.34 | |
| Neopolitan Mastiff | 16 | 7 | 51 | 22.56 | |
| Pug | 15 | 10 | 53 | 24.47 | |
| Canaan dog | 15 | 8 | 45 | 14.8 | |
| Miniatur schnauzer | 15 | 4 | 32 | 13.14 | |
| Bichon Frise | 15 | 4 | 19 | 10.67 | |
| Basenji | 13 | 4 | 14 | 7.61 | |
| Beagle | 12 | 10 | 31 | 17.83 | |
| Australian cattle dog | 11 | 5 | 18 | 10.65 | |

**Table 10-4 (continued)**

| Name of breed | Number of dogs assessed | Best score obtained | Worst score obtained[1] | Mean score of breed | Rank[2] |
|---|---|---|---|---|---|
| Bulldog | 10 | 10 | 88 | 41.8 | |
| Eskimo dog | 10 | 6 | 60 | 27.8 | |
| Hungarian Kuvasz | 9 | 10 | 65 | 26.89 | |
| Portugese water dog | 9 | 6 | 63 | 18.22 | |
| Bracco Italiano | 9 | 10 | 22 | 14.33 | |
| Estrela Mountain dog | 9 | 1 | 27 | 13.56 | |
| Pinscher | 9 | 6 | 18 | 12 | |
| Bull terrier | 9 | 4 | 12 | 8.56 | |
| Kooikerhondje | 8 | 7 | 25 | 11.88 | |
| Deerhound | 8 | 0 | 17 | 4.75 | |
| Basset Griffon Vendeen P.T. | 7 | 13 | 48 | 28.14 | |
| Grand Bleu de Gascogne | 7 | 7 | 54 | 19.57 | |
| Lakeland terrier | 7 | 3 | 9 | 6.86 | |
| Shih Tzu | 6 | 8 | 102 | 37.17 | |
| Swedish lapphund | 6 | 9 | 67 | 28.17 | |
| Schipperke | 6 | 9 | 47 | 16.83 | |
| Border terrier | 5 | 3 | 10 | 8.2 | |
| Griffon Bruxellois | 4 | 15 | 61 | 27.75 | |
| St Johns waterdog | 4 | 10 | 32 | 17 | |
| West Highland White | 4 | 7 | 14 | 10.25 | |
| Beauceron | 3 | 8 | 63 | 31.67 | |
| Bergamasco | 3 | 11 | 48 | 25 | |
| French bulldog | 3 | 8 | 49 | 23.33 | |
| Glen of Imaal terrier | 3 | 15 | 19 | 17.67 | |
| Spanish waterdog | 3 | 9 | 13 | 10.67 | |
| Hamilton stovare | 2 | 22 | 24 | 23 | |
| Dachshund (MLH) | 2 | 14 | 25 | 19.5 | |
| Dachshund (LH) | 2 | 8 | 27 | 17.5 | |
| American Cocker spaniel | 2 | 14 | 14 | 14 | |
| Welsh corgi (Cardigan) | 2 | 4 | 5 | 4.5 | |
| Borzoi | 2 | 0 | 2 | 1 | |
| Dogge de Bordeaux | 1 | 63 | | 63 | |
| Dachshund (WH) | 1 | 26 | | 26 | |
| Dandy Dinmont terrier | 1 | 20 | | 20 | |
| Dachshund (SWH) | 1 | 18 | | 18 | |
| Cesky terrier | 1 | 15 | | 15 | |
| Lhasa apso | 1 | 11 | | 11 | |
| Manchester terrier | 1 | 10 | | 10 | |
| Australian silky terrier | 1 | 9 | | 9 | |
| Chihuahua | 1 | 9 | | 9 | |
| Fox terrier (smooth) | 1 | 6 | | 6 | |
| Greyhound | 1 | 0 | | 0 | |
| Lafitte Paulette | 1 | 6 | | 6 | |
| Papillon | 1 | 6 | | 6 | |
| Lurcher | 1 | 4 | | 4 | |
| Lowchen | 1 | 3 | | 3 | |
| Scottish terrier | 1 | 7 | | 7 | |

[1] Maximum 106
[2] Beginning with the worst mean score.

The correct use of CHD scores for breeding selection has to take account of the prevailing situation within a breed:

1. Breeds in which no clinical cases of CHD occur require to breed only those animals with a score of 0 or a very low score to ensure that they remain trouble-free. They can readily do so because they have many animals whose scores are very low and there is little or no difficulty in rejecting from breeding those animals whose scores are approaching BMS.

2. Breeds where lameness from CHD occurs only occasionally still require to take steps to eliminate the problem and for them it is important to breed only from animals whose scores are specifically well below BMS, since to use those at BMS can be predicted to perpetuate the problems.

3. For those breeds in which clinical CHD is a regular occurrence it is even more important to effect selection at a score value that is markedly below BMS with an overall improvement being the objective and drastic action is called for.

In addition to calculating BMS, tables were compiled setting out the results achieved by a series of sires where not less than 20 of their offspring had been scored (Tables 10-5, 10-6, and 10-7). This was styled "Progeny Testing" and was intended to assist in the identification of how sires had contributed to the control of CHD, especially those that had produced progeny with low scores.

These tables must be viewed with caution since, of necessity, they require to make the assumption that the score points recorded for each of the nine features of the hip are of equal value although this has specifically never been claimed for the BVA/KC HD Scoring Scheme. In addition, the scores of the sires and of the dams are not stated although it is relevant information.

The tables, do, however, substantiate the claim that CHD has a polygenetic basis. They also give clear indication that all individuals, both male and female, that are being considered as potential breeding stock are required to be assessed individually if progress in the control of CHD is to be achieved.

It is not sufficient to rely solely upon the scores of the parents of an individual, or upon the sires known progeny record since it is well known that quite considerable differences in hip scores can occur even between the individuals of the same litter.

Overall, the creation of progeny test tables is liable to create unnecessary complications in the control of CHD which requires the persistent application of a straight forward, almost, simplistic, approach over a prolonged period.

Fortunately, many dogs that show x-ray evidence of CHD do not show significant clinical problems and can lead a normal life as domestic pets or even as gun dogs and so rejection from breeding does not require their destruction. Dog breeders are faced with many breeding selection problems of which CHD is only one example, but, it must be stressed that the ultimate responsibility for the control of defects rests squarely with breeders and the fact that CHD is known to create such serious problems in those animals that are clinically affected should affect their priorities.

## Results achieved in the UK in the control of CHD

It is far from simple to assess the overall results of the BVA/KCHD Scoring Scheme for a variety of reasons, but it is notable that the annual throughput of the scheme has risen constantly over the past 10 years. This indicates a continued interest in the scheme by the breeders. There is little doubt that the publication of scores on the kennel club registration certificates has materially assisted in promoting the scheme and it makes it possible for potential purchasers to ensure that the breeders have exerted care in selecting their breeding stock. The existence of the BMS has been, however, a mixed blessing. If employed with due regard to its background, the BMS can be of value, but there are still breeders who regard it as "the magic value" for breeding selection purposes, which is not true in most breeds.

"The breeding advice which is given to British dog breeders is that they should score all breeding stock and breed from the lowest scores consistent with other features that they are concerned with improving. They should attempt to score other stock that may not be used for breeding but which will add to the information on their bloodlines. The information given with sire tables is that breeders should breed from those sires with low progeny averages but that greater emphasis should be given to sires with sufficient progeny (at least 20 and ideally 40). They should also use sires whose averages are based upon more rather than fewer mates, other things being equal. Finally, they should seek to not only assess progeny mean but the distribution of those progeny. Sires which have a high percentage of progeny in the lower categories (0 to 5, 6 to 10, and 11 to 20) are preferable and those with a low percentage in the higher categories (over 31) are also to be preferred." Dr. M.B. Willis

### Table 10-5: Progeny tests for hip scores of German Shepheard Dog sires
For the whole period listed by score. Data current to March 10, 1997. (Data on the BVA/KC scores are produced by kind permission of Dr. M. B. Willis, geneticist.)

| Name of Sire (* scored) | Number of progeny | Dams[1] | Best[2] | Worst[3] | Mean[4] | %[5] 0–5 | % 6–10 | % 11–20 | % 21–30 | % 31–40 | % 41–50 | >51 |
|---|---|---|---|---|---|---|---|---|---|---|---|---|
| Lido v. grauen | 31 | 18 | 0 | 18 | 8.2 | 19 | 45 | 35 | 0 | 0 | 0 | 0 |
| Beaumonts charmer* | 23 | 14 | 3 | 29 | 10.5 | 26 | 26 | 39 | 9 | 0 | 0 | 0 |
| Sing sing of wadacre* | 21 | 11 | 4 | 28 | 11.2 | 14 | 38 | 43 | 5 | 0 | 0 | 0 |
| Iolanda dojan* | 25 | 13 | 5 | 22 | 11.7 | 12 | 36 | 40 | 12 | 0 | 0 | 0 |
| Metpol lincon* | 41 | 8 | 2 | 43 | 11.8 | 10 | 44 | 37 | 7 | 0 | 2 | 0 |
| Zandro v. trompetersprung* | 49 | 33 | 4 | 37 | 12.2 | 11 | 35 | 47 | 3 | 6 | 0 | 0 |
| Metpol ashley | 32 | 7 | 2 | 53 | 12.3 | 13 | 41 | 41 | 0 | 3 | 0 | 3 |
| Ghandi v arminius* | 25 | 16 | 2 | 41 | 12.4 | 12 | 40 | 32 | 12 | 0 | 4 | 0 |
| Ary v rohrenfurth | 22 | 14 | 4 | 50 | 12.8 | 9 | 36 | 45 | 5 | 0 | 5 | 0 |
| Gavington mascaro* | 24 | 12 | 6 | 37 | 13.4 | 0 | 33 | 58 | 0 | 8 | 0 | 0 |
| Cumnorhurst yoll* | 41 | 22 | 0 | 42 | 13.7 | 12 | 34 | 37 | 10 | 8 | 3 | 0 |
| Rebroc davos* | 26 | 15 | 3 | 43 | 13.7 | 9 | 35 | 46 | 9 | 0 | 4 | 0 |
| Iolanda tell* | 29 | 13 | 0 | 88 | 13.8 | 14 | 38 | 34 | 7 | 3 | 0 | 3 |
| Shadowsquad bruce* | 23 | 10 | 4 | 46 | 14 | 5 | 35 | 38 | 5 | 5 | 5 | 0 |
| Jumbo v adeloga* | 38 | 23 | 2 | 35 | 14.5 | 9 | 18 | 53 | 18 | 3 | 0 | 0 |
| Chanask edison* | 72 | 38 | 4 | 84 | 14.6 | 8 | 36 | 46 | 5 | 6 | 0 | 3 |
| Held v hirschel* | 50 | 30 | 3 | 61 | 14.9 | 12 | 36 | 34 | 10 | 2 | 2 | 4 |
| Ionimay shannan* | 99 | 62 | 2 | 88 | 14.9 | 10 | 29 | 45 | 9 | 3 | 3 | 3 |
| Shadowsquad caucasian* | 21 | 10 | 8 | 40 | 15 | 0 | 19 | 71 | 5 | 0 | 5 | 0 |
| Novem adagio of silkenwood* | 68 | 43 | 4 | 78 | 15.1 | 3 | 29 | 56 | 5 | 3 | 2 | 3 |
| Romeno nico* | 59 | 35 | 1 | 72 | 15.1 | 10 | 34 | 39 | 8 | 0 | 5 | 4 |
| Janshar zebedee* | 40 | 26 | 0 | 67 | 15.2 | 8 | 33 | 25 | 20 | 3 | 0 | 3 |
| Metpol totem* | 25 | 5 | 5 | 66 | 15.3 | 12 | 48 | 20 | 8 | 0 | 4 | 8 |
| Zac v adeloga | 61 | 35 | 0 | 76 | 15.3 | 13 | 28 | 43 | 8 | 4 | 5 | 2 |
| Kurtridge quando of videx* | 87 | 45 | 3 | 74 | 15.5 | 4 | 33 | 47 | 14 | 0 | 1 | 4 |
| Novem volka* | 34 | 18 | 5 | 71 | 15.5 | 8 | 28 | 47 | 12 | 3 | 0 | 3 |
| Bedwins quatro of jutone* | 57 | 35 | 3 | 63 | 15.8 | 2 | 26 | 58 | 7 | 0 | 0 | 7 |
| Moonwinds golden mahdi* | 78 | 52 | 0 | 95 | 15.8 | 8 | 39 | 37 | 8 | 2 | 1 | 6 |
| Mortoff marcus* | 24 | 13 | 6 | 46 | 15.8 | 0 | 42 | 33 | 13 | 8 | 4 | 0 |
| Calagran urko* | 54 | 29 | 5 | 69 | 15.9 | 5 | 26 | 57 | 2 | 7 | 2 | 2 |
| Romeno rolli* | 21 | 9 | 7 | 74 | 16 | 0 | 52 | 29 | 10 | 5 | 0 | 5 |
| Olderhill black wellie* | 23 | 13 | 1 | 55 | 16.2 | 5 | 30 | 43 | 13 | 4 | 0 | 4 |
| Greenveldt jago of nyrvana* | 49 | 24 | 0 | 51 | 16.3 | 6 | 31 | 43 | 10 | 2 | 4 | 4 |
| Rothick vinobe* | 25 | 15 | 1 | 46 | 16.3 | 36 | 12 | 28 | 4 | 4 | 16 | 0 |
| Kent v adeloga* | 27 | 16 | 3 | 55 | 16.4 | 8 | 26 | 48 | 4 | 7 | 4 | 4 |
| Kesyra hero* | 46 | 30 | 6 | 64 | 16.4 | 0 | 26 | 57 | 11 | 0 | 3 | 5 |
| Youkays putz of vidbar* | 28 | 15 | 6 | 61 | 16.4 | 0 | 29 | 46 | 14 | 4 | 0 | 4 |
| Videx yasso* | 24 | 13 | 4 | 62 | 16.5 | 4 | 12 | 63 | 16 | 0 | 0 | 4 |
| Anthrys morgan of jutone* | 29 | 18 | 4 | 57 | 16.8 | 4. | 31 | 52 | 4 | 0 | 4 | 7 |
| Donzarras nico of schutton* | 28 | 13 | 4 | 47 | 18.8 | 18 | 25 | 32 | 7 | 4 | 14 | 0 |
| Charisma of black knight* | 28 | 19 | 4 | 53 | 17 | 4 | 21 | 50 | 14 | 4 | 4 | 4 |
| Berwartstein enard* | 83 | 39 | 5 | 99 | 17.2 | 1 | 33 | 43 | 12 | 5 | 4 | 3 |
| Myter smokey blue warrior* | 32 | 13 | 4 | 49 | 17.2 | 4 | 25 | 53 | 4 | 3 | 12 | 0 |
| Salenze dexi* | 25 | 13 | 4 | 82 | 17.2 | 8 | 36 | 36 | 8 | 4 | 4 | 4 |
| Bedwins zamb | 24 | 14 | 4 | 72 | 17.3 | 12 | 34 | 30 | 13 | 0 | 9 | 4 |
| Vikkas pandorus* | 26 | 15 | 4 | 53 | 17.3 | 5 | 19 | 54 | 8 | 12 | 0 | 5 |
| Major force* | 29 | 8 | 4 | 54 | 17.6 | 5 | 24 | 48 | 7 | 14 | 0 | 5 |

**Table 10-5 (continued)**

| Name of Sire (* scored) | Number of progeny | Dams[1] | Best[2] | Worst[3] | Mean[4] | %[5] 0–5 | % 6–10 | % 11–20 | % 21–30 | % 31–40 | % 41–50 | % >51 |
|---|---|---|---|---|---|---|---|---|---|---|---|---|
| Lindanvale vegas* | 74 | 40 | 6 | 99 | 17.7 | 0 | 30 | 45 | 15 | 3 | 4 | 4 |
| Baldrick of conquell* | 50 | 25 | 3 | 67 | 17.9 | 5 | 38 | 36 | 9 | 2 | 5 | 9 |
| Bedwins siegaro* | 85 | 56 | 0 | 95 | 17.9 | 5 | 28 | 45 | 8 | 12 | 0 | 5 |
| Xaro v grundel at dunmonaidh* | 35 | 26 | 1 | 85 | 17.9 | 7 | 43 | 34 | 0 | 7 | 4 | 9 |
| Warrenways peron* | 28 | 18 | 6 | 93 | 18 | 0 | 32 | 46 | 11 | 4 | 0 | 6 |
| Arkov huhnegrab | 143 | 79 | 2 | 98 | 18.3 | 11 | 35 | 32 | 10 | 3 | 5 | 11 |
| Bedwins gildo* | 41 | 23 | 5 | 69 | 18.3 | 4 | 32 | 39 | 13 | 10 | 0 | 7 |
| Exl v batu* | 120 | 63 | 4 | 67 | 18.4 | 2 | 23 | 45 | 18 | 9 | 2 | 3 |
| Kesyra basko* | 38 | 26 | 2 | 76 | 18.7 | 5 | 24 | 47 | 11 | 5 | 0 | 8 |
| Laios v noort* | 158 | 74 | 0 | 85 | 18.7 | 8 | 30 | 37 | 9 | 7 | 3 | 10 |
| Ravenways lord luke* | 20 | 11 | 6 | 70 | 18.9 | 0 | 35 | 40 | 5 | 10 | 5 | 5 |
| Xero v grauen* | 53 | 31 | 6 | 91 | 18.9 | 0 | 17 | 62 | 9 | 4 | 4 | 3 |
| Jupaala quino* | 32 | 18 | 4 | 64 | 19.3 | 3 | 19 | 50 | 12 | 6 | 3 | 6 |
| Geshank z bethany* | 20 | 12 | 1 | 53 | 19.4 | 20 | 30 | 20 | 5 | 0 | 20 | 5 |
| Middross sonny* | 22 | 13 | 0 | 66 | 19.9 | 9 | 18 | 45 | 9 | 0 | 5 | 14 |
| Bedwins pirol* | 140 | 72 | 0 | 79 | 20 | 9 | 24 | 40 | 17 | 6 | 2 | 9 |
| Black knight of pembroke* | 27 | 12 | 5 | 57 | 20.1 | 4 | 19 | 30 | 22 | 15 | 7 | 4 |
| Blue fox of foxfold* | 27 | 7 | 2 | 74 | 20.1 | 7 | 22 | 44 | 7 | 11 | 0 | 7 |
| Saxon warrior of kingsmeadow* | 28 | 17 | 1 | 81 | 20.2 | 8 | 32 | 25 | 18 | 5 | 7 | 7 |
| Kemjon lex* | 30 | 18 | 3 | 106 | 20.3 | 7 | 20 | 47 | 10 | 3 | 7 | 7 |
| Vikkas rasputin* | 36 | 19 | 5 | 82 | 20.3 | 3 | 20 | 50 | 3 | 17 | 3 | 6 |
| Castor v altor* | 21 | 12 | 5 | 83 | 20.4 | 5 | 29 | 43 | 10 | 0 | 5 | 10 |
| Dux v burg esch* | 96 | 41 | 0 | 106 | 20.4 | 13 | 28 | 39 | 4 | 4 | 6 | 13 |
| Sagaro danzak* | 40 | 24 | 6 | 60 | 20.4 | 0 | 20 | 43 | 17 | 8 | 5 | 5 |
| Agro v wiesenborn | 104 | 58 | 0 | 99 | 20.5 | 13 | 31 | 33 | 5 | 6 | 2 | 12 |
| Quant v kirschental* | 52 | 31 | 5 | 80 | 20.5 | 5 | 31 | 40 | 4 | 3 | 8 | 11 |
| Romeno marksman* | 22 | 9 | 2 | 83 | 20.5 | 5 | 23 | 41 | 18 | 5 | 0 | 9 |
| Dillan am klooster bergen* | 30 | 18 | 3 | 91 | 20.7 | 11 | 23 | 36 | 14 | 4 | 4 | 11 |
| Kaisons kadet* | 26 | 8 | 5 | 76 | 20.9 | 4 | 23 | 35 | 23 | 4 | 4 | 8 |
| Shadowsquad krieg* | 24 | 12 | 6 | 85 | 21 | 0 | 42 | 25 | 12 | 12 | 0 | 9 |
| Middross panto* | 60 | 37 | 5 | 60 | 21.8 | 4 | 22 | 38 | 13 | 7 | 10 | 8 |
| Bedwins fedor* | 48 | 26 | 4 | 90 | 22.8 | 2 | 19 | 46 | 15 | 0 | 9 | 10 |
| Iemness atlas* | 25 | 17 | 7 | 101 | 22.8 | 0 | 28 | 48 | 0 | 4 | 12 | 8 |
| Raxmae tarot* | 22 | 8 | 4 | 97 | 23 | 5 | 36 | 23 | 13 | 5 | 10 | 9 |
| Sheroz bon jovi* | 29 | 17 | 1 | 63 | 23 | 14 | 10 | 31 | 17 | 7 | 14 | 7 |
| Greenstan canto* | 20 | 15 | 4 | 99 | 24.6 | 5 | 20 | 45 | 5 | 5 | 5 | 5 |
| Kingstown vegas of sagaro* | 22 | 16 | 1 | 75 | 24.9 | 5 | 18 | 36 | 18 | 0 | 9 | 14 |
| Jalinkas dax of jutone* | 20 | 12 | 5 | 105 | 25 | 5 | 35 | 30 | 0 | 10 | 5 | 15 |
| Tyeglen watz* | 21 | 12 | 8 | 76 | 25 | 0 | 5 | 46 | 23 | 14 | 9 | 5 |
| Natz v hirschel* | 70 | 44 | 8 | 90 | 26.6 | 0 | 10 | 39 | 23 | 6 | 10 | 11 |
| Kemjon natz cf jutone* | 27 | 16 | 2 | 92 | 28.6 | 13 | 18 | 30 | 19 | 8 | 4 | 18 |
| Gayvilles nilo* | 32 | 21 | 6 | 93 | 29.8 | 0 | 10 | 44 | 10 | 16 | 4 | 19 |
| Kelnik fergus* | 21 | 11 | 10 | 106 | 34.1 | 0 | 5 | 43 | 10 | 19 | 5 | 19 |

[1] Number of different dams producing these progeny.
[2] Lowest ( best) score among these progeny.
[3] Highest ( worst) score among these progeny.
[4] Mean progeny score (arithmetic mean).
[5] Percentage (nearest whole number) of scores progeny that fall within score categories. Only those sires with an axcess of 20 progeny were included.

### Table 10-6: Progeny tests for hip scores of Golden Retriever sires
For whole period listed alphabetically. Data current to February 14, 1997.
(Data on the BVA/KC scores are produced by kind permission of Dr. M. B. Willis, geneticist.)

| Name of Sire (* scored) | Number of progeny | Dams[1] | Best[2] | Worst[3] | Mean[4] | %[5] 0–5 | % 6–10 | % 11–20 | % 21–30 | % 31–40 | % 41–50 | >51 |
|---|---|---|---|---|---|---|---|---|---|---|---|---|
| Amberland black sabre* | 140 | 63 | 3 | 75 | 19.3 | 3 | 22 | 44 | 22 | 8 | 8 | 4 |
| Amberland sky hi* | 91 | 51 | 1 | 75 | 17.6 | 4 | 30 | 45 | 8 | 8 | 2 | 6 |
| Amirene adam* | 31 | 16 | 6 | 39 | 14.2 | 0 | 35 | 48 | 13 | 3 | 0 | 0 |
| Amirene king eider/davem* | 69 | 34 | 0 | 45 | 13.4 | 4 | 43 | 39 | 7 | 4 | 3 | 0 |
| Amirene liberator/delcott* | 36 | 21 | 1 | 74 | 15.2 | 6 | 58 | 14 | 11 | 3 | 6 | 3 |
| Amirene pacifique* | 27 | 17 | 8 | 54 | 16.8 | 0 | 41 | 30 | 22 | 4 | 0 | 4 |
| Ashlyn piper of canina* | 29 | 20 | 8 | 59 | 17 | 0 | 28 | 45 | 17 | 7 | 0 | 3 |
| Beaconholm bacchus* | 22 | 20 | 3 | 61 | 20 | 9 | 32 | 23 | 9 | 14 | 9 | 5 |
| Beaconholm duke* | 40 | 26 | 2 | 47 | 14.6 | 13 | 33 | 40 | 8 | 3 | 5 | 0 |
| Belway flick of flightline | 23 | 13 | 4 | 66 | 19.9 | 13 | 9 | 57 | 9 | 9 | 0 | 9 |
| Bethrob bracken* | 112 | 60 | 0 | 85 | 18.5 | 9 | 32 | 32 | 11 | 6 | 7 | 5 |
| Blakesley benjamin/westley* | 20 | 12 | 7 | 47 | 18.5 | 0 | 25 | 45 | 10 | 10 | 10 | 0 |
| Bolberry chacone/moorquest* | 56 | 30 | 4 | 61 | 18.9 | 2 | 27 | 46 | 11 | 7 | 2 | 5 |
| Brackengold hawk | 34 | 23 | 0 | 69 | 20.6 | 9 | 32 | 29 | 3 | 9 | 3 | 15 |
| Bramhills king of the castle* | 21 | 9 | 0 | 59 | 17.8 | 5 | 33 | 43 | 0 | 10 | 5 | 5 |
| bramhills pied piper* | 44 | 21 | 7 | 55 | 19.4 | 0 | 18 | 50 | 20 | 2 | 5 | 5 |
| Bridgefarm barleycorn* | 21 | 13 | 2 | 74 | 21.8 | 10 | 24 | 29 | 14 | 5 | 10 | 10 |
| Bryanstown gaucho* | 67 | 35 | 2 | 104 | 20.7 | 6 | 31 | 34 | 9 | 3 | 3 | 14 |
| Bryns guy of jamesmoor | 23 | 21 | 3 | 76 | 21 | 4 | 13 | 43 | 17 | 17 | 0 | 4 |
| Butleigh tally of tallygold* | 31 | 19 | 4 | 32 | 16 | 7 | 13 | 55 | 22 | 3 | 0 | 0 |
| Camrose fabius tarquin | 140 | 83 | 0 | 82 | 16.3 | 5 | 36 | 41 | 8 | 3 | 2 | 6 |
| Camrose fabius of davern* | 178 | 100 | 0 | 83 | 28.6 | 3 | 20 | 28 | 11 | 14 | 6 | 19 |
| Camrose tulfes interol* | 80 | 54 | 4 | 71 | 15.5 | 1 | 39 | 40 | 13 | 6 | 1 | 1 |
| Canina that entertainment* | 39 | 26 | 6 | 86 | 23.2 | 0 | 36 | 38 | 3 | 3 | 3 | 18 |
| Canina winter berry | 47 | 30 | 6 | 75 | 24.3 | 0 | 15 | 40 | 23 | 4 | 4 | 13 |
| Catcombe cheshire/m'green* | 21 | 13 | 8 | 31 | 15 | 0 | 24 | 62 | 10 | 5 | 0 | 0 |
| Catcombe cordoroy* | 30 | 22 | 4 | 67 | 24.6 | 3 | 20 | 20 | 37 | 10 | 3 | 10 |
| Cattryse mr rochester* | 66 | 29 | 2 | 99 | 25.5 | 2 | 9 | 44 | 15 | 11 | 12 | 8 |
| Chadzo secret admirer* | 31 | 16 | 5 | 65 | 22.6 | 5 | 19 | 39 | 13 | 6 | 6 | 13 |
| Chevanne free n easy* | 43 | 23 | 6 | 55 | 22 | 0 | 19 | 40 | 12 | 19 | 9 | 3 |
| Clancallum gregor mhor* | 44 | 22 | 6 | 80 | 21.8 | 0 | 23 | 45 | 9 | 9 | 2 | 12 |
| Coombstock disco dancer* | 22 | 13 | 6 | 49 | 21 | 0 | 18 | 45 | 14 | 14 | 9 | 0 |
| Comborough quartermaster* | 32 | 22 | 6 | 38 | 15.8 | 0 | 22 | 53 | 22 | 3 | 0 | 0 |
| Darris double o seven* | 27 | 16 | 4 | 44 | 17.8 | 8 | 22 | 37 | 22 | 4 | 8 | 0 |
| Darris star time at canina* | 22 | 16 | 7 | 59 | 18.3 | 0 | 32 | 45 | 9 | 5 | 5 | 5 |
| Davem figaro | 31 | 26 | 0 | 31 | 14.2 | 10 | 19 | 55 | 13 | 3 | 0 | 0 |
| Davem jacobin* | 26 | 12 | 8 | 62 | 17.1 | 0 | 19 | 65 | 4 | 8 | 0 | 4 |
| Davem quicksilver* | 68 | 29 | 5 | 54 | 15.2 | 2 | 40 | 40 | 12 | 3 | 3 | 1 |
| Deerflite clay* | 39 | 27 | 3 | 76 | 24.5 | 4 | 21 | 36 | 13 | 8 | 4 | 15 |
| Deerflite crescendo | 31 | 22 | 3 | 55 | 15.9 | 6 | 23 | 52 | 13 | 3 | 0 | 3 |
| Denmarella just a jester* | 35 | 24 | 4 | 61 | 26.1 | 3 | 9 | 34 | 20 | 14 | 14 | 6 |
| Dick of tugwood* | 28 | 16 | 7 | 71 | 17.8 | 0 | 18 | 61 | 11 | 7 | 0 | 4 |
| Earnfield teal* | 50 | 27 | 5 | 63 | 20.1 | 2 | 24 | 44 | 13 | 4 | 2 | 10 |
| Edgeley ensign* | 53 | 31 | 6 | 69 | 16.1 | 0 | 30 | 51 | 12 | 4 | 2 | 2 |
| Edgeley ere we go again* | 26 | 16 | 6 | 59 | 24 | 0 | 8 | 50 | 12 | 15 | 12 | 4 |
| Eilladale el dorado | 27 | 19 | 4 | 57 | 18.1 | 4 | 37 | 33 | 7 | 0 | 15 | 4 |
| Fenwood jagger at canina | 71 | 50 | 6 | 83 | 22 | 0 | 25 | 46 | 9 | 6 | 7 | 9 |
| Fernyvale rambler/pnecrest* | 41 | 17 | 5 | 47 | 15.3 | 2 | 37 | 41 | 12 | 5 | 2 | 0 |

### Table 10-6 (continued)

| Name of Sire (* scored) | Number of progeny | Dams[1] | Best[2] | Worst[3] | Mean[4] | %[5] 0–5 | % 6–10 | % 11–20 | % 21–30 | % 31–40 | % 41–50 | >51 |
|---|---|---|---|---|---|---|---|---|---|---|---|---|
| Flyngalee tigers eye* | 29 | 15 | 7 | 60 | 18.4 | 0 | 48 | 24 | 4 | 14 | 6 | 4 |
| Fourwinds bossanaova/l'ford* | 21 | 19 | 2 | 55 | 18.7 | 4 | 28 | 33 | 22 | 7 | 4 | 4 |
| Gaineda consclidator/s'sue* | 157 | 96 | 0 | 92 | 17 | 6 | 37 | 35 | 9 | 4 | 1 | 7 |
| Galalith crown prince* | 23 | 20 | 6 | 18 | 10.3 | 0 | 57 | 43 | 0 | 0 | 0 | 0 |
| Garbank special edition* | 57 | 28 | 5 | 40 | 14.4 | 2 | 32 | 49 | 9 | 9 | 0 | 0 |
| Gatchells sky at night* | 44 | 25 | 6 | 77 | 27.3 | 0 | 27 | 30 | 14 | 7 | 2 | 20 |
| Glennessa escapade | 26 | 11 | 2 | 67 | 16.9 | 12 | 23 | 46 | 4 | 8 | 0 | 8 |
| Goldcrest game of chance* | 31 | 14 | 6 | 75 | 24.4 | 0 | 7 | 45 | 26 | 13 | 0 | 10 |
| Goldwing saturn* | 21 | 9 | 11 | 54 | 22.6 | 0 | 0 | 52 | 33 | 10 | 0 | 5 |
| Golmas gioberti of siagar* | 26 | 14 | 8 | 67 | 18.5 | 0 | 35 | 38 | 12 | 4 | 8 | 4 |
| Goronne artful dodger b | 24 | 16 | 8 | 72 | 26.3 | 0 | 13 | 46 | 0 | 17 | 17 | 8 |
| Gunhills banjo of sansue* | 94 | 41 | 6 | 50 | 16.9 | 0 | 22 | 53 | 11 | 9 | 5 | 0 |
| Gwelo sinbad of tamsbrook* | 60 | 37 | 2 | 71 | 22 | 5 | 17 | 42 | 15 | 3 | 10 | 8 |
| Gyrima oliver | 52 | 34 | 4 | 67 | 21.5 | 8 | 23 | 38 | 8 | 4 | 8 | 12 |
| Gyrima scorpian* | 26 | 15 | 6 | 64 | 23.4 | 0 | 24 | 38 | 12 | 7 | 8 | 12 |
| Gyrima todmanton of dabess | 48 | 29 | 0 | 84 | 21.4 | 15 | 21 | 27 | 13 | 10 | 4 | 10 |
| Holway corbiere* | 65 | 30 | 0 | 36 | 11.1 | 7 | 54 | 31 | 8 | 2 | 0 | 0 |
| Holway trumpet | 44 | 25 | 2 | 41 | 13 | 9 | 36 | 39 | 14 | 0 | 2 | 0 |
| Hurricane chas of rayleas* | 20 | 14 | 6 | 77 | 16.4 | 0 | 25 | 60 | 10 | 0 | 0 | 5 |
| Jamescroft rheingold | 29 | 13 | 9 | 55 | 25.5 | 0 | 11 | 44 | 14 | 7 | 17 | 7 |
| Jamoon troika of ninell* | 25 | 14 | 8 | 62 | 20.1 | 0 | 16 | 60 | 4 | 12 | 4 | 4 |
| Jobeka jasper of nortonwood | 171 | 99 | 6 | 89 | 22.2 | 0 | 22 | 48 | 14 | 10 | 11 | 7 |
| Kidston daiquiri* | 27 | 19 | 5 | 64 | 22.3 | 4 | 22 | 37 | 11 | 11 | 5 | 11 |
| Lacons enterprise* | 61 | 30 | 4 | 86 | 22.8 | 5 | 16 | 37 | 18 | 6 | 10 | 8 |
| Laurenley landser of culray* | 41 | 21 | 7 | 78 | 24.6 | 0 | 34 | 26 | 13 | 5 | 5 | 17 |
| Lawnwoods swagman j* | 22 | 16 | 8 | 66 | 27.6 | 0 | 10 | 36 | 18 | 10 | 18 | 10 |
| Leithfield euryp des* | 20 | 11 | 6 | 65 | 20.6 | 0 | 20 | 50 | 20 | 0 | 0 | 10 |
| Linchael cartier of gloi* | 62 | 28 | 4 | 40 | 14.1 | 3 | 37 | 44 | 8 | 8 | 0 | 0 |
| Linchael casamayor* | 21 | 11 | 3 | 23 | 10.4 | 14 | 38 | 43 | 5 | 0 | 0 | 0 |
| Linchael conspiracy/ch'ne* | 68 | 32 | 6 | 73 | 19.6 | 0 | 22 | 47 | 12 | 10 | 3 | 6 |
| Linchael titan of camrose* | 65 | 40 | 5 | 69 | 15.5 | 3 | 43 | 40 | 11 | 2 | 2 | 5 |
| Linchael tortoiseshell/l* | 26 | 23 | 3 | 74 | 18.6 | 4 | 27 | 54 | 8 | 0 | 0 | 8 |
| Linchael vargas of motlaisa* | 37 | 25 | 6 | 79 | 17.3 | 0 | 41 | 38 | 11 | 5 | 0 | 5 |
| Lindys butterscotch m* | 21 | 9 | 7 | 73 | 22.3 | 0 | 24 | 38 | 19 | 5 | 5 | 10 |
| Lorinford lancelot* | 185 | 104 | 4 | 93 | 19 | 1 | 25 | 48 | 15 | 8 | 5 | 3 |
| Lovehayne betimoti of c* | 93 | 53 | 4 | 81 | 18.9 | 1 | 31 | 45 | 11 | 7 | 2 | 6 |
| Maunsfield star trooper* | 30 | 18 | 6 | 75 | 16.3 | 0 | 43 | 47 | 0 | 0 | 0 | 10 |
| Maurfield tuba smartie* | 61 | 26 | 5 | 63 | 17.9 | 1 | 26 | 49 | 13 | 5 | 4 | 4 |
| Meant to be at moorquest* | 95 | 48 | 2 | 73 | 22.1 | 4 | 24 | 35 | 14 | 9 | 8 | 8 |
| Melfricka ace in the hole* | 65 | 39 | 6 | 57 | 17.2 | 0 | 28 | 46 | 18 | 4 | 2 | 3 |
| Melfricka kudos rossb.* | 51 | 31 | 4 | 72 | 13.8 | 2 | 43 | 41 | 12 | 0 | 0 | 2 |
| Melfricka xmas wishes* | 51 | 30 | 4 | 70 | 19.3 | 2 | 22 | 43 | 22 | 4 | 6 | 2 |
| Melfricka zebediah* | 44 | 36 | 6 | 57 | 18.9 | 0 | 32 | 39 | 9 | 9 | 5 | 7 |
| Melfricka zed* | 79 | 37 | 4 | 50 | 16.8 | 3 | 30 | 40 | 15 | 8 | 3 | 0 |
| Milestone porthos* | 29 | 14 | 6 | 29 | 12.2 | 0 | 52 | 41 | 7 | 0 | 0 | 0 |
| Millwater laser* | 25 | 9 | 4 | 42 | 16.2 | 10 | 12 | 68 | 0 | 10 | 5 | 0 |
| Mjaerumhodas crusader* | 37 | 17 | 5 | 79 | 20.6 | 3 | 38 | 24 | 16 | 5 | 3 | 11 |
| Moorquest mugwump* | 56 | 31 | 2 | 69 | 20 | 7 | 25 | 36 | 7 | 12 | 7 | 5 |

## Table 10-6 (continued)

| Name of Sire (* scored) | Number of progeny | Dams[1] | Best[2] | Worst[3] | Mean[4] | %[5] 0–5 | % 6–10 | % 11–20 | % 21–30 | % 31–40 | % 41–50 | >51 |
|---|---|---|---|---|---|---|---|---|---|---|---|---|
| Motlaisa chalice of gold* | 26 | 15 | 7 | 80 | 30.8 | 0 | 15 | 23 | 23 | 8 | 12 | 19 |
| Mugs game at moorquest | 40 | 25 | 2 | 82 | 23.2 | 3 | 15 | 43 | 15 | 8 | 5 | 13 |
| Muskan mayerling/b'gold* | 42 | 27 | 8 | 48 | 18.9 | 0 | 21 | 50 | 10 | 15 | 5 | 0 |
| Muskan most likely* | 85 | 44 | 6 | 69 | 20.1 | 0 | 24 | 40 | 12 | 11 | 7 | 8 |
| Night romance of kenour* | 28 | 12 | 1 | 74 | 19.1 | 21 | 36 | 14 | 11 | 7 | 4 | 7 |
| Ninell rambruen* | 62 | 35 | 5 | 95 | 19.3 | 2 | 35 | 39 | 7 | 5 | 5 | 7 |
| Noravon trolius of camrose | 29 | 21 | 4 | 80 | 24.1 | 3 | 14 | 41 | 17 | 10 | 3 | 10 |
| Nortonwood checkmate* | 104 | 52 | 2 | 60 | 12 | 8 | 46 | 36 | 7 | 2 | 1 | 2 |
| Nortonwood faunus* | 51 | 31 | 0 | 52 | 14 | 10 | 38 | 36 | 8 | 5 | 2 | 2 |
| Nortonwood silvanus* | 135 | 70 | 4 | 52 | 18.4 | 2 | 24 | 45 | 17 | 5 | 7 | 2 |
| Nortonwood twain of rockwin* | 35 | 26 | 6 | 84 | 20.4 | 0 | 43 | 26 | 6 | 14 | 6 | 6 |
| Okus autumn adventurer* | 22 | 12 | 5 | 86 | 28.7 | 5 | 27 | 18 | 23 | 9 | 0 | 18 |
| Okus buccaneer* | 42 | 24 | 6 | 77 | 21.1 | 0 | 21 | 48 | 12 | 10 | 2 | 7 |
| Oystergold pandorina* | 20 | 10 | 7 | 64 | 20.6 | 0 | 20 | 40 | 30 | 5 | 0 | 5 |
| Papeta philosopher* | 65 | 33 | 5 | 39 | 12.7 | 2 | 46 | 42 | 7 | 5 | 0 | 0 |
| Paudell easter plantagenet* | 133 | 115 | 4 | 71 | 18.5 | 1 | 27 | 44 | 16 | 6 | 6 | 4 |
| Pinecrest pioneer of kidston* | 26 | 16 | 7 | 70 | 26 | 0 | 15 | 27 | 31 | 8 | 11 | 8 |
| Pinecrest salvador | 41 | 28 | 4 | 61 | 25 | 2 | 22 | 37 | 10 | 7 | 17 | 5 |
| Pitcote arcadian of garthfield | 108 | 75 | 4 | 70 | 19.4 | 2 | 18 | 49 | 13 | 7 | 4 | 7 |
| Pondcroft clannad* | 29 | 16 | 6 | 90 | 27.3 | 0 | 24 | 28 | 10 | 14 | 7 | 17 |
| Rachenco boomerang* | 20 | 12 | 6 | 43 | 17.9 | 0 | 30 | 40 | 15 | 10 | 5 | 0 |
| Rambleyne dominic of westley* | 29 | 18 | 4 | 47 | 13 | 4 | 52 | 38 | 4 | 4 | 0 | 0 |
| Rayleas caluimn* | 26 | 12 | 6 | 36 | 13 | 0 | 42 | 50 | 4 | 4 | 0 | 0 |
| Rayleas reema* | 73 | 44 | 9 | 84 | 27 | 0 | 3 | 38 | 25 | 17 | 6 | 13 |
| Record of yeo* | 26 | 20 | 4 | 44 | 18.4 | 4 | 27 | 38 | 12 | 12 | 8 | 0 |
| Ritzilyn cockney robin* | 77 | 42 | 5 | 78 | 18.3 | 2 | 19 | 48 | 18 | 4 | 4 | 3 |
| Ritzilyn macallister* | 23 | 13 | 7 | 46 | 19.9 | 0 | 12 | 52 | 17 | 13 | 5 | 0 |
| Ritzilyn renoir of satona* | 31 | 20 | 6 | 70 | 19.8 | 0 | 35 | 39 | 7 | 7 | 7 | 7 |
| Roksand oberon/westervane* | 33 | 24 | 2 | 47 | 15.8 | 3 | 39 | 33 | 15 | 3 | 6 | 0 |
| Rossbourne harvest gold* | 49 | 25 | 3 | 54 | 20 | 4 | 24 | 41 | 8 | 14 | 4 | 4 |
| Rossbourne just jaime | 20 | 10 | 8 | 51 | 14.8 | 0 | 35 | 50 | 10 | 0 | 0 | 5 |
| Rossbourne silvery sea* | 23 | 14 | 4 | 55 | 21.3 | 5 | 26 | 30 | 9 | 13 | 13 | 5 |
| Rossbourne trooper* | 41 | 22 | 4 | 64 | 17.5 | 2 | 22 | 51 | 12 | 7 | 0 | 5 |
| Rossmohr of clancallum* | 39 | 17 | 7 | 59 | 14.9 | 0 | 33 | 51 | 6 | 8 | 0 | 3 |
| Russway sunnie jim* | 26 | 14 | 9 | 85 | 26.8 | 0 | 12 | 38 | 15 | 19 | 4 | 12 |
| Rusty of the glen* | 20 | 17 | 7 | 87 | 25.1 | 0 | 35 | 25 | 10 | 10 | 5 | 15 |
| Sandusky bartholomew* | 25 | 17 | 7 | 80 | 27.1 | 0 | 24 | 24 | 16 | 12 | 8 | 16 |
| Sansue april joker* | 34 | 18 | 6 | 50 | 16.8 | 0 | 29 | 47 | 9 | 9 | 6 | 0 |
| Sansue castalian* | 169 | 90 | 3 | 71 | 19.4 | 4 | 36 | 28 | 13 | 7 | 6 | 9 |
| Sansue golden ruler* | 235 | 198 | 2 | 72 | 14.5 | 6 | 40 | 38 | 7 | 6 | 1 | 3 |
| Sansue royal flush/pyngold* | 38 | 18 | 7 | 83 | 22.5 | 0 | 29 | 39 | 11 | 5 | 5 | 11 |
| Shandeen sportsman p* | 60 | 29 | 2 | 95 | 21.7 | 5 | 28 | 27 | 17 | 7 | 12 | 5 |
| Shargleam ark royal* | 20 | 16 | 4 | 49 | 14.9 | 3 | 35 | 50 | 0 | 5 | 5 | 0 |
| Sherida sirdar* | 53 | 26 | 4 | 76 | 21.8 | 6 | 12 | 49 | 10 | 15 | 4 | 6 |
| Sinnheim sebastian* | 67 | 34 | 6 | 52 | 14.3 | 0 | 42 | 42 | 8 | 8 | 0 | 2 |
| Sinnheim toerag/kilgraston* | 25 | 15 | 5 | 29 | 13.3 | 5 | 32 | 52 | 12 | 0 | 0 | 0 |
| Skymaster at jamescroft* | 48 | 21 | 7 | 51 | 18.9 | 0 | 27 | 44 | 13 | 6 | 9 | 2 |
| Sootek dawn jest* | 34 | 20 | 1 | 84 | 18.3 | 9 | 20 | 44 | 6 | 15 | 3 | 3 |

**Table 10-6 (continued)**

| Name of Sire (* scored) | Number of progeny | Dams[1] | Best[2] | Worst[3] | Mean[4] | %[5] 0–5 | % 6–10 | % 11–20 | % 21–30 | % 31–40 | % 41–50 | >51 |
|---|---|---|---|---|---|---|---|---|---|---|---|---|
| Standerwick roland | 20 | 15 | 7 | 72 | 24.3 | 0 | 15 | 35 | 20 | 15 | 10 | 5 |
| Standerwick rumbustious* | 29 | 14 | 3 | 40 | 14.3 | 3 | 34 | 45 | 10 | 7 | 0 | 0 |
| Stanroph sailor boy* | 38 | 20 | 6 | 60 | 16 | 0 | 37 | 47 | 5 | 3 | 3 | 5 |
| Stanroph soldier boy* | 46 | 25 | 3 | 85 | 20.3 | 5 | 26 | 46 | 3 | 11 | 2 | 9 |
| Starmoss intrepid* | 25 | 15 | 6 | 72 | 16.7 | 0 | 56 | 20 | 8 | 8 | 0 | 8 |
| Stenbury sea laird of g.* | 36 | 20 | 3 | 35 | 12.2 | 6 | 50 | 31 | 11 | 3 | 0 | 0 |
| Stenbury sea tristram of c | 40 | 32 | 9 | 83 | 24.2 | 0 | 10 | 45 | 23 | 13 | 5 | 5 |
| Stirchley saxor* | 135 | 50 | 5 | 74 | 18.4 | 2 | 30 | 43 | 16 | 8 | 3 | 6 |
| Stirchley solomon* | 24 | 13 | 6 | 60 | 16.9 | 0 | 38 | 38 | 13 | 4 | 4 | 4 |
| Stradcot simon of crouchers | 21 | 13 | 8 | 32 | 19.1 | 0 | 19 | 29 | 38 | 14 | 0 | 0 |
| Styal scott of glengilde | 155 | 68 | 0 | 72 | 15.4 | 6 | 31 | 44 | 8 | 6 | 1 | 3 |
| Styal solamente/n wood* | 31 | 19 | 5 | 60 | 17.1 | 3 | 32 | 42 | 6 | 3 | 10 | 3 |
| Styal souvenir of nortonwood* | 37 | 19 | 4 | 78 | 22.4 | 5 | 24 | 27 | 19 | 5 | 5 | 14 |
| Sundar of sherida* | 33 | 19 | 7 | 50 | 23.4 | 0 | 15 | 39 | 15 | 15 | 15 | 0 |
| Sunspray solomon seal* | 28 | 18 | 7 | 57 | 19.6 | 0 | 25 | 46 | 14 | 4 | 0 | 11 |
| Tamarley top secret* | 25 | 13 | 6 | 54 | 17.6 | 0 | 28 | 40 | 20 | 8 | 0 | 4 |
| Teecons knight errant | 35 | 21 | 2 | 88 | 15.9 | 6 | 46 | 34 | 0 | 9 | 0 | 6 |
| Thenford gannymede/s'dusky* | 62 | 33 | 4 | 70 | 15.6 | 7 | 31 | 40 | 16 | 3 | 2 | 2 |

[1] Number of different dams producing these progeny.
[2] Lowest (best) score among these progeny.
[3] Highest (worst) score among these progeny.
[4] Mean progeny score (arithmetic mean).
[5] Percentage (nearest whole number) of scored progeny that fall within score categories. Only those sires with an excess of 20 progeny were included.

### Table 10-7: Progeny tests for hip scores of Newfoundland sires

For whole period ranked by mean score of progeny. Only those sires with an excess of 20 progeny were included. Data current to February 14, 1997. (Data on the BVA/KC scores are produced by kind permission of Dr. M. B. Willis, geneticist.)

| Name of Sire (* scored) | Number of progeny | Dams[1] | Best[2] | Worst[3] | Mean[4] | %[5] 0–5 | % 6–10 | % 11–20 | % 21–30 | % 31–40 | % 41–50 | % >51 |
| --- | --- | --- | --- | --- | --- | --- | --- | --- | --- | --- | --- | --- |
| Wellfont trampus* | 20 | 6 | 5 | 69 | 14.6 | 10 | 50 | 25 | 5 | 5 | 0 | 5 |
| Kelligrews carbonear* | 23 | 5 | 3 | 50 | 15 | 9 | 35 | 43 | 0 | 4 | 9 | 0 |
| Guay v soven* | 22 | 6 | 6 | 47 | 15.3 | 0 | 36 | 50 | 5 | 5 | 5 | 0 |
| Stormsail sacred spint* | 42 | 14 | 0 | 73 | 16.3 | 19 | 29 | 31 | 5 | 10 | 2 | 5 |
| Merrybear luige* | 71 | 26 | 0 | 80 | 20.4 | 6 | 27 | 39 | 8 | 10 | 4 | 6 |
| Culnor ebon nie* | 21 | 8 | 6 | 43 | 21 | 0 | 29 | 24 | 24 | 14 | 10 | 0 |
| Samson v soven* | 41 | 14 | 0 | 92 | 22.8 | 20 | 27 | 20 | 7 | 7 | 2 | 17 |
| Bouderee romani rokra* | 22 | 8 | 1 | 85 | 22.9 | 14 | 18 | 36 | 5 | 5 | 14 | 9 |
| Wellfont macillon* | 43 | 17 | 4 | 89 | 24.6 | 7 | 16 | 37 | 19 | 7 | 5 | 9 |
| Pouch coves repeat after me* | 34 | 13 | 7 | 84 | 25.7 | 0 | 32 | 32 | 9 | 6 | 0 | 21 |
| Harratons black piper* | 21 | 13 | 4 | 75 | 26.4 | 10 | 19 | 29 | 10 | 10 | 5 | 19 |
| Wellfont admiral* | 25 | 9 | 2 | 60 | 26.8 | 4 | 16 | 28 | 16 | 12 | 12 | 12 |
| Karazan yankee peddler | 23 | 14 | 4 | 88 | 36 | 9 | 9 | 22 | 13 | 4 | 17 | 26 |
| Asterion canis venatici* | 26 | 4 | 5 | 92 | 36.7 | 4 | 4 | 23 | 23 | 12 | 8 | 27 |
| La bellas winston* | 32 | 10 | 4 | 101 | 38 | 3 | 22 | 16 | 6 | 3 | 19 | 31 |
| Karazan rockafella* | 75 | 29 | 0 | 82 | 42.5 | 3 | 7 | 11 | 19 | 11 | 13 | 37 |
| Karazan bollinger* | 31 | 14 | 6 | 98 | 43.2 | 0 | 16 | 23 | 6 | 6 | 3 | 45 |
| Merrybear dunhill* | 29 | 10 | 6 | 104 | 44.3 | 0 | 10 | 17 | 7 | 17 | 7 | 41 |
| Tokeida outlaws treasure* | 32 | 22 | 7 | 72 | 24.6 | 0 | 19 | 41 | 16 | 3 | 13 | 9 |
| Tokeida starstealer* | 62 | 35 | 7 | 72 | 21.5 | 0 | 11 | 52 | 16 | 15 | 5 | 4 |
| Tugwood pirate* | 39 | 29 | 5 | 53 | 18.9 | 3 | 23 | 49 | 8 | 11 | 5 | 3 |
| Tugwood viking | 26 | 19 | 9 | 43 | 19.5 | 0 | 23 | 46 | 12 | 12 | 8 | 0 |
| Twilly apollo of davern* | 32 | 13 | 4 | 48 | 19 | 3 | 16 | 47 | 25 | 3 | 6 | 0 |
| Unavale fortune of okus* | 25 | 16 | 4 | 78 | 21 | 8 | 28 | 24 | 24 | 4 | 4 | 8 |
| Verdayne dandini of davern* | 49 | 35 | 4 | 82 | 18.2 | 2 | 16 | 57 | 16 | 4 | 0 | 4 |
| Westley jacob* | 100 | 56 | 6 | 72 | 20.2 | 0 | 24 | 41 | 17 | 5 | 6 | 8 |
| Westley munro of nortonwoo | 169 | 118 | 1 | 96 | 19.7 | 1 | 26 | 43 | 14 | 6 | 6 | 5 |
| Westley samuel* | 177 | 100 | 2 | 68 | 16.3 | 6 | 35 | 38 | 9 | 3 | 3 | 6 |
| Westley topic of sansue* | 25 | 18 | 1 | 42 | 13.6 | 12 | 44 | 24 | 12 | 4 | 4 | 0 |
| Winterknoll corylus* | 27 | 12 | 4 | 54 | 15.9 | 7 | 26 | 56 | 4 | 0 | 4 | 4 |
| Yeo mastermind* | 28 | 17 | 8 | 78 | 30 | 0 | 11 | 43 | 14 | 4 | 7 | 21 |

[1] Number of different dams producing these progeny.
[2] Lowest (best) score among these progeny.
[3] Highest (worst) score among these progeny.
[4] Mean progeny score (arithmetic mean).
[5] Percentage (nearest whole number) of scored progeny that fall within score categories.

In certain breeds, quite spectacular progress in the control of CHD has been made: e.g. The Newfoundland was noted to be very severely affected some years ago, but careful selection by the breeders of this relatively small breed society has a marked improvement in the status of the hips of many of the dogs produced. It is true that individual dogs that have high scores still turn up (Table 10-7), but they are now only a small proportion of all the animals bred rather than the majority as occurred some years ago. A similar situation applies to the Bernese Mountain Dog although, that breed was not so markedly affected in the first instance.

In some breeds it is possible to identify two distinct groups, those with low scores and those with high scores. This is most notable in the German Shepherd Dog (Table 10-3) and the Labrador Retriever and would appear to be the result of some breeders having a better appreciation of the significance of scoring than others.

The overall pattern changes constantly, with a general tendency to gradual improvement, but this occurs at a pace that is slower than is desirable. The BVA/KCHD Scoring Scheme remains an advisory one and it is entirely in the hands of the breeders to make proper use of the results of the scoring.

# Orthopedic Foundation for Animals, Inc.

E.A. CORLEY, DVM, PHD
Past Director
Orthopedic Foundation for Animals
2300 E. Nifong Blvd
Columbia, MO 652013856

The Orthopedic Foundation for Animals (OFA) is a private non-profit foundation that was formed on November 15, 1966. The following objectives have evolved over the past 30 years:
1. To collate and disseminate information concerning orthopedic and genetic diseases of animals.
2. To advise, encourage and establish control programs to lower the incidence of orthopedic and genetic diseases of animals.
3. To encourage and finance research in orthopedic and genetic disease of animals.
4. To receive funds and make grants to carry out these objectives.

In the US, OFA is recognized as the premier genetic registry for CHD and it houses the world's largest all breed database on the hip status. To fully appreciate what OFA is, how it operates, what it has accomplished, and its current mode of operation requires some understanding of its historical background.

National breed clubs are generally responsible for the creation of genetic disease registries, but the success of the registries may be credited to the dedicated efforts of one or two individuals from the club. The formation of the OFA to meet the perceived needs of breeders was no exception.

In 1963, John M. Olin, a noted philanthropist and avid sportsman, was appointed as chairman of the CHD committee of the Labrador Retriever Club of America. In this role, he became the primary force for development of a process to further the basic understanding of CHD and to better assist the breeder in control of CHD by providing the information necessary to make sound breeding decisions. Over 1964 and 1965, Olin called and funded a series of meetings of internationally known scientists from the disciplines of pathology, genetics, nutrition, skeletal development and veterinary practice. A select group of breeders and representatives of the American Kennel Club (AKC) were actively involved in the discussions. The results of these meetings are summarized as follows:
1. Basic research was needed. Biochemical changes associated with osteoarthritis, endocrine effects (particularly estrogen), the pathology of CHD associated with development of the hip joint, and better definition of the genetics of CHD were recommended as the immediate research direction.
2. The need for a standard protocol of radiographic evaluation of the hip status was recognized.
3. The need for a central organizational structure for funding research, maintaining the appropriate database, and provision of public service was defined. It was recognized that the efforts should not be limited to CHD or to the canine species.

The end result was creation of OFA with support from the Golden Retriever and German Shepherd Dog Clubs.

OFA and the John M. Olin Foundation provided much of the funding for scientists such as Drs. Wayne Riser, George Lust, and Sten-Erik Olsson for their early research of CHD. More recently, support has been provided for studies of joint laxity at Michigan State University, cineradiography studies of the dog in motion (Rachel Page Elliot), genetics of elbow dysplasia (Drs. Padgett, Mostosky, and Wind), and projects on epidemiology and genetics. OFA is particularly pleased to be associated with the Morris Animal Foundation and the American Kennel Club in providing support for molecular genetic research conducted at the University of Michigan and Michigan State University under the direction of Dr. George Brewer. Development of DNA technology and mapping of the canine genome will greatly enhance current techniques for diagnosis of genetic disease and will assist the breeder in control, or even elimination of some genetic diseases by better breeding selection.

To meet its public service obligation, a CHD control registry was formed in 1966 to provide a standard radiographic evaluation of the hip status and to maintain records on the evaluations over many generations. This registry was the first, and is the best known, of many registries operated by OFA. The hip registry recognizes those dogs deemed to be phenotypically normal, that is, no evidence of HD or Legg-Perthes disease was noted.

Data that were accumulated by OFA during the formative years indicated problems with the evaluation performed at 1 year of age (the false-negative diagnostic rate was unacceptably high), the hip scoring system was limited, and the issue of joint laxity as determined by palpation or stress radiography led to OFA sponsorship of the first international symposium on CHD in 1972. On the recommendations of this group of scientists OFA raised the age requirement to 24 months and established a 7-grade hip-scoring scheme that went into effect in 1974.

Table 10-8: Phenotypic distribution by year/s of birth – all breeds

| Born | Number | Excellent (%) | Good (%) | Fair (%) | Borderline (%) | Mild (%) | Moderate (%) | Severe (%) |
|---|---|---|---|---|---|---|---|---|
| 1980 | 127,315 | 7.8 | 56.0 | 17.7 | 1.1 | 8.8 | 7.2 | 1.4 |
| 1981–82 | 34,604 | 6.7 | 56.5 | 18.9 | 1.1 | 8.5 | 6.9 | 1.4 |
| 1983–84 | 47,919 | 7.9 | 53.8 | 19.0 | 1.0 | 9.1 | 7.7 | 1.5 |
| 1985–86 | 58,441 | 9.8 | 52.8 | 18.0 | 1.1 | 9.7 | 7.2 | 1.5 |
| 1987–88 | 66,585 | 10.5 | 52.7 | 18.3 | 1.4 | 9.1 | 6.6 | 1.5 |
| 1989–90 | 75,386 | 10.0 | 56.2 | 17.5 | 1.3 | 8.1 | 5.7 | 1.2 |
| 1991–92 | 76,052 | 11.5 | 59.2 | 15.5 | 1.1 | 6.9 | 4.8 | 0.9 |
| 1993–94 | 53,779 | 12.2 | 57.9 | 16.2 | 1.5 | 6.8 | 4.6 | 0.8 |

The issue of joint laxity as demonstrated by forcing the head of the femur away from the acetabulum was considered as experimental as data were not available to define the relationship of laxity demonstrated by force with the abnormal laxity associated with CHD.

Radiographs are voluntarily submitted to OFA for independent evaluation by three veterinary radiologists, each of whom independently classifies the hips as excellent, good, fair, borderline, mild, moderate or severe. The final report is the consensus of the three evaluations. Quality control data demonstrate that all three radiologists agreed on the consensus of normal or dysplastic in approximately 94% of the cases and agreed on the specific hip rating in approximately 80% of the cases. Affect of prior screening of the radiographs by attending veterinarians appears to remain constant over time and between breeds.

OFA evaluated 540,081 dogs from 221 breeds at 24 months of age or older between January 1, 1974 and December 31, 1996. The data represent findings in this specific population of dogs, a subset of the general population. There was no significant difference in frequency of dysplasia between males and females, but females tended to have a slightly higher frequency of dysplasia than males. All breeds with 35 or more submissions demonstrated some frequency of dysplasia. Breed risk for dysplasia in breeds with 100 or more submissions ranged from 70.8% in the Bulldog to 1.0% in the Schipperke. Breed data and other information may be accessed from OFA web page (http://www.offa.org).

The phenotypic distribution of the total OFA population is presented in Table 10-8. Results from the normal population are presented in Table 10-9. There has been a significant increase in dogs considered to be excellent and a corresponding decrease in dogs considered to be fair. There was no significant change in those considered to be good. The prior screening process has limited effect on the normal population; therefore, it can safely be stated that the hip status has significantly improved.

The results are even more dramatic when individual breeds are considered. Use of the standard position and evaluation procedures as the criteria for evaluation breeders can and have made significant progress in improving the hip status and in control of HD. Results from 26

Table 10-9: Normal phenotypic change by year/s of birth – all breeds

| Born | Total Number | Excellent Number | % | Good Number | % | Fair Number | % |
|---|---|---|---|---|---|---|---|
| 1980 | 103,747 | 9,960 | 9.6 | 71,262 | 68.7 | 22,525 | 21.7 |
| 1981–82 | 28,400 | 2,333 | 8.2 | 19,534 | 68.8 | 6,533 | 23.0 |
| 1983–84 | 38,649 | 3,786 | 9.8 | 25,759 | 66.6 | 9,104 | 23.6 |
| 1985–86 | 47,095 | 5,703 | 12.1 | 30,861 | 65.5 | 10,531 | 22.4 |
| 1987–88 | 54,308 | 7,016 | 12.9 | 35,103 | 64.6 | 12,189 | 22.4 |
| 1989–90 | 63,135 | 7,551 | 12.0 | 42,365 | 67.1 | 13,219 | 20.9 |
| 1991–92 | 65,577 | 8,725 | 13.3 | 45,058 | 68.7 | 11,794 | 17.9 |
| 1993–94 | 46,460 | 6,584 | 14.2 | 31,151 | 67.0 | 8,725 | 18.8 |

**Table 10-10: Trends in hip dysplasia breeds with more than 1000 evaluated dogs born in or before 1980 compared to dogs born in 1986–87 and 1993–94**

| Breed | Rating total dogs | 1980 (%) | 1986–87 (%) | 1993–94 (%) | change 1980 to 1993–94 (%) |
|---|---|---|---|---|---|
| Afghan Hound | Excellent | 24.3 | 34.4 | 30.3 | +24.7 |
|  | Dysplastic | 5.5 | 8.3 | 4.1 | -25.5 |
|  | Total Dogs | 2.768 | 314 | 122 |  |
| Akita | Excellent | 7.5 | 15.9 | 20.5 | +173.3 |
|  | Dysplastic | 17.5 | 17.2 | 10.1 | -42.3 |
|  | Total Dogs | 2.208 | 1.242 | 975 |  |
| Alaskan Malamute | Excellent | 10.4 | 18.2 | 20.0 | +92.3 |
|  | Dysplastic | 14.1 | 12.3 | 8.1 | -42.6 |
|  | Total Dogs | 3.816 | 863 | 581 |  |
| Australian Shepherd | Excellent | 10.5 | 14.0 | 14.5 | +38.1 |
|  | Dysplastic | 8.6 | 6.9 | 4.8 | -44.2 |
|  | Total Dogs | 2.248 | 1.158 | 1.678 |  |
| Brittany Spaniel | Excellent | 5.7 | 6.8 | 7.7 | +35.1 |
|  | Dysplastic | 20.3 | 18.7 | 10.3 | -49.3 |
|  | Total Dogs | 2.824 | 926 | 845 |  |
| Chesapeake Bay Retriever | Excellent | 5.9 | 10.1 | 12.3 | +108.5 |
|  | Dysplastic | 25.5 | 24.0 | 18.4 | -27.8 |
|  | Total Dogs | 1.783 | 663 | 665 |  |
| Doberman Pinscher | Excellent | 12.5 | 19.9 | 17.9 | +43.2 |
|  | Dysplastic | 8.2 | 6.3 | 4.5 | -45.1 |
|  | Total Dogs | 2.415 | 797 | 702 |  |
| English Springer Spaniel | Excellent | 7.0 | 7.3 | 7.8 | +11.4 |
|  | Dysplastic | 20.2 | 16.3 | 9.6 | -52.5 |
|  | Total Dogs | 1.914 | 687 | 651 |  |
| English Setter | Excellent | 3.3 | 8.2 | 8.9 | +169.7 |
|  | Dysplastic | 28.5 | 15.6 | 11.6 | -59.3 |
|  | Total Dogs | 1.605 | 548 | 473 |  |
| Great Dane | Excellent | 6.2 | 11.3 | 13.9 | +124.2 |
|  | Dysplastic | 13.4 | 12.3 | 9.5 | -29.1 |
|  | Total Dogs | 2.219 | 495 | 490 |  |
| Golden Retriever | Excellent | 1.8 | 3.2 | 4.7 | +161.1 |
|  | Dysplastic | 23.4 | 23.8 | 16.6 | -29.1 |
|  | Total Dogs | 18.170 | 7.784 | 6.918 |  |
| German Shepherd Dog | Excellent | 2.5 | 3.1 | 3.3 | +32.0 |
|  | Dysplastic | 20.7 | 22.8 | 16.8 | -18.8 |
|  | Total Dogs | 12.810 | 6.284 | 6.453 |  |
| Gordon Setter | Excellent | 3.8 | 8.9 | 9.8 | +157.9 |
|  | Dysplastic | 25.9 | 21.4 | 19.2 | -25.9 |
|  | Total Dogs | 1.142 | 439 | 256 |  |
| German Shorthaired Pointer | Excellent | 19.6 | 21.9 | 24.4 | +24.5 |
|  | Dysplastic | 7.5 | 6.0 | 2.6 | -65.3 |
|  | Total Dogs | 1.449 | 640 | 706 |  |

### Table 10-10 (continued)

| Breed | Rating total dogs | 1980 (%) | 1986–87 (%) | 1993–94 (%) | change 1980 to 1993–94 (%) |
|---|---|---|---|---|---|
| Irish Setter | Excellent | 5.0 | 9.0 | 12.1 | +142.0 |
| | Dysplastic | 15.1 | 12.8 | 9.2 | -39.1 |
| | Total Dogs | 3.954 | 534 | 371 | |
| Labrador Retriever | Excellent | 10.4 | 16.0 | 17.7 | +70.2 |
| | Dysplastic | 14.5 | 13.6 | 11.5 | -20.7 |
| | Total Dogs | 15.342 | 9.861 | 12.331 | |
| Norwegian Elkhound | Excellent | 5.4 | 4.0 | 8.1 | +50.0 |
| | Dysplastic | 24.8 | 26.6 | 10.9 | -56.0 |
| | Total Dogs | 1.031 | 248 | 148 | |
| Newfoundland | Excellent | 3.3 | 6.5 | 9.8 | +197.0 |
| | Dysplastic | 32.4 | 25.0 | 17.8 | -45.1 |
| | Total Dogs | 1.888 | 928 | 732 | |
| Poodle | Excellent | 7-7 | 9-0 | 10.7 | +39.0 |
| | Dysplastic | 17.3 | 15.8 | 8.7 | -49.7 |
| | Total Dogs | 2.404 | 893 | 903 | |
| Rottweiler | Excellent | 4.0 | 7.6 | 10.4 | +160.0 |
| | Dysplastic | 24.0 | 23.5 | 17.0 | -29.2 |
| | Total Dogs | 6.869 | 10.057 | 7.247 | |
| Rhodesian Ridgeback | Excellent | 13.9 | 19.4 | 22.2 | +59.7 |
| | Dysplastic | 12.2 | 7.0 | 2.4 | -80.3 |
| | Total Dogs | 1.198 | 527 | 603 | |
| Samoyed | Excellent | 8.1 | 7.9 | 11.9 | +46.9 |
| | Dysplastic | 13.8 | 11.0 | 9.2 | -33.3 |
| | Total Dogs | 4.182 | 1.051 | 564 | |
| Old English Sheepdog | Excellent | 7.4 | 14.6 | 14.5 | +95.9 |
| | Dysplastic | 23.6 | 20.4 | 8.4 | -64.4 |
| | Total Dogs | 4.876 | 553 | 332 | |
| Sibirian Husky | Excellent | 24.2 | 38.0 | 35.0 | +44.6 |
| | Dysplastic | 2.7 | 2.1 | 0.9 | -66.7 |
| | Total Dogs | 4.689 | 972 | 571 | |
| Vizsla | Excellent | 12.1 | 16.0 | 17.0 | +40.5 |
| | Dysplastic | 10.4 | 8.3 | 3.8 | -63.5 |
| | Total Dogs | 1.646 | 486 | 607 | |
| Weimaraner | Excellent | 12.7 | 20.9 | 22.4 | +76.4 |
| | Dysplastic | 12.1 | 10.5 | 5.3 | -56.2 |
| | Total Dogs | 1.680 | 526 | 700 | |

breeds with 1000 or more evaluations of dogs born in 1980 are compared in Table 10-10.

Breeds with a high percent participation have demonstrated great progress. OFA has access to the stud books and thus complete breeding data on the Portuguese Water Dog (PWD) and Shar Pei (SP) and reported on the progress made by these breeds. Over 90% of the breeding pairs of the PWD and over 40% for the SP were evaluated by OFA. CHD declined from 24.0% to 17.0% over 4 years in the PWD study and from 20.9% to 6.6% over 11 years in the SP study even though some breeders from both breeds continued to breed dysplastic dogs. The progress was high considering the fact that heritability estimates based on parent-progeny were $0.30 \pm .06$ for the PWD and $0.31 \pm .05$ for the SP. It appears that persistent and consistent use of OFA evaluations will result in improved quality of the normal hip and a corresponding decrease in the frequency of CHD.

While genetic registries are effective, for those that follow the program, organizations such as the AKC must rethink their role in animal health. There are clear indications that movement in this direction is occurring. Issues such as dealing with dog identification, assuring stud book integrity, providing genetic research support, rethinking the requirements for registration and dog recognition, and education of the public is each being dealt with in a limited fashion. Breeders, breed clubs, the veterinary profession, and the genetic registries must continue to challenge dog owners to have the breeding animals evaluated by an accepted test method as it has been demonstrated that as the number of dogs evaluated for CHD increases, the number of normal dogs used in a breeding program increase and there is a corresponding increase in normal progeny produced. Currently, less than 5% of all dogs registered by AKC are evaluated by OFA and an even smaller percentage is evaluated by other registries.

# Control of CHD in Switzerland

Dr. Mark Flückiger, Dipl. ECVDI
Department for Internal Veterinary Medicine
Section of Diagnostic Imaging
University of Zurich
Switzerland

## History

Hip dysplasia is seen in most breeds of dog, varying only in frequency and the level of severity. The diagnosis is based on radiographic findings, but the radiographs are not interpreted throughout the world according to the same criteria. As a result, a variation in assessment of the same radiograph among nations is not uncommon. This conflict in radiographic evaluation is also well known to be present among evaluators even within the same national evaluation center. This is despite early efforts to develop a uniform assessment protocol. The hip interpretation training of the examiners in the various European countries differs widely and ranges from experienced radiologists or surgeons, to practitioners chosen at random. Often no specialty training is required for these reviewers and in some countries, breed club representatives are sporadically allowed to interpret radiographs. In Switzerland, with the installation of a CHD screening program in the mid-60s, radiographs have been exclusively read by faculty members from the two universities in Zurich and in Bern ever since.

## New protocol

It was because of the apparent lack of a uniform internationally standardized analysis protocol that the dysplasia assessment protocol was modified. The aim was to develop a protocol that would be simple and thorough and yet would cover all commonly examined breeds and forms of dysplasia in a manner comprehensible both to the examiner and to the dog owner and would permit placement of the results into one of the five FCI dysplasia grades. To be operable, the system needs to be: (1) objective and simple, (2) reproducible, (3) able to yield a correct interpretation in all breeds, (4) able to conform with FCI recommendations, (5) user friendly, and (6) applicable even to radiographs of suboptimal quality. Further, the protocol should permit a direct comparison between the different existing protocols. The newly developed protocol was designed to combine the FCI's recommendations with the methodically more exact British model. In contrast with the British version with nine radiographic parameters that were scored ranging from 0 to 6 (with one exception), in the proposed system only six parameters were specified and graded on a point scale ranging from 0 to 5 with 0 indicating normal and 5 indicating a severely pathologic parameter. The six parameters are described (Table 10-11) along with the radiographic criteria (Table 10-12), and a grading key (Table 10-13).

**Table 10-11: Parameters used for radiographic evaluation of hips**

1. Norberg Angle
2. Relation of femoral head center to the dorsal acetabular edge
3. Character of the craniolateral acetabular edge
4. Character of the cranial subchondral acetabular bone
5. Character of the femoral head and neck
6. Presence of a Morgan-Line

It is important to understand that any system of evaluation must recognize changes associated with early joint laxity as well as the later changes of arthrosis. In our scheme, the first two criteria evaluate the nature of the fit between femoral head and acetabulum. The first criterion quantifies the Norberg angle while the second criterion describes the relationship between the center of the femoral head and the dorsal acetabular edge. The degree of femoral head subluxation strongly influences scoring of these two parameters as does acetabular depth. Criteria three and four are parameters reflecting changes of secondary arthrosis within the acetabulum. The third criterion describes the appearance of the craniolateral acetabular edge and indicates a range of appearance from that of an edge parallel and congruent to the edge of the femoral head to a flattened and finally expanded acetabular cup with the presence of bony exostoses. The fourth criterion evaluates the thickness and uniformity of the cranial subchondral acetabular bone and indicates the distribution of load between the articular surface of the femoral head and the cranial acetabular cup. Criteria five and six are parameters indicating changes of secondary arthrosis of the femoral head and neck. The fifth criterion evaluates modeling of the femoral head and the femoral neck and the sixth criterion examines for a specific bony response, enthesophytes, on the caudal aspect of the femoral neck at the transition zone from the femoral head to the femoral neck.

Thus, in dogs judged to be minimally dysplastic, changes are only noted in the first two parameters and changes of arthrosis are virtually absent. In dogs with more severe arthrosis, two patterns may be present: the first two parameters may predominate or there is elevation of the scores of the third to sixth criteria. Thus, no single parameter is

## Table 10-12: Radiographic criteria for canine hip dysplasia grading CHD[1]

| Score point | Norberg Angle (JS = Joint Space) | Relation FHC/DAE*, Width of Joint Space (JS) | Craniolateral Acetabular Edge (CAE) | Cranial Subchondral Acetabular Bone | Femoral Head (H), Femoral, Neck (N) | Morgan-Line |
|---|---|---|---|---|---|---|
| 0 | 105° or more | FHC medial to DAE (>2 mm), JS narrow | Parallel to femoral head | Fine, even | H: round, smooth N: well demarcated | Not visible |
| 1 | 105° or more, but JS widened slightly, or 100°–104°, but JS narrow | FHC medial to DAE (2mm) JS minimally divergent | Horizontal on lateral 1/4 | Even or thickened cranially | H: round N: poorly demarcated (cylindrical) | Edged shoulder on view with limbs flexed (Position 2) |
| 2 | 100°–104° | FHC superimposed on DAE, JS slightly divergent | Slightly flattened, or mild exostosis | Slightly thickened laterally, slightly reduced medially | H: slightly flattened N: mild exostosis | Fine linear spur (up to 1 mm wide) |
| 3 | 90°–99° | FHC lateral to DAE (5 mm), JS moderately divergent | Moderately flattened, mild exostosis, two part surface | Moderately thickened laterally, moderately reduced medially | H: moderately flattened N: mild exostosis | Well defined spur (up to 3 mm wide) |
| 4 | 80°–89° | FHC lateral to DAE (6–10mm), JS markedly divergent | Markedly flattened, moderate exostosis | Markedly thickened laterally, may not be present medially | H: moderately flattened N: moderate exostosis | Broad irregular spur (>3mm wide) |
| 5 | <80° | FHC lateral to DAE (>10mm), or luxation | DAE absent, acetabulum markedly deformed | Blending with lateral pelvic rim or absent | H: severely deformed N: massive exostosis | Spur incorporate in or superimposed by general exostosis |

**Classification:** Joints are graded individually
Each parameter is scored from 0 to 5, Scores are then added up
0 points representing the best score, 30 points the worst for a single joint
CHD grade is assessed based on the worse of the two hip joints

*FHC = Femoral Head Center; DAE = Dorsal Acetabular Edge

## Table 10-13: Correlation between numerical score and FCI grading scheme (based on the worse of the two coxofemoral joints)[1]

| Total score per hip joint | Degree of CHD (according to FCI) | |
|---|---|---|
| 0–2 | A | Normal, no evidence of hip dysplasia |
| 3–6 | B | Borderline case, transitional case |
| 7–12 | C | Mild CHD |
| 13–18 | D | Moderate CHD |
| >18 | E | Severe CHD |

[1] FLÜCKIGER M, LANG J, BINDER H, BUSATO A, BOOS J.
Die Bekämpfung der Hüftgelenksdysplasie in der Schweiz. Ein Rückblick auf die vergangenen 24 Jahre. Schweiz Arch Tierheilkd 137: 243-250, 1995.

a specific indicator of CHD since both joint laxity and secondary arthrosis may be present. Following is a more specific discussion of the six criteria used in judgment of the hip joint.

The first parameter evaluates the position of the femoral head within the joint cup, the depth of the joint cup, and the position of the joint cup opening relative to the body's sagittal plane. Dogs with a sagittally positioned cup but a strongly inclined femoral neck may develop a normal hip joint despite having a small Norberg angle. In contrast to the other parameters, the Norberg angle offers the advantage of being measurable. Its influence on the variability of the final score is strong and only surpassed by the second parameter. Two types of malpositioning during radiography strongly influence this measurement. Pelvic rotation around its long axis results in a smaller Norberg angle measurement on the hip joint that lies closer to the table surface. Pelvic rotation around its transverse axis is caused by forcing the femora in a position parallel to the tabletop. The result is that the projected point of intersection between the dorsal and the cranial acetabular edge is moved medially resulting in lower angle readings that are false.

Measurement of the second parameter is affected by the degree of subluxation of the femoral head, shape of the acetabular roof, and depth of the acetabulum and is easily quantified. According to the FCI's rules, it is only applied to define grade B dysplasia. Based on our results, this is the most sensitive parameter and is essential for evaluation of all grades of dysplasia. Assessed separately, this parameter influences the variability of the final result more strongly than any other parameter. The recession of the dorsocranial acetabular edge is indicative of femoral subluxation. Therefore, shape of the acetabular edge and degree of femoral head coverage constitute the earliest radiographically detectable indicators of dysplasia. Our findings support the hypothesis that joint instability promotes progression of secondary changes within the hip joint since it is the dorsocranial part of the acetabular edge that is poorly developed. Tilting of the pelvis around its long axis may lead to change and misinterpretation of the acetabular roof shape.

Parameter three indirectly reveals subluxation of a femoral head when the dog is bearing weight. Stress views are usually required for exact quantitation of the degree of subluxation. In the healthy coxofemoral joint, the articular surface of the acetabulum is congruent with the articular surface of the femoral head. The width of the joint space is uniformly narrow except in the area of the fovea capitis. In a lax coxofemoral joint during locomotion, large forces deform the dorsocranial acetabular edge resulting is eventual development of secondary arthrosis. This parameter qualifies as the third most important parameter and is the most sensitive factor in the detection of arthrosis. In dogs with moderate to severe dysplasia, it is the leading factor in the variability of the score assigned to the joint.

The fourth parameter reflects the effects of forces exerted on the subchondral bone during movement and is an established criterion in the diagnosis of secondary arthrosis. Subchondral bone may respond to an increase in pressure by bony buildup that is viewed on the radiograph as a thickening of the radiodense line of the subchondral bone. Therefore, thickening of the subchondral bone at the craniolateral acetabular edge is an indication of high pressure and a tendency of the femoral head to subluxate under load. In severe joint laxity with persistent subluxation of the femoral head, subchondral bone plate thickness begins to decrease craniomedially due to the reduced load at this site. This parameter is not mentioned as criterion in the FCI's recommendation, but it rates as an arthrosis-associated parameter based on our results. Its contribution to the final score is variable and is dictated by the level of arthrosis.

Parameters five and six address secondary changes involving the femoral head and neck consisting of deformation and spurs of new bone formed on the craniomedial or caudolateral edge of the femoral head. The finding of spurs results in the hip being judged as dysplastic following the FCI recommendation. The sixth parameter scores more frequently and in higher numbers in lax hip joints than in tight ones. It is therefore considered an indicator of joint laxity. It can be missed if the femora are not sufficiently rotated internally. Use of insufficient radiographic exposure can also result in an inability to detect the Morgan-Line.

Parameters five and six are influenced by positioning of the femora. It is recommended that the flexed hind limb position is modified: the tarsi are held together and raised 30 to 40 cm above the tabletop. In this position, the femora are viewed in a mediolateral projection and early spur formation at the cranial and caudal aspects of the femoral head and neck interface can readily be estimated.

Use of this method of radiographic examination allows for a scoring of even slight differences in severity of dysplasia of CHD based on objectively defined parameters. The system takes into account the recommendations of the FCI and could be used in central and northern Europe without having to modify prevalent grading. It can be substituted for the too detailed British system since the same principle of analysis is used. This system

Table 10-14: Comparison of different grading schemes for CHD (Final grading is based on the worse hip joint.)

| FCI | Germany | UK (1 joint) | Switzerland | Sweden | USA (OFA) |
|---|---|---|---|---|---|
| A, Normal hip | A1 | 0 | 0 | 0 | Excellent |
|  | A2 | 1–3 | 1–2 | 0 | Good |
| B, Bordeline | B1 | 4–6 | 3–4 | 1 | Fair |
|  | B2 | 7–8 | 5–6 | 1 | Borderline |
| C, Mild HD | C1 | 9–12 | 7–9 | 2 | Mild |
|  | C2 | 13–18 | 10–12 | 2 | Mild |
| D, Moderate HD | D1 | >18 | 13–15 | 3 | Moderate |
|  | D2 |  | 16–18 | 3 | Moderate |
| E, Severe HD | E1 |  | 19–21 | 4 | Severe |
|  | E2 |  | 22–24 | 4 | Severe |

As a general rule no dog scoring D or E may be used for breeding in Switzerland. A substantial number of Swiss breed clubs further restrict or even ban the use of dogs scoring C for breeding. Some tolerate only A-dogs for breeding.

even enables a classification of CHD into seven grades as proposed by the OFA, thus, a transferal to the classification system used in the United States is possible. A proposal for conversion of current international CHD grades is summarized indicating the international applicability of this new system (Table 10-14).

We are convinced that the internationally uniform application of a clear and structured assessment protocol based on objective criteria would be advantageous for dog breeders and potential dog buyers because it would become possible to: (1) evaluate joints for CHD more reliably, (2) compare more accurately the frequency and severity of CHD in different countries and for various breeds, (3) evaluate and compare results and efficacy of the various CHD eradication programs, and (4) understand more clearly the meaning of a certain grade of dysplasia particularly when intended for use as a breeding animal in the country of origin.

## Current status

In Switzerland, CHD is diagnosed in more than 40% of all purebred dogs that are evaluated despite a 30-year eradication program. This program has diminished the severity and the prevalence of the disease. However, a steady improvement of coxofemoral joint quality has not been achieved and CHD remains common especially among dogs of popular breeds. Multiple factors are responsible for the slow progress. In addition to the lack of standardized analysis of radiographs as discussed above, the conventional VD positioning that is used in diagnosis does not truly reflect the genetic make-up of a dog. While this positioning permits accurate identification of secondary arthrosis, it does not correctly evaluate for joint laxity. Another reason for the continued high prevalence of CHD is the continued use of dysplastic dogs and their offspring for breeding. Obviously, radiographic screening cannot help under such conditions.

The use of only A and B graded dogs for breeding with an efficient ban on all dysplastic dogs would cause a remarkable decline in the frequency of CHD. This has been noted throughout the world in closed breeding colonies such as those for guide dogs.

Unfortunately, current CHD programs are more a type of "current CHD status" programs rather than "CHD eradication" programs. This is particularly true in the UK, in the USA, for many French clubs, and for Eastern and Southern Europe. Since hardly any consequences relative to breeding are drawn from the radiographic results. This situation is somewhat better in Germany and Switzerland since no dogs graded D or E may be used for breeding, and in some breeds, even no dogs graded C.

## Stress studies

The conventional VD positioning of the patient in dorsal recumbency or Olsson position remains the standard worldwide, however, it is not a physiologic position and most dogs resist this form of positioning. Therefore, it can only be implemented in the majority of dogs when under general anesthesia or deep sedation. The presence of secondary arthrosis can be evaluated quite reliably by this technique, however, the determination of joint laxity is unreliable. This method of positioning results in a spiral tensioning of the non-elastic joint capsule which itself leads to repositioning of a subluxated femoral head back into the acetabular cup. In addition, the relation of femoral head and acetabular cup tends to be affected by the traction applied to the limbs.

Yet, laxity is assumed to be the primary causative factor in CHD and often is the only indication of dysplasia in the younger dog. The continued prevalence of CHD may at least be partially due to the fact that the degree of hip joint laxity as an indicator of dysplasia is not evaluated reliably when using conventional positioning for the examination. A study was designed to evaluate a new, more reliable method of judging the quality of the dog's hip joint using a more appropriate stress radiographic technique that more closely simulates the forces on the hip joint during locomotion.

Joint laxity has been evaluated using a variety of stress techniques. They all have as a similar goal the production of a radiograph that permits evaluation of the lateral displacement of the femoral head. It is possible to obtain this information through the use of a fulcrum device positioned between the limbs with the application of a medially directed force on the stifles. This positioning results in a lateral displacement of the femoral heads. Initially this technique was recommended with the limbs fully extended but this position again resulted in a twisting and stretching of the fibers in the capsule, resulting in an incomplete determination of the maximal joint laxity.

Badertscher (1977) reported a "half axial view" that would have avoided this drawback, but the technique was not published in a scientific journal and, therefore, it was not placed into use in most hip examinations. His recommendation was to place the dog in dorsal recumbency with the femora at a 45 angle to the tabletop. Placement of a wooden fulcrum on the pelvic symphysis and adduction of the stifle joints resulted in lateral subluxation of the femoral heads in the affected dog. Later, Smith, et al (1990) determined a distraction index (DI) by comparison of a compression and distraction radiograph. Both studies were made with the femora raised approximately 90° off the tabletop. DI was defined as the ratio of the distance from the center of the femoral head to the center of the acetabulum divided by the radius of the femoral head. A DI of less than 0.3 is found in a dog with normal hips whereas a dog with a DI of over 0.4 will develop CHD or is considered to carry a disposition for CHD.

Both of these stress techniques test only for lateral movement of the femoral head, and yet the load on the acetabulum is in a craniodorsal direction. Since the first radiographic changes are visualized at the craniodorsal acetabular edge, the perfect stress technique should permit detection of femoral head displacement in this direction. Smith's technique of compression/distraction requires some training and customized tools to accomplish and is thus unlikely to be accepted widely throughout the profession.

Thus, the described stress techniques were modified and tested on more than 300 dogs. With the newly recommended technique, femoral head dislocation is achieved by placement of the dog in dorsal recumbence with the thorax in a Styrofoam trough with the femora at a 60° angle with the tabletop. The stifles are adducted and flexed and the tibiae used as a lever in placement of a moderate force directed craniodorsally at the time of radiographic exposure. This positioning is similar to that used in performing the Ortolani maneuver and results in a similar displacement of the femoral head in a dorsocranial and lateral direction. The technique is especially attractive since no special tool and only a brief special operator training is required. A subluxation index (SI) was created in a manner similar to the distraction index (DI) used by Smith. The kVp values need to be increased by 10 to 12 when compared to settings used with the standard ventrodorsal positioning because of the increase in thickness of muscle tissue as a result of the hind limb positioning.

Unequal pressure placed on the tibiae results in excessive tilting of the pelvis and a non-diagnostic study. However, the effect of slight pelvic malpositioning on the final interpretation was found to be virtually negligible. Quality of patient positioning can be evaluated by comparison of the size and shape of the foramen obturatoria. Early studies by Smith showed that an already small force applied resulted in near maximal subluxation of the femoral head during radiography.

It must be noted that all types of radiographic studies using a stress technique are only as valuable as the examiner intends. Fraudulent manipulation of the techniques is easy to accomplish and could not be detected on the resulting radiograph.

Evaluating the relationship between the degree of subluxation and the CHD grade, two critical SI values, 0.3 and 0.5, respectively, could be defined. Only 71% of those dogs graded normal or borderline and, even worse, only 32% of all dogs graded mildly dysplastic have truly stable hip joints reading an SI of not more than 0.3. Of the dogs with a SI value over 0.5, 95% were CHD graded C to E, deemed dysplastic (Table 10-15). This seems to confirm the concept of defining an upper limit of maximally tolerable joint laxity when scoring a hip joint as normal. It remains important to understand that any stress technique using flexed hind limbs and standardized distraction will yield specific degrees of tolerable subluxation

**Table 10-15: Realtion between CHD grade and SI value (indexing) in 302 dogs**
(Dogs grading C were subclassified in C1 and C2 – see Table 10-14)

| SI | A | B | C1 | C2 | D | E | Total |
|---|---|---|---|---|---|---|---|
| <0.3 | 40 | 67 | 21 | 10 | 1 | 0 | 139 |
| >0.3–0.5 | 9 | 33 | 25 | 23 | 28 | 6 | 124 |
| >0.5 | 1 | 1 | 6 | 11 | 18 | 2 | 39 |
| Total | 50 | 101 | 52 | 44 | 47 | 8 | 302 |

CHD-Grade, corresponding number of dogs

(an SI that should be considered within normal limits) for a given population of dogs or a particular breed.

Assuming that coxofemoral instability and arthrosis are undesirable findings in breeding dogs, only those CHD graded A or B, with a SI of maximum 0.3 should be accepted for breeding.

## Summary

The persistent problem of CHD has been attacked in two different directions in our hospital in the hope that a combined effort can make a difference in how this crippling disease affects dogs. The evaluation of hip radiographs has been strictly standardized resulting in a more consistent grading. Furthermore, the use of a stress view has been shown to more accurately detect joint laxity in dogs that were earlier being passed and recommended for breeding. Combining these two methods will result in optimized selection of CHD-free breeding stock.

In the future, all energy should be focused at encouraging progeny testing and the implementation of a modern breeding value estimation (BVE) program which would allow a more precise determination of the breeding value of a specific dog for a specific disease (ie, CHD). Such programs are highly successful in farm animal breeding and are also used in many dog breeds in Germany quite successfully. The BVE becomes most valuable when all offspring are radiographed, or when randomly selected offspring are evaluated. The remarkable advantage over the current selection mode is that a dog's breeding value is: (1) only mildly dependent upon his own conformation ($h2$ approximately 0.4) and (2) the value is constantly changing with increasing data information from related dogs. Thus, it is possible that a dog may loose breeding credibility after a few litters with poor quality hips, however, the dog may increase in breeding credibility as an increasing number of litters with excellent hips are produced.

Another method that would influence the frequency of CHD is to limit the currently unrestricted use of male dogs for breeding. If the quality of a breeding dog was ascertained after production of 20 puppies, it would be possible to remove the dog from breeding activity if the quality became undesirable or below average. There is no reason to use a male excessively while females are used in only a limited manner and are taken out of breeding after a few years.

# The Institute for Genetic Disease Control in Animals (GDC)

An open registry for multiple diseases in all breeds of dogs.

PAUL W. POULOS JR., DVM, VET. MED. DR., DAVCR
Executive Director and Chief Executive Officer, GDC
Box 222
Davis, California, USA

## Introduction

The concept of the open registry was pioneered in Scandinavia through the cooperation between the Swedish Kennel Club (SKK) and concerned veterinarians who realized that the only way to control hereditary disease was to know the genotype rather than the phenotype alone, and that this could only be accomplished when concerned breeders were willing to share genetic information in an open and unbiased manner. Once the registry was established, cooperation in this system allowed for a decrease in the prevalence of HD in Sweden from 46% to 23% in 13 years, a 50% reduction.

Encouraged by the results in Sweden, Dr. Alida Wind, with support from Barbara and Martin Packard, called together an international group of veterinary surgeons, radiologists, geneticists and academicians who met in Davis, California in the summer of 1989. As a result of this meeting, two entities were born: The International Elbow Working Group (IEWG) and The Institute for Genetic Disease Control in Animals (GDC). Originally sponsored by a single breed club, The Bay Berners, the GDC now boasts the support of many clubs and breeds as will be demonstrated below. Thus, from this humble beginning in the summer of 1990, the GDC was born as a non-profit organization dedicated to the better health of dogs through the reduction of heritable diseases that could be eliminated, or greatly reduced in the population, thereby reducing the pain and suffering of our canine companions. The GDC began by offering an open registry for orthopedic diseases that were known to be heritable, namely HD, elbow dysplasia, and osteochondrosis. However, this registry has the breadth and capacity to expand to include any heritable disease that is requested by any breed club.

Although GDC was modeled after the Swedish orthopedic registry, that is where the similarity ended. GDC is concerned with the genotype of the entire family and does not limit itself to a single genetic disease but looks at as many diseases within a breed as are requested by any supporting breed club. For example; it was the Poodle Club of America (PCA) working with the Genodermatosis Research Foundation that requested that the GDC establish an open registry for Sebaceous Adenitis, the world's first soft tissue genetic registry. This registry now has cooperation and registration from poodle breeders in the United States, Canada and Australia. It was also the PCA that voted unanimously to support and establish an open eye registry to include the heritable eye diseases of all breeds. We are currently reprogramming our computer so that the recording of data on eye diseases will be more breed-specific.

Since the establishment of the GDC in 1990 and the requests of the PCA, several other breed clubs have come forward with both support and requests for expansion of the original orthopedic registry. In 1993, the Cairn Terrier Club of America requested the establishment of open registries for Legg-Perthes disease, craniomandibular osteopathy, and medial patellar luxation. These registries are currently utilized by many breeds in which these diseases exist and have a similar mode of inheritance. In 1994, the Bernese Mountain Dog Club of America established the world's first open tumor registry for their breed and we currently register dogs which have a positive diagnosis of Histiocytosis or Mastocytoma.

## Currently maintained open genetic registries

The following are examples of genetic diseases for which the GDC currently maintains open genetic registries. In these diseases, the mode of inheritance and the age of onset are known and there is an accepted method of diagnosis.

Hip dysplasia
Elbow dysplasia
    Joint incongruity
    Fragmented medial coronoid process
    Ununited anconeal process
    Osteochondrosis of the medial humeral condyle
Osteochondrosis
Legg-Perthes disease
Craniomandibular osteopathy
Medial patellar luxation
Sebaceous adenitis

Hereditary eye diseases
Globoid cell leukodystrophy

In other diseases such as diabetes mellitus, lateral patellar luxation, and intervertebral disc disease there is a method of diagnosis but criteria have not been established relative to the mode of inheritance or the age of onset. In these examples, the data must be established by some acceptable means such as test mating or the establishment of a research database (RDB). All information, along with a signed release on both affected and unaffected individuals is placed in a GDC research data base until sufficient data is collected to establish the criterion that is missing. Once this is accomplished, the research database will automatically be converted to an open registry at the suggestion of the GDC board and with the approval of the sponsoring club.

In 1997 the first cardiac disease registry was established for tricuspid valve dysplasia of Labrador Retrievers, and in 1999 we established a subaortic stenosis (SAS) registry for the Bernese Mountain Dog. These registries were developed with the support of diplomates of the American College of Veterinary Cardiology. We will continue to add other breeds to these registries as requests are received and will continue to add other cardiac registries as they are requsted and approved.

In 1997 the Dalmatian Club of America sponsored a deafness registry for all breeds. There is a test to determine deafness, and once a panel of experts reached agreement on how the data should be collected, the registry was opened.

## Examples of existing research data bases

### Idiopathic Epilepsy of Irish Setters, Labrador Retrievers and Bernese Mountain Dogs
This is a disease of great concern in many dog breeds. Unfortunately the mode of inheritance is unknown and there is no specific diagnostic test. The establishment of a research data base is essential to gain an understanding of epilepsy. Until a definitive diagnostic test is developed, the diagnosis will depend upon ruling out other causes of seizures. This will be based on criteria developed by a panel of experts. The resultant data will be evaluated by a principal investigator to determine if the patient meets established criteria to be placed in the hereditary epilepsy data base for that breed.

### Chondrodysplasia (Dwarfism) of Great Pyrenees
This is a skeletal disease that affects growing dogs of this breed. A research database has been established by the Great Pyrenees Club of America.

### Tumors
There are a group of tumors that have not yet been proven to be heritable. A research database has been established by the Bernese Mountain Dog Club of America.

### Medial and lateral patellar luxation
This is currently maintained for Great Pyrenees, Chinooks and Belgian Shepherd Dogs.

### Portosystemic shunts
Portosystemic shunts were added to our list of data bases in 1994 and all terrier breeds were included in this data base in 1997.

## Sebacious Adenitis (SA)

Although there is an open registry for Sebacious Adenitis (SA) of poodles the disease is not proven to be genetic in other breeds, therefore, in 1998 we established a research data base for SA in all breeds.

## Examples of registries that are in the progress of being developed

### Hypothyroidism
This disease is clouded by controversy because of the many physiologic interactions that may occur between other disease processes and with some medications. Therefore the GDC is currently working with the Society of Veterinary Endocrinologists to develop a research database that will not only establish diagnostic criteria to be used in the separation of hereditary hypothyroidism but also provide useful information on other aspects of the disease. Material from an AKC sponsored conference on hypothyroidism is being utilized in the establishment of this registry. In addition to a hypothyroid protocol, the material from this conference should greatly aid in the in the establishment of comparable research databases for both Addison's and Cushing's diseases.

## The concept of open versus closed, or confidential, registries

An open genetic disease registry is a data bank of genetic history for any breed and for specific genetic diseases. In an open registry owners, breeders, veterinarians, and scientists can trace the genetic history of any particular dog once that dog and close relatives have been registered. In order to control genetic diseases the prevalence of the disease within the breed and in any particular bloodline must be known. This information is only available when data from both normal and abnormal individuals is submitted to the registry in a manner that reduces bias. This is accomplished when conscientious breeders, in order to improve the health and well being of their breed, submit all information, including litter registration, to an open registry regardless of the anticipated outcome. In our open registry, our computer automatically links information about each dog with other relatives in the registry.

In general, data in the GDC registry is available to people who need support and information in the selection of breeding dogs, the correct selection of which will lead to a reduction of genetic disease in a kennel or in the breed. All information must be used in accordance with ethical breeding standards and is released upon receipt of a written request, on specific animals for a nominal fee, in order for the breeder to make knowledgeable selection of mates whose bloodlines indicate a reduced risk of producing genetic disease. This information is available only because the owner has signed a release so that their dog may be placed in the open registry.

A closed registry, on the other hand, gives only phenotypic information. You know that the individual is free of signs of the disease, but you can not know if his/her parents, siblings, half siblings or progeny are affected. It is well known that the mating of phenotypic unaffected dogs may result in offspring that are affected, unaffected, or a combination of both.

## Advantages of an open registry

Registry with the GDC will give phenotypic data at one year of age for most orthopedic diseases. In late onset diseases such as progressive retinal atrophy (PRA) and sebaceous adenitis (SA) certification is yearly until the age of late onset is reached. The availability of genotypic data depends upon the degree of participation by breeders, breed clubs and the dog owning public. As GDC grows, more and more information will be available within a breed and specific lines.

GDC produces the KinReport that contains information to enable conscientious breeders to make educated decisions regarding selection of breeding animals. In order to provide the greatest amount of information, we must know the affected animals because there is no doubt that these individuals carry the genes; however, only by being able to discern the prevalence of the disease(s) in a family can we begin to know how heavily concentrated any disease is within that family.

The RDB is a valuable tool for scientists studying any of the diseases for which a RDB has been established. In part this is because of the wealth of information that is available within the KinReports to study the heritability of disease. In addition families can be identified with high and low incidence of a disease. This is an invaluable tool for those scientists who are searching for the genetic markers of the disease. Further, there is the scientific symbiosis that exists between finding the gene and therapy. This information may be transferable from the dog to the human and visa versa. A perfect example of this is Globoid Cell Leukodystrophy of Cairn and West Highland White Terriers. Here the gene and genetic tests were first found in humans and our canine friends are reaping the benefit. The next step may well be that a drug will be found that will save the lives of both children and dogs.

GDC will eventually become a clearing house for genetic information for scientists working on diseases such as lateral patellar luxation, epilepsy, juvenile renal disease, bloat, hypothyroidism, Cushing's and Addison's disease and other diseases yet to become requested registries or research data bases.

It has been said that there are less than 200 veterinary geneticists worldwide. Therefore, it is now more important than ever that the veterinary profession become well informed about genetic disease and the means of control. It will be the task of the family veterinarian to inform the owner and breeder of the more than 300 canine genetic diseases that have already been identified. Some scientists suspect upwards of 1,000 diseases may exist. Veterinary schools must be encouraged to increase the awareness of veterinarians to this problem through continuing education and inclusion of veterinary geneticists on the faculties rather than to rely on schools of agriculture to teach veterinarians only the basics of genetics without dealing with the genetic diseases about which they will need to inform their clients.

## Common questions asked of GDC

*1. Why does the GDC register hip and elbow dysplasia at 1 year of age and the OFA registers the same diseases at 2 years of age?*

As previously stated the GDC was established based on the Swedish open registry which had a proven track record in reducing the incidence of HD from 46% to 23% in thirteen years using evaluation at 1 year of age. In all other countries the accepted age of evaluation is between 12 and 18 months. (The only organization in the world that currently requires certification to wait until two years of age is the OFA.)

Although the question concerns the evaluation of pelvic radiographs between the ages of 1 and 2 years, a more important consideration should be whether or not to use the GDC open registry since it will give genotypic information on the entire family rather than only the phenotype of the dog in question.

A reality of medicine is that all diagnostic tests (procedures) including radiographs have a degree of error that must be accepted. Indeed, variability of analysis due to different observers (inter-observer variation) is equal to the difference between the number of false normals at 12 months of age; thus it is the human factor and not the age that keeps us from a higher level of competence. In order to compensate for inter-observer variation, we at GDC request re-evaluation at 2 years of age of borderline cases and withhold certification until that time.

### 2. Should anesthesia, tranquilization or hand restraint be used in obtaining pelvic radiographs?

General anesthesia is by far the best method of restraint for orthopedic evaluation because it allows for accurate positioning of the patient while allowing personnel to be as far away from the primary beam as possible when the radiographic exposure is made. Proper positioning on the first attempt will decrease the cost of retake examinations, decreased radiation exposure of personnel, and help to assure that the films are not returned to the client as being unacceptable for interpretation. Today with the availability of new means of sedation and muscle relaxation, including various combinations of drugs, hand restraint is not an acceptable technique.

### 3. How can your veterinarian keep a copy of the film for his records and send the original film to a registry that must keep the film that is sent to them?

A radiograph is the property of the practice and an integral part of the medical records. The client does not own the film. The primary veterinarian does. In some states it is required that the veterinary practice maintain films as part of their medical records for at least five years and in some states even longer.

An exact duplicate of the film that is to be sent can be made by placing two films in the cassette and making the exposure with an increase of 10 kVp over the amount noted in the technique chart. This technique is the least expensive, costing only the amount of an additional film and its processing. A second film could also be exposed at the time of examination or a duplicate film could be made at a local hospital. In some cases a duplicate film can be requested from the registry, in this case the cost is usually about $10 per film.

### 4. Who can certify eye examinations for the open registry?

Eyes can only be certified by a member of the American College of Veterinary Ophthalmology. It is best if a certification examination for open registry is requested on a Canine Eye Registry Foundation (CERF) form. The owner's copy of that examination, or a copy of both sides of the owner's copy, is sent to the GDC with the proper application form and check. All finding are registered and when appropriate, the GDC issues a certificate of unaffected that is valid for one year. In the event of an affected diagnosis, the check is returned with the notice of registration.

### 5. Who procures the skin biopsies for the sebaceous adenitis registry?

The skin biopsy is done by the primary care veterinarian in a manner described in the SA application. The biopsy, with the appropriate form and fees, is then sent to one of the dermato-pathologists who has been selected to perform the evaluation of the histology slides. Their names and addresses can be found on the form.

### 6. Who procures the tissue biopsies or necropsy material for the tumor registry?

Biopsies are normally performed in the referring veterinarian's office. Anyone performing a biopsy or necropsy can send the appropriate samples accompanied by the GDC tumor form to one of the Pathologists listed on the form.

### 7. Is there any means of verification of accuracy of records?

Yes, an owner can request the GDC records on their dog(s) at any time in order to verify accuracy of that information.

### 8. In cases of disputed diagnosis is there any recourse?

Yes, there is a protocol for appeal. Appeals are handled on an individual basis depending on the specific registry involved. There is no charge for an appeal.

## Philosophy

No fee is charged for recording data on affected animals. The ultimate goal of the registry is to include as many affected animals as possible with their four generation pedigrees in order to have the maximum genetic pressure on reducing the incidence of any genetic disease. Therefore, the inducement for submitting affected animals is a priority of the GDC and should be for any contributor in order to claim the prize of improved genetic health of the breed or line.

Litter rates are an important part of the inducement package. A reduced fee is charged for any registry when an entire litter is submitted at one time. The inclusion of the entire litter into the KinReport adds substantially to the value of the resultant report.

The concept of open registries has been supported by many prominent veterinary educators and geneticists. The following are just a few quotes to demonstrate the importance of the open registry concept:

In a paper entitled "Champions and Genetic Disease," Professor Heinrich Binder of the Veterinary Faculty at the University of Zurich concluded: "Successful breeders are rightfully proud of their accomplishments and generally are not willing to show their hand. To a great extent, the facilitation with breeding lies in the desire to achieve perfection by "working" with the strong and weak points of one's breeding stock. In the past, "success" was measured primarily on external traits with high heritability. Therefore, the individual breeder could depend on a high probability for success by selecting according to past experience with his own dogs. In light of an ever increasing occurrence of diseases, it would be a grave mistake to continue to treat ones own breeding stock as an individual unit and to only share information selectively. Such actions will lead to the downfall of any breed. To refuse the collection and sharing of progeny data on every stud dog or to provide incomplete information out of fear that a "top dog" may loose value (which very well could happen) is genetically and morally wrong. A successful attack on breed disposed diseases requires the cooperative efforts of all breeders and expert coordination by a central organization. This is the only way in which an increase in genetic breed problems can be averted."

In 1987, Dr. Donald Patterson, Professor of Medicine and Chief of Medical Genetics at the University of Pennsylvania, School of Veterinary Medicine, wrote an article for the AKC Gazette in which he proposed the establishment of "The Canine Genetic Disease Information System." That system is scheduled to become available to veterinarians on a computer disc in 1997. He went on to state that the next step should be the establishment of a "comprehensive certification for genetic diseases." That next step has been taken. The GDC has offered a "comprehensive certification for genetic diseases," since 1990.

According to Dr. George Padgett, a pathologist at the University of Michigan School of Veterinary Medicine, dogs now suffer more frequently from genetic diseases than any other animals, including humans. In fact, up to 70% of some breeds are affected. He further states, "Using GDC's resources, the countries dog lovers could easily reduce genetic disease by ten to twelve percent per year. With the knowledge we have right now, in a decade we could cut the rate of disease to five percent from its present thirty to seventy percent."

According to Dr. William D. Schall, Professor of Small Animal Medicine and Surgery at Michigan State University, it costs American dog owners at least $2 billion a year to treat genetic diseases in man's best friend.

"One essential component of the genetic constitution of any breed is that those same genes in different forms are present in every other breed. Thus, breed specific solutions apply across all breeds and clubs can deservedly celebrate victories in any breed." James W. Edwards, PhD.

Anyone wishing information or application forms for specific registries that the GDC operates can obtain them from:

GDC
PO Box 222
Davis, CA 95617

Telephone or Fax: 530-756-6773

http://www.vetmed.ucdavis.edu/gdc/gdc.html

## References

BINDER H.; Champions and Genetic Diseases; SFBB Newsnote, February 1996, pp. 5-8

EDWARDS JAMES W.; American Kennel Club Parent Club Conference, October 20-22, 1995

HEDHAMMAR Å.; "Breeding healthier dogs in Sweden," Tijdschrift voor Diergeneeskunde, Vol. 116, April 1991, Supplement pp. 76-78.

PADGETT G.; Please Join the Fight to Eradicate Genetic Disease in Dogs. A Special Appeal to America's Pet Industry. Institute for Genetic Disease Control Document, January 2, 1997.

PADGETT G.; Control of canine Diseases, Howell Book House, Simon & Schuster Macmillan, 1998.

PATTERSON D.; Pure Bred Dogs/American Kennel Gazette, July, 1987.

SCHALL W. D.; Proceedings, American Kennel Club's "Molecular Genetics and Canine Genetic Health Conference," October 7-8, 1994.

# Hip dysplasia diagnosis - the use of distraction radiography

GAIL K. SMITH, VMD, PHD
Department of Clinical Studies
School of Veterinary Medicine
University of Pennsylvania
3850 Spruce Street
Philadelphia, PA 19104-6010

A stress-radiographic diagnostic method for early (4 months) detection of susceptibility to HD has been developed and tested at the University of Pennsylvania over the past 14 years (Smith 1994, 1997). The method requires the dog to be under deep sedation or general anesthesia and incorporates two views with the dog in supine position and hips at neutral (stance phase) flexion/extension angle. A compression view is made with the femoral heads fully seated in the acetabula and a distraction view is obtained by levering a custom-designed distractor between the legs at the level of the ventral pelvis creating maximal lateral displacement of the femoral heads (Smith, et al 1990). Along with the new positioning, a new measurement method was developed to quantitate the relative degree of femoral head displacement from the acetabulum in either the compression or distraction views. The new measurement method utilizes an index from 0 to 1 with 0 being a fully congruent hip, as seen in the compression view and 1 representing the most extreme joint laxity as might be seen in the distraction view of hips that are virtually luxated. The distraction index (DI) is a ratio scale, meaning a hip with a DI of 0.6 shows twice the laxity of a hip with a DI of 0.3. The following discussion summarizes pertinent research findings in support of the new stress-radiographic method.

## Mechanical testing

Mechanical testing instrumentation was designed and machined to evaluate the biomechanics of hip stability, including a newly discovered hydrostatic phenomenon, and to explore the role of passive hip laxity in overall hip stability (Heyman, et al 1993). The first part of the study involved mechanical testing of cadaver canine hips to reveal the range of flexion/extension, adduction/abduction, and internal/external rotation associated with maximal passive laxity of the hip joint. This information was critical for optimizing the new distraction method particularly regarding quality assurance and repeatability from one examiner to another. Relative to the plane of the pelvis, the optimal range of hip position was found to be between 10° of flexion and 30° of extension, between 10° and 30° of abduction, and between 0° and 10° of external rotation. Any deviation out of this range caused a precipitous decrease in lateral displacement of the femoral head from the acetabulum. In fact, mechanical data from cadaver hips positioned in the standard extended, internally rotated, OFA orientation demonstrated a minimum 50% reduction in measurable hip laxity, corroborating earlier necropsy observations that the winding up of the joint capsule had a profound effect on apparent hip laxity (Smith, et al 1990).

Mechanical testing of cadaver hips also showed that the load/displacement behavior of passive hip laxity was sigmoidal rather than linear. Translated, this meant that in the design of a stress radiographic method, it was unnecessary to quantitate the actual distractive force applied to the hip because individuals of differing strength could expect to create similar measurable joint displacements in anesthetized or heavily sedated animals. That is, mechanical testing results suggested method repeatability should be very high, both within examiner and between examiners as long as applied loads were above the recognized critical minimum (approximately 20n).

## Clinical data

### Hip laxity comparisons

In a population of purebred dogs (n = 142), hip laxity in the standard OFA radiographic view was compared with hip laxity from the distraction view. The distraction radiograph was found on average to reveal 2.5 times more joint laxity than the standard hip extended radiograph (Smith, et al 1990). The distraction view always revealed more laxity than the hip-extended view and often showed obvious measurable laxity when the hip-extended view showed none (Smith, et al 1995).

### Correlation of laxity to osteoarthrosis (OA)

An analysis of passive hip laxity and the coexistence of OA in a cross-section of large and giant breed dogs (mean age 28 months, n = 227), showed hip laxity from the distraction radiographic view to be highly correlated with the radiographic appearance of OA. Particularly striking was the observation that tight hips were highly unlikely to show evidence of OA. As laxity increased, there was an associated increase in the probability for hip OA. Interestingly, no hip with a distraction index less than 0.3 showed radiographic evidence of OA. However, not all dogs having hip laxity greater than 0.3 demonstrated evidence of OA.

In the same sample of dogs, the correlation of hip laxity with hip OA from the standard hip-extended radiograph also yielded a statistically significant, though weaker, correlation. Unlike the distraction method however, there was no recognizable threshold of joint laxity below which no dogs were found to have hip OA. That is, although OA susceptibility clearly decreased with hip tightness on the standard radiographic view, there was no practical range of joint laxity at which hips could be considered non-susceptible to OA. Similar to patterns observed for the distraction method, not all loose-hipped dogs showed radiographic evidence of OA even though the mean age of this population was 28 months.

From these data it was theorized that hip laxity was divisible into two forms: 1) passive hip laxity, which is the relative looseness of the hip joint as measured in the sedated dog absent of active muscle contracture or weight bearing, and 2) functional hip laxity, the pathological form of hip laxity, occurring during weight bearing and ultimately leading to OA. While functional hip laxity is clearly of greatest diagnostic interest, there currently are no means to measure it. Passive hip laxity, on the other hand, is a readily measurable quantity and since it was shown in this study to be a prerequisite for functional laxity, it was considered a risk factor for OA or, loosely defined, perhaps a carrier state. In other words, passive hip laxity was necessary for OA but not alone sufficient to cause OA. Importantly, however, dogs having hip distraction index less than 0.3 were true negatives for HD within the span of the study (Smith, et al 1993). Dogs with DI greater than 0.3 were considered to have hip hyperlaxity, and were OA susceptible even though phenotypically normal on the standard hip-extended radiograph (Smith, et al 1995).

## Breed-specific passive hip laxity and susceptibility to OA

Breeds of dogs known to have a very low frequency of HD (<1%) were found to have uniformly tight hip joints on distraction radiography. In fact, the mean passive laxity for racing greyhounds and performance-bred Borzois was significantly tighter than breeds of dogs commonly afflicted with HD, such as German Shepherd Dogs, Golden Retrievers, and Rottweilers (p<0.0001). Greater than 98% of all Borzois and Greyhounds had distraction indices less than 0.3 with some being as tight as 0.08 (Smith, et al 1992). This finding supported the hypothesis mentioned above that 0.3 was a biological threshold separating normal, disease-free hips from hips susceptible to OA. In contrast, using the standard hip-extended procedure to determine joint laxity, there were no statistically significant differences in breed-specific joint laxity nor was a disease threshold identified.

## Repeatability of distraction index over time and the prediction of OA

In a 3-year longitudinal evaluation of more than 140 dogs followed from 4 months of age, the DI was shown to be clearly more repeatable over time than either the Norberg angle or the OFA-type score (Smith et al 1993). Four-month DI correlated highly with 6 month, 12 month, and 24 month DI (intraclass correlation coefficients of 0.87, 0.82, and 0.85, respectively). Lower ranges of correlation coefficients over the same intervals were 0.40 to 0.55 for the Norberg angle and 0.06 to 0.29 for the OFA score. Early DI was shown to correlate better with the development of OA than Norberg angle or OFA score. Statistical analysis using a logistic regression model confirmed that of the variables measured, DI at an age as young as 4 months was the best predictor of OA probability and that the strength of the prediction improved when the analysis was done at 6 months or 1 year (Smith, et al 1993 b). Specifically, German Shepherd Dogs were found to have 6.3 times higher probability to show OA than other dogs in the sample. Further, for German Shepherd Dogs, each 0.1 increase in DI was associated with a 4.1-fold increase in the risk of OA, supporting the hypothesis that "tighter hips are better hips." A subsequent study of Rottweilers confirmed the patterns of OA where again DI was the only significant predictor of risk for hip OA. Each 0.1 increase in DI however, was associated with only a 2.9 fold increase in OA risk, lower than that for German Shepherd Dogs. Accordingly, compared to Rottweilers, German Shepherd Dogs had 6.4 times more risk of developing OA. This might suggest either that the German Shepherd Dogs are more sensitive to passive hip laxity, or alternatively, that Rottweilers are laxity-tolerant and therefore relatively OA resistant (Popovitch, et al 1995). These data emphasized the need to develop similar logistic regression curves for all popular breeds of dogs to permit valid application of the distraction index as a selection criterion. Such a need underscores the importance of a nationwide database to study the relationship of passive hip laxity to OA on a breed by breed basis.

A separate study of 45 8-week-old German Shepherd Dog puppies was conducted to learn whether hip laxity at an age younger than 16 weeks would also be predictive of disease susceptibility (Smith, et al 1998). Results in this sample of puppies revealed that hip laxity at 8 weeks of age is not sufficiently reliable to use in a predictive sense. Preliminary evidence, however, from other centers suggests that some breeds of dogs may demonstrate joint laxity and disease susceptibility at an age earlier than 16 weeks. For the present, however, it is recommended that dogs should not be evaluated before 16 weeks of age and that follow-up radiography to confirm the 16 weeks laxity should be done at 6 months or 1 year of age.

### Relationship of OFA Score to DI

Hips were evaluated in a population of 65 large-breed dogs both by the official OFA radiographic process and by the compression/distraction stress-radiographic method (Smith, et al 1992). An analysis of the distribution of DI scores corresponding to the seven OFA scoring categories revealed several interesting findings. All dogs graded as having mild, moderate, or severe HD by the OFA had corresponding DI scores above 0.3 (mean DI 0.55), indicating excellent agreement of the two scoring methods relative to disease phenotpyes. That is, all dogs that the OFA judged to have dysplasia were clearly in the hip hyperlaxity category (OA susceptible) as judged by the distraction method. The converse, however, was not true. Of the dogs having hips judged excellent by the OFA, 50% had DI scores in the OA susceptible category, above 0.3 (mean DI 0.3). Further, 66% of the dogs judged to be good and 100% of the dogs judged fair by the OFA had DI scores greater than 0.3 (mean DI 0.35 and 0.50, respectively). Therefore a high percentage of dogs that were officially approved for breeding by OFA subjective scoring had hip laxities corresponding to OA susceptibility. Whether dogs with hip hyperlaxity actually express OA within their lifetimes or not may be of little importance if in their genetic makeup they carry or have the potential to transmit the susceptibility for OA to their offspring. It is this very fundamental association between hip laxity and susceptibility of OA that we feel is not addressed by the current OFA diagnostic method and which perhaps explains the poor progress in reducing HD frequency after 31 years of application of OFA score as a selection criterion.

### Heritability of passive hip laxity

Studies of HD heritability, or more specifically of passive hip laxity heritability, are ongoing. All estimates of heritability to date are presently limited to the German Shepherd Dog and Labrador Retriever breeds. Heritability of passive laxity is a property of the population under study and therefore it must be calculated for each breed. An upper limit of a trait's heritability is the intra-class correlation coefficient of repeatability over time and, this correlation coefficient for German Shepherd Dogs in the sample mentioned above was between 0.67 and 0.74, an extremely high upper limit. Similar support is derived from regression analysis of litter mean DIs plotted against mid-parent mean DIs which has yielded estimates of laxity heritability for the German Shepherd Dog from 0.42 to 0.65 and an upper limit for the Labrador Retrievers of 0.92. Although heritability analyses are still incomplete, these early results are promising that the heritability of passive laxity (and therefore the likelihood for OA) will be much higher than the low heritability estimate of 0.22 for HD as diagnosed by the standard hip-extended method (Leighton, et al 1977). If so, the use of the distraction index as a selection criterion can be expected to result in more rapid progress in reducing the incidence and severity of HD.

Our most rigorous estimates of heritability of passive hip laxity are derived from analyses of the full pedigree from the closed populations of dogs bred and raised by The Seeing Eye, Inc. Using a derivative free restricted maximum likelihood procedure that incorporates the full pedigree structure among dogs, we have recently reported the heritability of passive hip laxity to be 0.46 in the GSD and 0.46 in the labrador retriever (Leighton, et al 1998).

### PennHIP

In the spring of 1993, the University of Pennsylvania Hip Improvement Program (PennHIP) was established as a collaborative effort of academic and private-practice veterinarians to facilitate the controlled transfer of technology to multiple centers for public utilization. The program was designed to fulfill many objectives, the primary one being to reduce the frequency of HD. Data from participants are compiled in a large medical database and are used to investigate genetic aspects of passive hip laxity both individually and by breed. The approximately 16,000 dogs evaluated thus far must be expanded many fold to address the numerous breed-specific questions and concerns of breeders. Through periodic monitoring and reporting of the success of this method, as it becomes more widely available, it is planned that the scientific integrity of this technology will be maintained (Smith 1997).

In the United States and Canada, pet owners or dogs breeders desiring to have their animals evaluated by the PennHIP system, can be referred to one of the PennHIP Network Members. For veterinarians interested in training and participating in PennHIP, the current minimum recommended requirements include a 300mA radiographic unit and an automatic film processor. PennHIP information including training programs or an updated list of certified PennHIP members may be obtained by contacting Synbiotics Corporation at 11-11 Via Frontera, San Diego, CA 92127 (telephone 800-228-4305 or 619-451-3771).

# References

HEYMAN SJ, SMITH GK, COFONE MA. A biomechanical study of the effect of coxofemoral positioning on passive hip joint laxity in the dog. AJVR 54: 210-215, 1993.

LEIGHTON EA, LINN JM, WILLHAM RL. et al. A genetic study of canine hip dysplasia. AJVR 38:241-244, 1977.

LEIGHTON EA, SMITH GK, BIERY DN, HOLLE DM, MCNEIL M, GREGOR TP, PATTERSON D. Heritability of hip joint distraction index and a hip joint quality score among German Shepherd Dogs and Laarador Retrievers in a closed breeding colony. JAVMA In Press 1999.

POPOVITCH CA, SMITH GK, GREGOR TP, SHOFER FS. Factors affecting the risk of developing hip degenerative joint diseae and ocmparison of hip dysplasia susceptibility in Rottweiter and German Shepherd breeds. JAVMA 206:648-650, 1995.

SMITH GK. Distraction Radiography for Hip Dysplasia Diagnosis: University of Pennsylvania Hip Improvement Program. Proceedings of the 1994 Annual Scientific Meeting of the Veterinary Orthopedic Society, Snowbird/Alta, p45-50, 1994.

SMITH GK. Canine Hip Dysplasia: Advances in Diagnosis. submitted to JAVMA 210: 1451-1457, 1997.

SMITH GK, BIERY DN, GREGOR TP. New concepts of coxofemoral joint stability and the development of a clinical stress-radiographic method for quantitating hip joint laxity in the dog. JAVMA 196:59-70, 1990.

SMITH GK, GREGOR TP, BIERY DN, RHODES WH, REID CF. Hip dysplasia diagnosis: A comparison of diagnostic methods and diagnosticians. Proceedings of the 1992 Annual Scientific Meeting of the Veterinary Orthopedic Society, Keystone, CO, p20, 1992.

SMITH GK, GREGOR TP, RHODES WH, BIERY DN. Coxofemoral joint laxity from distraction radiography and its contemporaneous and prospective correlation with laxity, subjective score, and evidence of degenerative joint disease from conventional hip-extended radiography in dogs. AJVR 54:1021-1042, 1993.

SMITH GK, POPOVITCH CA, GREGOR TP. Evaluation of factors contributing to the risk of developing degenerative joint disease associated with canine hip dysplasia. JAVMA 206:642-647, 1995.

SMITH GK, HILL CM, GREGOR TP, OLSON K. Reliability of the hip distraction index in two-month-old German Shepherd Dogs. JAVMA 212:1560-1563, 1998.

# Control of elbow dysplasia in Sweden

Lars Audell, DVM
Radiology Consultant
Gudby Gård
194 92 Upplands Väsby
Sweden

An important offspring of the HD program in Sweden is the Elbow Dysplasia Control Program. During the last 20 years elbow joint lesions have become of great concern in some breeds of dogs. In Sweden it became evident in the early 1980's that lameness originating from the elbow joint lesions caused more problems than HD in Bernese Mountain Dogs and Rottweilers. A research screening program was started in 1978, and it developed into a central elbow arthrosis control program in 1983.

To this date, over 50,000 dogs of (120) breeds have had elbow radiographs scrutinized and classified by the same radiologist and the results have been registered and computerized at the Swedish Kennel Club (SKK). Elbow as well as hip joint radiographs have now become a routine examination in the veterinary practices and many clinicians as well as breeders prefer to perform both examinations at the same time. This is usually when the dogs are between 12 to 16 months of age. The amount of data is now large enough to allow estimations of incidence and heritability of elbow disease in some of the most affected breeds.

In contrast to the various HD programs in operation throughout the different countries of the world, through the efforts of the International Elbow Working Group, the programs controlling elbow dysplasia are almost identical. The Swedish program is based on the protocol established by this group. This includes the following concepts:

1. The dogs must be over 1 year of age at examination and be permanently tattooed to have radiographs of the elbows classified as being free of disease. The minimum age of 1 year is recommended although it is known that a limited number of dogs can develop elbow arthrosis caused by dysplasia even up to the age of 3 years. Younger dogs can be included in the program if they show signs of lameness since, if positive, there is a great risk that they will not return for another examination at an older age. The purpose is to identify the majority of affected dogs as early as possible and prevent them from being used in breeding programs.

2. No films are evaluated unless the owner has signed a paper stating that they give permission for all radiographs to be registered and stored at the SKK and that the results of the examination are open. The owners usually receive the results within a week, but the results are also sent to breed clubs where they are published. Information concerning the results can be obtained from the SKK.

3. Only one radiograph of each elbow in the flexed lateral position is used for evaluation. It is necessary that the anconeal process of the ulna be clearly visible since the periarticular osteophytes on this process are usually the earliest and the easiest detected signs of arthrosis in the majority of dogs regardless of the etiology of the arthrosis. It is difficult to clearly identify fragmented coronoid process and joint incongruity except by the detection of the secondary changes associated with the arthrosis.

4. The radiographs are evaluated as normal. If arthrosis is present, it is classified into three categories to provide the owners with additional information. A radiograph classified with minimal arthrosis (grade 1) has clearly visible osteophyte formation less than 2 mm in size in one or more of five specific locations. A radiograph classified with moderate arthrosis (grade 1) has larger osteophytes, between 2 and 5 mm, while those classified with severe arthrosis have osteophytes over 5 mm in height in one or more of the specific locations.

5. To encourage owners to submit as many studies as possible into the program and in particular to submit studies with arthrosis, all radiographs of dogs with more than minimal arthrosis are evaluated and registered without cost.

6. Because all radiographs are evaluated by the same radiologist, it is important to have an appeal panel that can adjudicate any problems. This panel consists of radiologists from Finland, Norway, and Denmark.

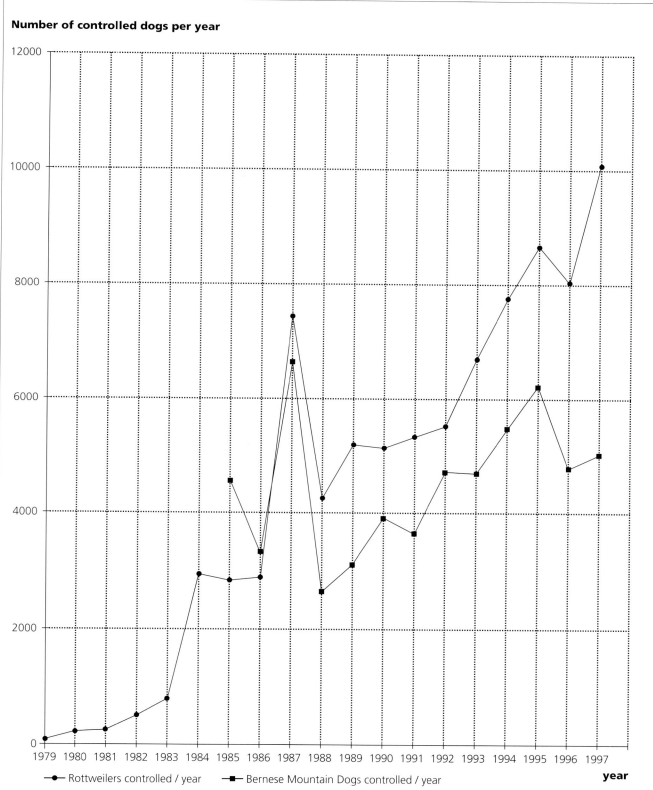

**Figure 10-5** The total number of dogs that were controlled for elbow dysplasia from 1979 to 1997. The number of specific breed, Bernese Mountain Dogs, that were controlled for elbow dysplasia from 1985 until 1997 is included.

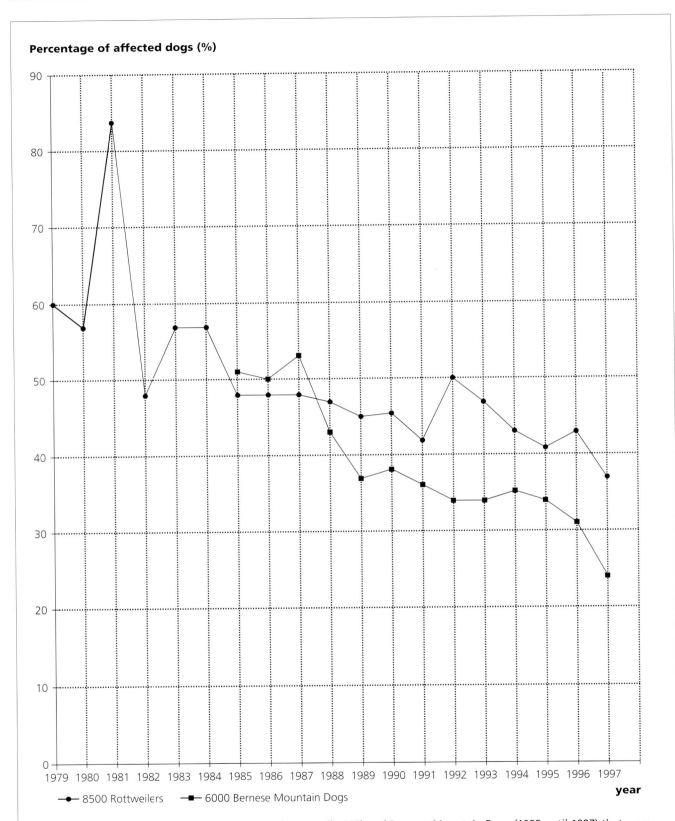

**Figure 10-6** The percentage of Rottweilers (1979 until 1997) and Bernese Mountain Dogs (1985 until 1997) that were affected with elbow dysplasia. Note the decrease in the percentage affected.

## Results

The frequency of elbow examinations in the most controlled breeds was tabulated for the period between 1978 until 1988 and for the single year of 1993 (Table 10-16).

**Table 10-16: Frequency of elbow examination in seven breeds from the period of 1978 until 1988 compared with the single year 1993**

| Breed | Number radiographed 1978-1988 (average number per year) | 1993 |
|---|---|---|
| Bernese Mountain Dog | 120 | 468 |
| German Shepherd Dog | 18 | 1929 |
| Golden Retriever | 8 | 1768 |
| Grosser Schweizer Sennen | 5 | 37 |
| Labrador Retriever | 31 | 1278 |
| Newfoundland | 7 | 183 |
| Rottweiler | 136 | 669 |

As seen from the number of dogs examined, the owners, breeders, and veterinarians have rapidly increased their interest in the program. The total number of dogs radiographed in 1994 was near 8000 and this exceeded 10,000 in 1997 (Figure 10-5). This is thought to be due to the breeders understanding that a decrease in affected offspring results in fewer dogs that require surgery or eventual euthanasia. The veterinarians have accepted the program readily, particularly since the radiographic technique is much easier to perform than that used for the evaluation of the hip joints. Also, the evaluation of the elbow radiographs is simpler with a resulting evaluation that is easier to understand and without the disagreement often found in evaluations of hip studies.

The first breed in the program was the Rottweiler, which after a few years was followed by the Bernese Mountain Dog. Today between 70% and 80% of all dogs of these breeds that are registered by the SKK have the status of their elbows controlled. In the last 5 years, an increasing interest in the program has been noticed from breeders of Retrievers and working German Shepherd Dogs.

Early results indicate that a decrease in frequency of elbow arthrosis is seen in the most controlled breeds. This is especially evident in the Bernese Mountain Dogs in which the percentage of affected dogs has declined from 52% in 1985 to a level of 24% in 1997. While the decline is less prominent in the Rottweiler breed, the percentage of affected dogs has still declined from a level of 57% in 1984 to a level of 37% in 1997 (Figure 10-6). Data suggests that the progeny from affected parents have around two times higher frequency of elbow arthrosis as compared to the progeny of parents classified as normal. The heritability estimates lie within the range of 0.25 and 0.45, which clearly indicates that the frequency of arthrosis can be decreased with selective breeding.

## References

AUDELL L. Heredity of elbow dysplasia: Can elbow dysplasia be controlled by judicious breeding. AAHA Scientific Proceedings 730-733, 1990.

SWENSON L, AUDELL L, HEDHAMMAR Å. Prevalence and inheritance of and selection for elbow arthrosis in Bernese Mountain Dogs and Rottweilers in Sweden and benefit: cost analysis of a screening and control program. JAVMA 210:215-221, 1997.

# International Elbow Working Group (IEWG)

Dr. Mark Flückiger, Dipl. ECVDI
Department for Internal Veterinary Medicine
Section of Diagnostic Imaging
University of Zurich
Switzerland

## Structure and purpose

In the late-70s, alarming results were reported from elbow examinations of Norwegian and Swedish Rottweilers and Bernese Mountain dogs. Between 48% and 58% of them were reported to be affected by elbow arthrosis (Grøndalen 1979). A Swiss study on 77 nonselected Bernese Mountain dogs demonstrated a 40% prevalence of elbow arthrosis (Bienz 1985). As a result, breeders and veterinarians from many countries became interested and concerned about diseases of the elbow. In 1989 an international group of surgeons, radiologists, geneticists, clinicians, and dog breeders formed the International Elbow Working Group (IEWG). Subsequent annual meetings were held in conjunction with the meetings of large veterinary organisations such as the American Animal Hospital Association (AAHA), the World Small Animal Veterinary Association (WSAVA), the International Veterinary Radiology Association (IVRA), the American College of Veterinary Radiology (ACVR), the British Small Animal Veterinary Association (BSAVA), and the European College of Veterinary Surgeons (ECVS). IEWG meeting reports were published in the JAVMA (197:1269, 1990 and 205:1376, 1994).

The IEWG is structured as an international mailing list membership group. The purpose of the IEWG is to offer a forum for meeting and discussion to researchers, practicing veterinarians and breeders interested in canine elbow dysplasia or elbow disease (ED). The main goal of the IEWG is to coordinate internationally the efforts to reduce the prevalence and the severity of ED and to disseminate the available information on canine ED and its prevention to all dog breeders and to the veterinary profession world wide. The IEWG is interested in all aspects of ED including clinical aspects, diagnosis, treatment, prognosis, etiology, mode of transmission, prevention, and data collection. Special emphasis is placed on the analysis of progeny data for the objective assessment of both mode and degree of heredity of ED. To reach its goal the IEWG provides a structured method of diagnosis and disease control. Guidelines for the establishment of registries for the diagnosis of elbow dysplasia and the recording of both affected and normal dogs are available from the IEWG. The group is dedicated to avoid the cumbersome divergence of diagnostic modes and breeding recommendations as evolved in the various CHD programs worldwide.

In 1997, the IEWG board was reorganized. Continental or regional representatives were assigned. Their duty is to collect relevant data on ED and to establish or stay in contact both with ED researchers and breed club representatives within their region. Further cooperation between IEWG, WSAVA, and kennel club authorities is planned and will lead to the production of an explanatory ED booklet for the dog owner and a guide to the radiographic interpretation of the canine elbow joint. Currently the guide offered by Wind and Doval (1994) provides a useful information for interpretation of mediolateral radiographs.

## Definition of elbow dysplasia

Elbow dysplasia (ED) is defined as a developmental malformation of the elbow joint in the growing dog that often occurs bilaterally. The predominant abnormality is probably the inadequate development of the ulnar trochlear notch, which is too small to encompass the humeral trochlea (Weis 1983, Wind 1986). Depending on the age of the animal at which the anomaly occurs, either UAP or FCP may result. This may explain why some dogs only demonstrate an elbow joint incongruity and a resulting osteoarthrosis while others demonstrate articular fragmentation and a more severe pattern of disease (Weis 1983, Wind 1989). One of more of the following primary lesions may be the cause of elbow dysplasia: (1) malformed, fissured, or fragmented medial coronoid process (FCP), (2) ununited anconeal process (UAP), (3) osteochondrosis of the medial humeral condyle (OCD), (4) incongruity of articular surfaces, (5) articular cartilage anomaly, and (6) mineralization of soft tissue caudal to the medial humeral condyle. Malformation leads to elbow arthrosis, which may induce chronic pain during the growing stage or later in life. Often only the arthrosis is recognized by commonly used diagnostic techniques.

## Heritability of ED

Breeding records showed that the prevalence of elbow dysplasia in first-degree relatives of affected dogs was significantly higher than in the general population indicating that genetic factors are involved (Guthrie and Pidduck 1990). Statistical analysis of data showed that ED in the Labrador Retriever is heritable (Studdert, et al 1991). Breeding of affected dogs has shown to produce disease in the offspring at a rate of 50% or greater (Audell 1990; Swenson, et al 1997). Diagnosis could, in most instances, be made from elbow radiographs taken in fully flexed lateral position (Grøndalen 1990). Heritability of ED depends on the period of time and the group of dogs examined and may reach 40% (Swenson, et al 1997).

## Screening registry guidelines and radiographic diagnosis

The IEWG encourages the formation of screening programs in order to find families with low prevalence of the disease. Currently radiographic screening is considered to be the method of choice for mass screening of dog breeds at risk. In breeds with an increased risk for ED radiographic screening should be established both for dams and sires and also for as many non-preselected offspring as possible. Statistical analysis of the collected radiographic diagnoses will provide information on the genetic quality of the potential breeding stock. From such data, a breeding value can be calculated for any individual dog. Building a valuable database requires the cooperation of determined dog owners, their veterinarians and breed clubs, as well as geneticists and statisticians.

The IEWG developed the following guidelines for those establishing elbow arthrosis screening registries: (1) Radiographs of both elbows should be evaluated, (2) Radiographs should be made using a non-grid, tabletop, technique, (3) Each elbow should be radiographed at least in a flexed position with an elbow opening angle of 30° to 45°. (A craniocaudal 15° pronated projection is recommended in dogs radiographed before 2 years of age.), (4) Radiographs should be marked permanently with the dog, owner, veterinary clinic or hospital making the radiographs, and examination date, (5) Permanent evaluation of the status of the elbow joints should be made after 12 months of age but (6) Preliminary evaluation of the status of the elbow joints can be made at less than 12 months of age, (7) No dog of a breed at risk for ED should be used for breeding prior to elbow screening. (8) All information on ED should be collected in a database open both to public and to dog breeders as a valuable source of information for selective breeding.

In the event of early elbow lameness radiographs should be made at any age of the dog. Radiographs of these puppies should be submitted for registration in the database, which then can be used for statistical analysis. It should be noted that dogs that have no clinical signs and are evaluated to be normal at less than 12 months of age might later develop prominent arthrosis.

The number of projections used for scoring should be noted on the examination report. If possible the report of the status of the elbow joints should include a diagnosis of the cause of the elbow disease such as the presence of: (1) an ununited anconeal process, (2) fragmented coronoid process, (3) OCD of the humeral condyle, or (4) only the presence of osteoarthrosis. Recording of additional data within the registry may include the: (1) clinical signs, (2) diet, (3) rate of skeletal growth, (4) and data derived from surgical exploration or necropsy examination. A system of appeal should be established within the registry in the event the owner or veterinarian questions the radiographic evaluation. Radiographs should be archived for future scientific analysis. The fee for registering a dog and for evaluating and recording the status of the elbow joints should be at a rate that encourages owner participation in the registry. The IEWG suggests that no charge be made for the recording of studies of dysplastic dogs (those scoring 2 or 3, as described below).

Evaluation of radiographs and scoring of the severity of the changes is currently based on the Swedish model proposed by Audell (1990). These guidelines are discussed by the FCI and the WSAVA as the official standard for elbow screening in purebred dogs. They provide an international standard, that can be used for official exchange and reciprocal acceptance of film scoring.

Diagnosis is based on findings on a mediolateral radiograph of the flexed elbow. Any finding on an additional projection should be included in the final grading.

Classification reflects the degree of secondary joint disease or the presence of a primary lesion and covers 4 groups, graded 0 through 3:

| Score | Degree of arthrosis | Radiographic findings |
|---|---|---|
| 0 | No arthrosis | Normal |
| 1 | Mild arthrosis | Osteophytes of less than 2 mm and/or obvious step radius/ulna and/or sclerosis ulnar trochlear notch |
| 2 | Moderate arthrosis | Osteophytes of 2 to 5 mm high |
| 3 | Severe arthrosis | Osteophytes of more than 5 mm high or evidence of primary disease such as UAP, FMCP, OCD or previous elbow surgery |

Recent studies prove that a substantial number (up to 10%) of ED is not diagnosed when a mediolateral projection only is evaluated (Lang 1995, Hazewinkel 1995). Additional projections such as a craniocaudal 15° pronated one for detection of incongruence or OCD are recommended for all dogs.

## Breeding recommendations

Reduction of ED prevalence can be expected by eliminating affected animals from breeding. Breeding should be restricted to animals with normal elbows or ED grade 1 at worst, while animals scoring grade 2 or 3 should not be used for breeding. In Rottweilers, grade 1 dogs rarely develop clinical signs (Read 1997). Reduction of ED-prevalence within a population is feasible if the above mentioned recommendations are followed. It can be accelerated by breeding only ED-free dogs. There is no established positive correlation between the prevalences of CHD and ED.

Establishing a breeding value estimation program, at least for male dogs, is highly recommended as a powerful tool to further reduce the prevalence of ED in purebred dogs (Benning 1993).

Secretary of the IEWG:
Barbara Packard
12640 La Cresta Drive
Los Altos Hills, CA 94022-2511
USA
Telephone and fax 650-941-7848

## References

ANOMYMOUS. Elbow group recommends protocol. JAVMA 205:1376-1377,1994.

ANOMYMOUS. Canine elbow arthrosis registries encouraged. JAVMA 197:1269,1990.

AUDELL L. AAHA Scientific Proceedings pp730-733,1990.

BENNING R. Department of Animal Breeding, Univ of Giessen, 35390 Giessen, Germany, 1993.

BIENZ H. Thesis, University of Zurich,Vet.Med.Faculty, 1985.

GRØNDALEN J. Arthrosis in the elbow joint of young rapidly growing dogs, Nord.Vet.Med. 31; 62-68; 69-75; 212-218; 520-527, 1979.

GRØNDALEN J, GRØNDALEN T. Arthrosis in the elbow joint of young rapidly growing dogs V A pathoanatomical investigation. NordVet Med 33:1-16, 1981.

GRØNDALEN J. Arthrosis in the elbow joint of young rapidly growing dogs VI. Interrelation between clinical, radiographical and pathoanatomical findings. NordVet Med 34:65-75, 1982.

GRØNDALEN J. Arthrosis in the elbow joint of young rapidly growing dogs.VII Occurrence in the Rottweiler dogs. NordVet Med 34:76-82, 1982.

GRØNDALEN J. Elbow Screening Programs – Radiographic positioning: presented at the 1990, IEWG , San Francisco CA.

GRØNDALEN J. Personal communication,1990.

GUTHRIE A, PIDDUCK HG. Heritability of elbow osteochondrosis within a closed population of dogs. J Sm Anim Pract 31:93-96,1990.

HAZEWINKEL H. IEWG meeting, Constance, Proceedings pp29-32,1995.

LANG J. IEWG meeting, Constance, Proceedings pp37-38,1995.

READ RA. IEWG meeting, Birmingham, Proceedings pp7-8.1997.

STUDDERT VP, LAVELLE RB, BEILHARZ RG, MASON TA. Clinical features and heritability of osteochondrosis of the elbow in Labrador retrievers. J Sm Anim Pract 32:557-563,1991.

SWENSON L, AUDELL L, HEDHAMMAR Å. Prevalence and inheritance of and selection for elbow arthrosis in Bernese Mountain Dogs and Rottweilers in Sweden and benefit: cost analysis of a screening and control program. JAVMA 210:215-221, 1997.

WEIS M. Thesis, University of Zurich,Vet.Med.Faculty,1983.

WIND AP. Elbow incongruity and developmental elbow diseases in the dog. Part I. JAAHA 22:711-724, 1986.

WIND A, DOVAL J. GDC, Box 222, Davis, CA. 95616, USA, 1994.

# Index

**Bold for figure.**

Acetabuloplasty – 193
Anatomy
    distal ulna – 97, **98**
    elbow joint – 51, **52, 53**
    femoral head – **3, 130, 131**
    hip joint – **124,** 125, **126, 127, 157**
    lumbosacral region – 215
    shoulder – **26, 27**
    stifle joint – 232, **234**
    talus – 240
    whole body – **2**
Antiversion, femoral neck – 162
Arthrosis – see osteoarthrosis
Arthrography
    shoulder joint – 28, **30, 33, 36**
Aseptic necrosis femoral head – 176, **177, 178**
Aseptic necrosis femoral head, steroid induced – 177, **179**

Badertscher view – 140
Bardens' technique – 120
Bicipital tenosynovitis – 22, 34, **36**
Breeds affected
    elbow dysplasia – 42
    hip dysplasia – 112
    medial coronoid process disease – 79
    osteochondrosis of humeral condyle – 87
    osteochondrosis of humeral head – 21
    osteochondrosis of sacrum – 227
    osteochondrosis of talus – 244
    spinal canal stenosis – 228
    transitional lumbosacral vertebrae – 226
    ununited anconeal process – 70

Cartilaginous flap – 7
Calcium level – 13
Cauda equina syndrome – 214
Chemonucleolysis – 221
Clinical signs
    elbow dysplasia – 48
    femoral condyle osteochondrosis – 231
    hip dysplasia – 113
    humeral condyle osteochondrosis – 88
    humeral head osteochondrosis – 24
    lumbosacral disease – 117, 212, 220
    medial coronoid process disease – 79
    retained distal ulnar cartilage core – 97
    talus osteochondrosis – 239
    transitional lumbosacral vertebral segment – 118, 212, 220
    ununited anconeal process – 73
Chondrodysplasia
    elbow – **45, 46**
    hip joint – **45**
Congenital hip luxation – **174**
Conservative treatment
    humeral head osteochondrosis – 35

    medial coronoid process disease – 85
    retained distal ulnar cartilage core – 106
    ununited anconeal process – 76

Decompressive laminectomy – **221**
Diagnosis
    general – 16
Diaphyses – 3
Diet – 12
Differential diagnosis
    elbow dysplasia – 61
    femoral condyle osteochondrosis – 236
    hip dysplasia – 175
    humeral condyle osteochondrosis – 89
    humeral head osteochondrosis – 34
    lumbosacral disease – 220
    medial coronoid process disease – 84
    retained distal ulnar cartilage core – 106
    talus osteochondrosis – 243
    ununited anconeal process – 76
Discography – 218, **219**

Elbow dysplasia
    clinical signs – 48
    definition – 9
    differential diagnosis – 61
    etiology – 46
    heritability – 14
    history – 41
    physical examination – 51
    prognosis – 67
    radiographic diagnosis – 61
    treatment – 65
Elbow joint
    anatomy – **52, 53, 82**
    congenital luxation – **47**
    chondrodysplasia – **45**
    developmental diseases – 44
    osteoarthrosis – **44**
Enthesophyte – 12
Epidurography – 217
Epiphyseal dysplasia
    humeral head – **34**
Epiphyses – 3
Epiphyseal growth plate – 5
Etiology
    elbow dysplasia – 46
    hip dysplasia – 111
    osteochondrosis – 6
Excision arthroplasty – 194

Femoral head and neck ostectomy – 194, **195**
Femoral neck
    antiversion – 162, 164
    retroversion – 162, 164
Flückiger view – 140
Fragmented medial coronoid process – 54

Genetics
    horse – 15
    role of – 14
Greater trochanteric repositioning – 193
Growth rate – 12

Heritability
    elbow dysplasia – 68
    femoral condyle osteochondrosis – 237
    general – 14
    hip dysplasia – 14, 197
    humeral condyle osteochondrosis – 90
    humeral head osteochondrosis – 37
    medial coronoid process disease – 86
    transitional lumbosacral vertebrae – 226
    retained distal ulnar cartilage core – 107
    sacral osteochondrosis – 227
    spinal canal stenosis – 228
    talus osteochondrosis – 244
    ununited anconeal process – 77
Hip dysplasia
    acetabulum – 126
    anatomy – 125
    antiversion, femoral neck – 162, 164
    Bardens' technique – 120
    bilabiation – 155
    breeds affected – 112
    clinical signs
        general – 113
        puppy – 113
        preadolescent – 114
        young dog – 115
        adult dog – 117
    compression–distraction views – 141
    definition – 9, 109
    diagnosis
        influence of age – 172
        influence of breed – 172
    differential diagnosis – 175
    distraction index – 142
    dorsal acetabular rim view – 143
    femoral head – 126
    femoral neck – 130
    Flückiger view – 140
    greater trochanter – 131
    heritability – 14, 197
    hip joint – 128
    history – 109
    inclination of femoral neck – 158
    joint laxity – 118, 147
    modeling patterns – 156
    Morgan Line – 144, 152
    norberg angle – 128, 149
    ortolani technique – 121
    pelvic conformation – 165
    pelvic symmetry – 167
    physical examination – 118

prevalence – 112
prognosis – 197
radiographic changes, grading – 168
radiographic diagnosis – 143
radiographic views – 131
retroversion, femoral neck – 162, 164
soft tissue changes – 110
subchondral sclerosis – 154
treatment
    conservative – 184
    medical – 185
    surgical – 186
Histological section
  humeral head – **6, 7**
History
  elbow dysplasia – 41
  hip dysplasia – 109
  lumbosacral disease – 210
  medial coronoid process disease – 77
  osteochondrosis of femoral condyle – 231
  osteochondrosis of humeral condyle – 87
  osteochondrosis of humeral head – 21
  osteochondrosis of talus – 239
  retained distal ulnar cartilage core – 95
  ununited anconeal process – 71
Humeral condyle, osteochondrosis
  clinical signs – 88
  differential radiographic diagnosis – 89
  general – 87
  heritability – 90
  history – 87
  physical examination – 88
  prognosis – 90
  radiographic diagnosis – 89
  treatment – 90
Humeral head, osteochondrosis
  anatomy – 27
  clinical signs – 24
  differential radiographic diagnosis – 34
  general – 21
  gross lesion – 23
  grading of lesions – 31
  heritability – 37
  history – 21
  physical examination – 26
  prognosis – 37
  radiographic diagnosis – 27
  treatment – 35, 36

Inclination of femoral neck – 158
Infectious arthritis hip joint – 180, **181, 182**
Intertrochanteric derotational varus osteotomy – 192
Intertrochanteric lateralization procedure – 193

Labrador retriever
  frequency of disease – 249
Lumbosacral disease
  anatomy – 215
  cauda equina syndrome – 214
  chemonucleolysis – 221
  clinical signs – 212
  discography – 218
  epidurography – 217
  history – 210
  medical treatment – 220
  myelography – 218
  physical examination – 214
  radiographic diagnosis – 216

  stress radiography – 216
  surgical treatment – 221
Medial coronoid process disease
  clinical signs – 79
  differential radiographic diagnosis – 84
  general – 77, **78-80,** 83, 84
  heritability – 86
  history – 77
  physical examination – 80
  prognosis – 85
  radiographic diagnosis – **66**, 80
  treatment
    conservative – 85
    surgical – 85
Metaphyseal growth plates – 3, 8
Morgan Line – 144, 152, **153**
Myelography – 218

Neck lengthening of the proximal femur – 193
Norberg angle – 128, 144

Ortolani technique – 121
Ossification centers
  distal ulna – 98
  elbow joint – 54
  hip joint – 157
  shoulder joint – 26
  stifle joint – 232
  talus – 240
Osteoarthrosis
  definition – 10
  elbow – **44, 59, 60, 64, 85**
  shoulder – 33
Osteoblasts – 3
Osteochondritis dissecans, definition – 4, 5
Osteochondroma
  definition – 35
  shoulder joint – 32, 35
Osteochondrosis
  heritability – 14
  horses – 13
  humeral condyle – 87
  humeral head – 21, **23-25**
Osteochondrosis, definition – 4
Osteochondrosis femoral condyle
  anatomy – 232
  clinical signs – 231
  differential diagnosis – 236
  general – 231, 235, 236
  heritability – 237
  physical examination – 232
  prognosis 237
  radiographic diagnosis – 233
  treatment – 236
Osteochondrosis humeral condyle
  clinical signs – 88
  differential diagnosis – 89
  general – **86-88**
  heritability – 90
  history – 87
  prognosis – 90
  radiographic diagnosis – 89
  treatment – 90
Osteochondrosis sacrum
  general – 226
  heritability – 227
  radiographic diagnosis – 227

Osteochondrosis talus
  anatomy – 240
  clinical signs – 239
  differential diagnosis – 243
  general – 239, 242, 243
  heritability – 244
  physical examination – 239
  prognosis – 244
  radiographic diagnosis – 241
  treatment – 244
Osteoclasts – 3

Panosteitis – **66**
Pectineus surgery – 187
Phosphorus level – 13
Physeal fracture femoral neck – **180**
Physical examination
  elbow dysplasia – 51
  femoral condyle osteochondrosis – 232
  hip dysplasia – 118
  humeral condyle osteochondrosis – 88
  humeral head osteochondrosis – 26
  lumbosacral disease – 212
  medial coronoid process disease – 79
  retained distal ulnar cartilage core – 97
  talus osteochondrosis – 239
  ununited anconeal process – 74
Pig – 16
Premature physeal closure – **63**
Primary arthrosis hip joint – 183
Prognosis
  elbow dysplasia – 67
  femoral condyle osteochondrosis – 237
  general – 16
  hip dysplasia – 197
  humeral condyle osteochondrosis – 90
  humeral head osteochondrosis – 37
  lumbosacral disease – 223
  medial coronoid process disease – 85
  retained distal ulnar cartilage core – 107
  talus osteochondrosis – 244
  ununited anconeal process – 77
Protein level – 13
Radiograph
  elbow dysplasia – **11, 48, 57, 58, 60, 61, 62**
  distal ulna – **99**
  hip dysplasia – 10, 116, 129, 136, 138, 140, 142, **145-148,** 150, 152, **154-156, 158-160,** 164, 165, 169, 172, 173,
  retained distal ulnar cartilage core – **9**
  transitional lumbosacral segment – **168**
Radiographic diagnosis
  elbow dysplasia
    differential diagnosis – 61
    general – 58
  femoral condyle osteochondrosis – 233
  hip dysplasia – 143
  humeral condyle osteochondrosis – 89
  humeral head osteochondrosis – 27
  lumbosacral disease – 220
  medial coronoid process disease – 80
  retained distal ulnar cartilage core – 98
  sacral osteochondrosis – 227
  spinal canal stenosis – 228
  talus osteochondrosis – 241
  transitional lumbosacral vertebrae – 223
  ununited anconeal process – 74
Radiography
  distal ulna – 100

elbow joint – 54, **55, 56**
hip – 131
    Badertscher view – 140
    compression–distraction views –141
    dorsal acetabular rim view – 143
    Flückiger view – 140
    standing position – 139
    ventrodorsal "frog" leg view – 136
    ventrodorsal wedge view – 138, 148
    ventrodorsal view – 133
lumbosacral region – 216
    stress radiography – 216
shoulder – **28**
stifle joint – 233
tarsus – 241
Retained distal ulnar cartilage core
  anatomy – 97
  clinical signs – 97
  differential radiographic diagnosis – 106
  general – 95, 96, **100-103**
  heritability – 107
  history – 95
  physical examination – 97
  prognosis –107
  radiographic diagnosis – 98
  treatment
    conservative – 106
    surgical – 106
Retroversion, femoral neck – 162, 164

Sacral osteochondrosis – **210**, 226
Sarcoma
  elbow – **65**

pelvis – **194**
Significance of disease – 16
Skeletal development – 3
  shoulder – 26
Spinal canal stenosis – 209, 213, 227, 228
Stenosis spinal canal – 209, 213, **217**
Stress radiography – 216
Surgical treatment
  femoral condyle osteochondrosis – 237
  humeral condyle osteochondrosis – 58
  humeral head osteochondrosis – 36
  lumbosacral disease – 220
  medial coronoid process disease – 85
  retained distal ulnar cartilage core – 106
  talus osteochondrosis – 244
  ununited anconeal process – 76

Tension relief procedures – 188
Total hip replacement – 196, **198**
Transitional lumbosacral vertebrae
  definition – 223
  general – 211
  heritability – 226
  radiographic diagnosis – **222**, 223, **224, 225**
Treatment
  conservative
    elbow dysplasia – 65
    femoral condyle osteochondrosis – 236
    hip dysplasia – 184
    humeral head osteochondrosis – 35
    lumbosacral disease – 220
    medial coronoid process disease – 85
    retained distal ulnar cartilage core – 106

talus osteochondrosis – 244
ununited anconeal process – 76
general – 16
medical
  hip dysplasia – 185
  lumbosacral disease – 220
surgical
  elbow dysplasia – 65
  femoral condyle osteochondrosis – 237
  hip dysplasia – 186
  humeral condyle osteochondrosis – 90
  humeral head osteochondrosis – 36
  lumbosacral disease – 220
  retained distal ulnar cartilage core – 106
  talus osteochondrosis – 244
  ununited anconeal process – 76
Triple pelvic osteotomy – 189

Ununited anconeal process
  clinical signs –73
  differential radiographic diagnosis – 76
  general – 69, **70-75**
  heritability – 77
  history – 71
  physical examination – 74
  prognosis – 77
  radiographic diagnosis – 74
  treatment
    conservative – 76
    surgical – 76

Valgus deformity femoral neck – **176**
Vitamin d level – 13

F.C. STADES · M. WYMAN · M.H. BOEVÉ · W. NEUMANN
# Ophthalmology for the Veterinary Practitioner

Here is the comprehensive volume you need to more accurately diagnose the majority of ophthalmic disorders you will encounter in your clinic. Heavily illustrated with 185 brilliant color photos and 209 ink drawings, all of striking quality, the text organizes information logically by eye part or condition in a format that offers easy access even during hectic situations. Recommendations rely on typically available equipment and a minimum of advanced specialty training.

Each chapter features a brief introduction to the morphology and physiology of the specific ocular structure, followed by abnormalities according to pathogenesis. Sections cover congenital anomalies, environmentally based disorders, inflammatory processes; and degenerative, autoimmune, and neoplastic diseases.

Problems that present most commonly receive the most attention, making this volume essential to everyday practice.

**Includes:**
- Clinical and differential diagnostic procedures
- Diagnostics and therapy for eye diseases
- Ocular emergencies
- Orbital and periorbital structures
- Lacrimal apparatus
- Conjunctiva and nictitating membrane
- Eyelids
- Conjunctival adhesions
- The globe
- Cornea and sclera
- Intraocular pressure and glaucoma
- Anterior uvea
- Lens and vitreous
- Fundus and optic nerve
- Breed predisposition and hereditary eye diseases

204 pages, 394 illustrations · 8 ½ X 11", Hardcover · ISBN 3-87706-488-4 · $ 98.00

JOE P. MORGAN · JOHN DOVAL · VALERIE SAMII
# Radiographic Techniques: The Dog

You and your staff can produce consistently high-quality radiographs. This easy-to-use book is designed to keep everyone in the clinic up-to-date on the latest standards for patient positioning. Includes all of the views necessary to complete a given anatomic study. Plus space for writing personal notes about successful in-clinic techniques.

Refer to concise, list-format descriptions that specify correct placement and central beam direction. Detailed drawings further clarify each recommendation, and additional illustrations show the anticipated radiographic outcome.

Particular emphasis is placed on the pelvis, hip joint, and femur as well as the head and spine, because of the difficulty in making a radiographic diagnosis in those areas and the need to produce films taken from multiple angles.

Reader-friendly book layout enables quick location of a desired view and straight-forward interpretation of the positioning and immobilization required to obtain that view radiographically. Recent innovations in patient restraint are clearly illustrated. Added "Comments" are particularly valuable for veterinary technicians and students.

**Includes:**
- General introduction
- Thorax
- Abdomen
- Head
- Mandible
- Pharyngeal studies
- Spine, Occipitoatlantoaxial region,
- Cervical region,
- Cervicothoracic region,
- Thoracic region,
- Thoracolumbar region,
- Lumbar region,
- Lumbosacral region,
- Pelvic region
- Nasal passages, paranasal sinuses, maxillary region
- Dental studiies
- Forelimb
- Scapula
- Shoulder
- Humerus
- Elbow
- Antebrachium
- Carpus, metacarpus, digits
- Hindlimb
- Femur
- Stifle
- Tibia and fibula

268 pages, 200 drawings · 5 ½ X 8 ¼", Hardcover · ISBN 3-87706-524-4 · $ 48.00

**4 Easy Ways to order for U.S.A. and Canada!**
CALL TOLL FREE: 888-880-0328
FAX: 802-864-7626
ONLINE: sva.orders@aidcvt.com
MAIL: PO Box 30, Williston

schlütersche
Hans-Böckler-Allee 7
D-30173 Hannover
Fax: +49-511-8550-3600